CRITICAL INTERVENTIONS IN THE ETHICS OF HEALTHCARE

Medical Law and Ethics

Series Editor
Sheila McLean, Director of the Institute of Law and Ethics in Medicine,
School of Law, University of Glasgow

The 21st century seems likely to witness some of the most major developments in medicine and healthcare ever seen. At the same time, the debate about the extent to which science and/or medicine should lead the moral agenda continues, as do questions about the appropriate role for law.

This series brings together some of the best contemporary academic commentators to tackle these dilemmas in a challenging, informed and inquiring manner. The scope of the series is purposely wide, including contributions from a variety of disciplines such as law, philosophy and social sciences.

Other titles in the series

The Jurisdiction of Medical Law
Kenneth Veitch
ISBN 978-0-7546-4944-1

Law, Mind and Brain
Edited by Michael Freeman and Oliver R. Goodenough
ISBN 978-0-7546-7013-1

Speaking for the Dead
The Human Body in Biology and Medicine
D. Gareth Jones and Maja I. Whitaker
ISBN 978-0-7546-7452-8

Altruism Reconsidered
Exploring New Approaches to Property in Human Tissue
Edited by Michael Steinmann, Peter Sykora, and Urban Wiesing
ISBN 978-0-7546-7270-8 (forthcoming)

The Child As Vulnerable Patient
Protection and Empowerment
Lynn Hagger
ISBN 978-0-7546-7252-4 (forthcoming)

Critical Interventions in the Ethics of Healthcare

Challenging the Principle of Autonomy in Bioethics

Edited by

STUART J. MURRAY
Ryerson University, Canada

and

DAVE HOLMES
University of Ottawa, Canada

ASHGATE

Published by
Ashgate Publishing Limited
Wey Court East
Union Road
Farnham
Surrey, GU9 7PT
England

Ashgate Publishing Company
Suite 420
101 Cherry Street
Burlington
VT 05401-4405
USA

www.ashgate.com

British Library Cataloguing in Publication Data
Critical interventions in the ethics of healthcare :
challenging the principle of autonomy in bioethics. -
(Medical law and ethics)
1. Medical laws and legislation 2. Medical ethics
3. Autonomy (Philosophy)
I. Murray, Stuart J. II. Holmes, Dave
344'.041

Library of Congress Cataloging-in-Publication Data
Critical interventions in the ethics of healthcare : challenging the principle of autonomy in bioethics / edited by Stuart J. Murray and Dave Holmes.
p. ; cm. -- (Medical law and ethics)
Includes bibliographical references and index.
ISBN 978-0-7546-7396-5 (hardback)
1. Medical ethics. 2. Bioethics. I. Murray, Stuart J. II. Holmes, Dave, 1967- III. Series: Medical law and ethics.
[DNLM: 1. Bioethical Issues. 2. Delivery of Health Care--ethics. WB 60 C934 2009]

R724.C8247 2009
174.2--dc22

2009006723

ISBN: 978-0-7546-7396-5 (hb)
ISBN: 978-0-7546-9122-8 (E-book)

FSC Mixed Sources
Product group from well-managed forests and other controlled sources
www.fsc.org Cert no. SGS-COC-2482
© 1996 Forest Stewardship Council

Printed and bound in Great Britain by
TJ International Ltd, Padstow, Cornwall

Contents

List of Figures

List of Tables

Notes on Contributors

Susan Abbey, MD, FRCPC, is the Director of the Program in Medical Psychiatry at the University Health Network and the Head of Psychosocial Services in the Multi-Organ Transplant Program at the University Health Network. She is an Associate Professor in the Department of Psychiatry at the University of Toronto.

Bradley Bryan is the Director of the Technology and Society Program and a Visiting Professor in Political Science at the University of Victoria. He has written *Perilous Participation: Democracy, Autonomy, and Power in an Age of Expertise* (UBC Press, forthcoming), and is at work on a book on biotechnology and political subjectivity, entitled *Code Dependency: Biotechnology and the Vocation of Biopolitics*. Other recent publications include "Approaching Others: Aristotle on Friendship's Possibility," *Political Theory*; "Reason's Homelessness: Rationalization in Bentham and Marx," *Theory and Event* (2003); and "Property as Ontology: On Aboriginal and English Conceptions of Ownership," *Canadian Journal of Law and Jurisprudence* (2000).

Sarah Burgess is Assistant Professor in the Department of Communication Studies at the University of San Francisco. She is currently working on a manuscript tentatively titled *Standing Before the Law: Recognition, Power, and the Limits of Identity,* a project that investigates how we might perform a critique of the practices of power in and through which legal recognition takes place.

David L. Clark is Professor in the Department of English and Cultural Studies and Associate Member of the Health Studies Program at McMaster University, where he teaches courses on Continental philosophy, contemporary critical theory, narratives of illness, and the discourses of HIV/AIDS. He has published research on a wide variety of subjects, ranging from the representation of the surgical separation of conjoined twins, to the question of addiction in philosophical modernity, to the ethical treatment of animals. Recent published work includes: *Bodies and Pleasures in Late Kant* (Stanford University Press, forthcoming); "Speaking of HIV/AIDS: Some Reflections on the Local Faces of the Epidemic" (with Anna G. Joong), *McMaster University Medical Journal* (2008); and "On Being 'the Last Kantian in Nazi Germany': Dwelling with Animals after Levinas." He is currently completing two projects: *Towards a Prehistory of the Post-Animal: Kant, Levinas, and the Regard of Brutes*, and *Mourning Schelling: On the Remains of Idealism*.

Marion Doull has an MHSc in Health Promotion and is currently completing her PhD in Population Health at the University of Ottawa. Her research interests include adolescent sexual health, reproductive rights, and HIV/AIDS. Her doctoral thesis, entitled "Girl Power? Contextualizing Positive Sexual Health Among Heterosexual Canadian Adolescents – An Exploration of Gendered Power Dynamics and the Social Determinants of Health," examines the gendered dynamics of power and positive sexual health among Canadian adolescents.

Twyla Gibson is Assistant Professor of Culture and Technology in the Faculty of Information at the University of Toronto, where she teaches graduate seminars on media theory, information ethics, and bioinformatics. She holds an MA and PhD in Philosophy of Education and a BA in Philosophy and Religious Studies from the University of Toronto. She pursued postdoctoral research in the Departments of Classics and History at the University of Michigan at Ann Arbor. As a researcher at THiiNC Health Canada, she developed an ethical framework for dealing with privacy issues associated with genetic information for the Canadian Biotechnology Secretariat. Since 1991, she has been a senior research associate specializing in assessments of acquired brain injury at Robert D. Katz and Associates Rehabilitation Medicine in Toronto.

Dave Holmes is Professor in the Faculty of Health Sciences (School of Nursing) and Faculty of Medicine (Department of Psychiatry) at the University of Ottawa and Researcher at the University of Ottawa, Institute of Mental Health Research (Forensic Psychiatry Program). After completing his PhD in Nursing, he completed a postdoctoral fellowship in Health Care, Technology and Place – a CIHR Strategic Interdisciplinary Research Training Program – at the University of Toronto. To date, he has received research funding, as principal investigator, from CIHR, SSHRC, and various nursing associations and hospitals, to pursue a research program focusing on risk management in the fields of Public Health and Forensic Nursing. His research interests include critical analysis of health and social care, epistemology, and sociopolitical aspects of nursing and allied health care professions.

Patricia McKeever is a health sociologist. She holds the Bloorview Kids Foundation/University of Toronto Chair in Childhood Disability Studies, Bloorview Research Institute, and is Professor in the Lawrence S. Bloomberg Faculty of Nursing, University of Toronto. Her research program addresses sociospatial, philosophical, and policy aspects of disability and chronic illness. Her areas of expertise include policy analysis, interdisciplinary scholarship, contemporary social theory and philosophy, and qualitative research methods. She has taught multiple interdisciplinary graduate courses and has supervised graduate students from a range of academic disciplines and health science professions.

Stuart J. Murray is Assistant Professor of Rhetoric and Writing in the Department of English and the School of Graduate Studies at Ryerson University, Toronto. He teaches in the Faculty of Arts and in the York University/Ryerson University Joint Graduate Program in Communication and Culture. He received his PhD in Rhetoric from the University of California, Berkeley, after which he held a Social Sciences and Humanities Research Council of Canada Postdoctoral Fellowship in the Department of Philosophy at the University of Toronto. His research interests include the philosophy of technology, philosophy and rhetoric, Foucault, biopolitics, and bioethics. He is currently working on a manuscript on biopolitics and thanatopolitics, tentatively titled *The Living from the Dead.*

Michael Orsini is Associate Professor in the School of Political Studies at the University of Ottawa. His research interests are in the area of health policy and politics, in particular, the role of interest groups and social movements in policy processes, and in discursive approaches to public policy. He recently co-edited a collection with Miriam Smith, entitled *Critical Policy Studies* (UBC Press, 2007). He has also published articles in *Social Policy and Administration*, the *Canadian Journal of Political Science*, *Social and Legal Studies*, and *Policy and Society*, among others.

Jennifer M. Poole is Assistant Professor at Ryerson University's School of Social Work, Toronto. A graduate of the Department of Public Health Sciences at the University of Toronto (where she completed her PhD under contributor Ann Robertson), her research explores notions of recovery in health and mental health, taking up theoretical, practical, and policy concerns. Current projects focus on the experiences of psychiatric survivors, older adults, and heart transplant recipients, but her other interests include mental health, health promotion, chronic illness, critical pedagogy, contemporary social theory, and qualitative research. She hails from Montreal.

Ann Robertson is Professor at the Dalla Lana School of Public Health, University of Toronto, where she teaches in the PhD Program in Social Science and Health. Her major research interest is in applying a critical social science perspective to the analysis of prevailing discourses on health, risk, and illness. In 2002–03, Dr Robertson received a Canadian Institutes of Health Research (CIHR) Career Transition Award to study bioethics and public health genetics at the University of Cambridge. Following this, she has taken a leadership role in facilitating a Public Health Ethics initiative at the University of Toronto. She is also the coordinator of and an instructor in a public health ethics module of an ongoing bioethics capacity-building project in southern Africa, funded by the Fogarty International Center, National Institutes of Health (USA).

Heather Ross, MD, MHSc, FRCP (C), is Associate Professor of Medicine at the University of Toronto and Director of the Cardiac Transplant Program at Toronto

General Hospital. She received her medical degree from the University of British Columbia and completed her cardiology training at Dalhousie University in Canada. Dr Ross completed her postdoctoral fellowship in cardiac transplantation at Stanford University, and earned her Masters Degree in Bioethics from the University of Toronto. Dr Ross served as the President of the Canadian Society of Transplantation in 2005, and as an executive member of the International Society for Heart and Lung Transplantation from 2002 through 2005, and is now the Secretary Treasurer. She is associate editor for the *American Journal of Transplantation* and *Journal of Heart and Lung Transplantation*. Currently, she is an executive member of the Canadian Cardiovascular Society and sits on the Board of the Academy of the Canadian Cardiovascular Society. She is the Florence and Reuben Fenwick Family Professor in Advanced Heart Failure and Deputy Director of the Multi-Organ Transplant Program.

Christabelle Sethna is Associate Professor in the Institute of Women's Studies and the Faculty of Health Sciences at the University of Ottawa. She is an historian who researches and publishes in the history of sex education, contraception, and abortion, receiving funding from the Social Sciences and Humanities Research Council of Canada (SSHRC) for her study on the history of the birth control pill and its impact on young single women in Canadian universities between 1960 and 1980. She is currently Principal Investigator for another SSHRC-funded research project on the travel women undertake to abortion clinics in Canada.

Margrit Shildrick is Reader in Gender Studies at Queen's University Belfast, and Adjunct Professor of Critical Disability Studies at York University, Toronto. Her research interests lie in postmodern feminist and cultural theory, bioethics, body theory, and critical disability studies. She is the author of *Embodying the Monster* (Sage, 2002), and *Leaky Bodies and Boundaries* (Routledge, 1997), and joint editor of *Ethics of the Body* (MIT Press, 2005) with Roxanne Mykitiuk; and *Feminist Theory and the Body* (Edinburgh University Press, 1999) and *Vital Signs* (Edinburgh University Press, 1998) both with Janet Price. Recent articles include work on Derrida, Foucault, Lacan, and Deleuze in relation to disability.

Deborah Lynn Steinberg is Reader in the Department of Sociology, University of Warwick (UK). She has a BA in Women's Studies from the University of California at Berkeley, an MA in Women's Studies from the University of Kent (UK), and a PhD in Cultural Studies from CCCS (Centre for Contemporary Cultural Studies), University of Birmingham (UK). Her research interests revolve around three key areas: cultures of science, feminist media studies, and mourning and politics. Her books include: *Blairism and the War of Persuasion* (2005); *Mourning Diana: Nation, Culture and the Performance of Grief* (1999); *Bodies in Glass: Genetics, Eugenics and Embryo Ethics* (1997); and *Border Patrols: Policing the Boundaries of Heterosexuality* (1997).

Roanne Thomas-MacLean is Associate Professor in the Department of Sociology and Co-director of the Qualitative Research Centre at the University of Saskatchewan. Prior to her appointment there, she completed a postdoctoral fellowship in interdisciplinary primary health care research. Her interests focus on the exploration of chronic illness, particularly, cancer and its implications for people's everyday lives. She holds a Canadian Institutes of Health Research (CIHR) / Saskatchewan Health Research Foundation New Investigator Award.

Kim Walker's career spans acute clinical paediatric nursing, senior academic and management positions in hospitals, higher education, and the professional colleges. His scholarly interests lie in critiquing the prevailing orthodoxies and regimes of truth that influence the operations and strategies of the healthcare system and those who work in it. He is currently in a conjoint professorial appointment between St Vincent's Private Hospital, a not-for-profit acute care surgical hospital, and Australian Catholic University, where he conducts research into clinical and ethical governance.

Shelley Wall, MScBMC, PhD, is a practising biomedical artist specializing in patient education. She is on faculty in the Biomedical Communications program, Institute of Medical Science, University of Toronto, and at the Institute of Communication and Culture, University of Toronto Mississauga, where she teaches courses in biomedical visualization and writing. In addition to her freelance practice, she has worked as a staff multimedia developer for The Hospital for Sick Children in Toronto, Canada. Her research interests include patient education, health literacy, web-mediated health information, and representations of sex and gender in medical visualization.

Acknowledgements

Several of the contributions in this volume were first presented as part of a public lecture series at the University of Toronto in the fall of 1995. "'What is Life?' Lecture Series on Bioethics and Bioinformatics" was sponsored by the Faculty of Information and the Department of Philosophy, and was held in conjunction with an undergraduate course in critical bioethics taught by Stuart Murray.

Dave Holmes and Stuart Murray would like to acknowledge the support of the Social Sciences and Humanities Research Council of Canada (SSHRC). Dave Holmes would also like to thank the Faculty of Health Sciences at the University of Ottawa for granting a sabbatical year during which this book was edited. Special thanks to John Appleby, whose patient work at various stages of the manuscript has been indispensable. We would also like to thank Natalya Androsova.

Introduction: Towards a Critical Bioethics

Stuart J. Murray and Dave Holmes

The contributions gathered in this volume represent part of a growing movement that seeks to intervene in the dominant ways that bioethics is understood and practised. The need for new and critical approaches to bioethics does not merely reflect recent theoretical scholarship, but is at the heart of unprecedented advances in biotechnology, coupled with current trends in healthcare management and delivery. This is all the more pressing as bioethics itself has been institutionalized as an integral part of mainstream medical management and administration. Written from a variety of disciplinary perspectives, these contributions variously suggest that traditional modes of bioethics are proving incommensurable with burgeoning biotechnologies, medical management systems, and the emergent conceptions of the "self" that have arisen in their midst.

An intervention is called for in times of breakdown or crisis. In the popular sense of the term, to undergo an intervention is to be reminded that we are not autonomous creatures, that our actions affect others and extend in myriad ways into the world around us. To intervene is not necessarily to condemn; the one who intervenes claims only to be unable to continue to live with the way things are. Each of these contributions makes such a claim, reminding us that bioethics is, in its most immediate sense, an ethics of non-autonomous life—of the *bios*—and that what is at stake here are the terms of a liveable life, a good life, and all this might entail. Arguably, mainstream or professional bioethics—from the classroom to the clinic—has forsaken this insight, with all its ambivalence, for an instrumental logic or a set of normative principles that promise consistency, efficiency, and ready implementation. Ironically, these principles often are held to be logically "self-evident" and thus in the last instance constitute a matter of faith that obviates the need for any bioethical reflection in the first place. Indeed, the harsh critic might say that this is the surreptitious goal of bioethics-as-usual: to evacuate ethical decision-making of its ambivalence and discomfort, and to offer a set of best-practice guidelines to produce ethical "outcomes," to pre-empt lawsuits, and to safeguard the putative goodness of one's good conscience.

What, then, is a "critical" approach to bioethics? This is an increasingly vexing question because bioethics has become such an integral part of mainstream medical management, and healthcare discourse such an integral part of daily life, that it is difficult to imagine a space from which to wage a critique. While bioethics was originally inspired by sociopolitical and counter-cultural movements in the

1960s, including civil rights and feminism, the terms of bioethical debate have grown increasingly corporate, abstract, and legalistic. Bioethics has become what McKinnie (2004) has referred to as an "affirmative institution": pro-capitalist, pro-technology, and pro-governmental. As M.L. Tina Stevens argues, bioethics has become a "midwife" to the implementation of technologies: "The bioethics 'movement' … assisted in transforming alarm over exotic technologies into a situation in which ethical experts manage problems—problems generated by technologies seen, ironically, as value-neutral in their creation" (2000, xiii). Consequently, critical questions that take account of power and its effects are virtually impossible to formulate, since these discourses have been neutralized and their language has been supplanted by the depoliticized Newspeak of the "ethical expert" and "manager." Without an analysis of power and its complexities, mainstream bioethics is ill-equipped to consider social, political, or even economic issues in any robust manner. To begin to wage a critique, we must call into question and resist the reductive binary logic that tends to inform mainstream bioethics: theory/practice, mind/body, subject/object, nature/culture, and so on. Moreover, critics must seek to understand the many broader contexts—sociopolitical, socioeconomic, historical, cultural—that provide the conditions under which mainstream bioethical principles have become authoritative, if not hegemonic. Finally, critique will mean that we work together to find a conceptual vocabulary that will allow us to interrogate the "expert" authoritarianism of bioethics without ourselves adopting a simple antiauthoritarianism (see Murray et al. 2008).

To offer a critique of bioethics is not to suggest that the field is unified or monolithic. Along with professional philosophers, we might dismiss any serious consideration of religious faith-based ethics and distinguish among several more or less systematic bioethical concepts and "methodologies." Deontologists, such as the philosopher Immanuel Kant, base ethical conduct on rules or duties derived from logical principles, rather than from the consequences of an individual's actions. In contradistinction, consequentialists, including utilitarians, weigh consequences or effects and hope to maximize the presumably calculable utility of ethical decisions, often summed up as the pursuit of "the greatest good for the greatest number." On the other hand, virtue ethics, which hearkens back to Aristotle, finds its basis in the virtuous traits that make up an individual's character (*ethos*); here virtue is defined most often in accord with social values and practical wisdom (*phronēsis*), both of which are socio-historically contingent. Finally, the most popular approach today is principlism, which holds that all human beings share a common morality that can be parsed into a set of ethical principles meant to govern action.

With the exception, perhaps, of virtue ethics—which is rarely taken seriously in the clinic or the classroom—the approaches above presume that human reason plays the central role in ethical decision-making. Thus, while bioethics is neither conceptually nor methodologically monolithic, its various strands nevertheless take for granted the truth of personhood or subjectivity as it is derived from Enlightenment reason—including the belief that the individual is a free, autonomous, and rational agent. In other words, the conventional subject of bioethics is presumed to be a stable and coherent self, sovereign in its ethical judgements. The roots of this modern subject stretch back to the early seventeenth century, when philosophers, such as René Descartes, began to conceive of the self as abstract reason ("I think, therefore I am"), a mind divorced from the body (which was soon regarded as "property").

Nowhere is this cognitivist conceit better demonstrated than in principlism. To offer one example, we turn to Beauchamp and Childress, whose book *Principles of Biomedical Ethics* is an industry standard, spanning over thirty years and six editions. They assert:

> All persons living a moral life grasp the core dimensions of morality. They know not to lie, not to steal others' property, to keep promises, to respect the rights of others, not to kill or cause harm to innocent persons, and the like. (2009, 2–3)

This suggests that to live is, in some sense, no different than to know, that ontology and epistemology are of the same order—or better, that the epistemic principles that stand as "bioethics" emerge naturally, as it were, from the kind of life that one leads—provided that this life is "a moral life." This begs the ethical question: what, then, qualifies a life as "moral" if not those epistemic principles that would organize that life *ex post facto*? It turns out that the "common morality," as Beauchamp and Childress call it, is understood as "universal" not by virtue of our common living-together, but according to particular rational principles that have been universalized and presumed to be natural and necessary. In other words, these values are assumed to be trans-historical and trans-cultural structures, yet immanent to one's "moral" livingness. It is on the basis of this problematic assumption that they derive their four well-known bioethical "principles": respect for autonomy, nonmaleficence (do no harm to others), beneficence (benefit others), and justice.

While these four principles are not reducible to the first ("respect for autonomy"), each of them ultimately must presume the existence of a modern subject/agent founded in rational autonomy. Arguably, even "respect for autonomy" presumes autonomy not just on the part of the one whose autonomy is respected, but also on the part of the one who respects (respect, almost by definition, would be invalid without it). Derived from the Greek *auto-* (self or own) + *nomos* (law), "autonomy" has come to describe the way that the self is conceived as governing or conducting itself. Thus, the self is considered to be fully autonomous only when it governs itself according to rational principles that have been conventionally recognized as such. One might be recognizably "human," but one is not considered fully autonomous when ruled by emotions or bodily urges; such an individual might forfeit certain "rights" and risks being ostracized socially and politically. Rational autonomy therefore presumes that one acts and is acted upon in a very particular way. In the medical context, rational autonomy is a strange convention in part because its philosophical underpinnings continue to be dualistic, founded in a binary logic that sees agency as a mental activity of free will, and bodies no more than resistant, brute matter or a heap of "spare parts." From the patient's perspective, we might ask: who—or what—acts, and who—or what—is acted upon? The clinician can be said to act, is the agent who is presumed to know, and yet acts in myriad ways—through words and deeds, through argument and physical actions, in and through bodies, affecting other bodies. And what is the relation between the patient and the patient's body? Does the patient act? Is the patient acted upon? Or is it the body that undergoes the action—the action of the patient's own body's genes, for example, or of a virus, a drug, a surgeon's scalpel, the persuasive regulatory force of the healthcare leviathan, the insurance industry, loved ones? Could we not declare each of these agents "autonomous," obedient to—and demanding—a particular logic?

So when, from within this nexus, the patient "consents" to a medical procedure, is this an act of the patient's sovereign and free will, based on rational knowledge, or does the body not also "consent" or resist, in its own way, ambivalently, perhaps? We need only reflect on the body in illness and pain to understand that the rational and coherent subject is a conventional fiction: in practice, this subject is fragmentary, radically uncertain, contradictory, and embodied. Any "autonomous" decision takes place between the patient and a vast healthcare complex in the face of which the patient can hardly be said to be "rational" or "free." Moreover, ethical decision-making is also self-reflective, which means that it involves the patient's self-relation—often a relation of emotional and intellectual doubt, in which the subject's "autonomy" is questionable at best. After all, the terms of the patient's self-understanding will surely call upon a wide range of possibly alien(ating) discourses, from genetics, biomedicine, and risk management, to popular literature, personal narratives, and infomercials promoting everything from a cleaner colon to a better sex life—even the desire for "good health" is highly wrought and discursive. The gap that opens up in the subject's ethical self-relation cannot be bridged by positive knowledge alone: it is also—and perhaps primarily—both an affective space and a relational space that is marked by intersubjective relations of care. Must we presume that these relations and actions are rational (or even reasonable) and that those who, in some sense, "do" them, as well as those to whom, in another sense, they are "done," are governing themselves accordingly? It is too simple to say that the patient "wilfully" cedes autonomy since the will itself is implicated. And is any of the patient's ambivalence mitigated if we now call that patient a "client"? Does this "empower"? Or are we just looking for new ways to try to instantiate this person's putative autonomy? Who will judge? Will bioethics decide, will it govern this governance, and if so, how, and according to whose terms? And how will we ensure that the demand for autonomy is not itself experienced as a kind of violence when autonomy is the *sine qua non* of personhood, dignity, rights, and full "citizenship"?

The contributions in this volume variously suggest that there is something wrong in the way that bioethics asks—or refuses to ask—these questions: the intelligibility of its discourse presumes a model of rational autonomy that is intrinsically problematic, even if it were not also fast becoming obsolete. Several contributions here point to recent advances in biomedical technology in order to demonstrate how rational autonomy is deeply troubled; others point to the operation of healthcare complexes themselves, from academe to the clinic; still others draw on recent philosophy, political theory, and cultural studies to make their case. The challenge, of course, is how to imagine an ethics that need not seek recourse to an autonomous, rational, liberal subject. In other words, if we dispense with rational autonomy, what then could serve as the foundation (if this is the right metaphor) for ethics? How might we conceive of responsibility without our current understanding of personhood and free will? This is no small challenge because our terms bear the weight of history and its ossified conventions; there is considerable resistance when it comes to remaining genuinely open to the new. And yet if we glance beyond medicine, we can begin to see that nearly every facet of life in the West presumes—and relies on—the fiction of this modern, rational, autonomous subject: our legal and judicial systems, so-called "free market" capitalism, democracy, and education, to name just a few. In coming years, these pillars of Western culture will need to be overhauled to keep pace with advances in the biosciences. Thus, we face a moment of crisis and breakdown. Presuming that ethics is a relation, the terms of this relation are not yet invented; we hope to chart what is an emerging field of inquiry, one that will have implications not just for healthcare but for post-industrial economies, consumer culture, militarism, law—all forms of governance that presume the givenness of an autonomous, rational subject.

The four sections of this volume should in no way imply that there are only four kinds of interventions into mainstream bioethics-as-usual. We have sought interdisciplinary and thought-provoking contributions; our aim is to foster further dialogue in the field. Each of the four parts reflects a distinct sphere in which the terms of ethical self-relation and autonomy are called into question. These include biomedicine in the clinical setting, the biopolitical dimensions of healthcare, representations of gender and the body, and cultural constructions of biomedical subjectivity. In each of these spheres, we find that the fiction of the liberal, autonomous subject is repeatedly (re)constituted; however, we argue that these spheres are also sites of ethical resistance, productive ambivalence, crisis, and intervention. The contributions gathered in each part seek to deconstruct the authoritative grip of rational autonomy operating within each sphere to intervene in the debates, to engage the reader's imagination, and to suggest new terms for ethical relationality.

The chapters in Part I, "Clinical Interventions," take a critical look at clinical bioethics. Each begins in the clinical setting, discussing a concrete instance in which the principle of autonomy is in crisis. The first chapter is a passionate contribution by Kim Walker, written from the perspective of a nurse and an academic. Walker tells the story of his sister, Donna, from the moment she is diagnosed with terminal breast cancer. To what extent, he asks, does it make sense to speak of Donna as an autonomous subject? And how do we locate the personal and highly affective narrative of the patient/client/subject within the dominant discourse of evidence-based practice (EBP)? While EBP has strongly influenced the clinical healthcare agenda across the discursive territories of policy, research, and scholarship, Walker contends that in practice EBP's much touted ideal of patient autonomy and "patient-centeredness" cannot be realized. His contribution dramatizes the ethical tension between academic and clinical discourses, on the one hand, and a deeply existential and affective narrative, on the other. If the terms of these discourses are incommensurable, Walker suggests it is just this irreconcilable tension that the patient is forced to navigate. A critical bioethics would abandon the onerous language of autonomy and the logic of EBP within contemporary acute care practice, and turn instead to a reappraisal and a reinstatement of case-based healthcare decision-making.

The chapter by Jennifer M. Poole and her colleagues presents novel and potentially disturbing research on cardiac transplantation. Poole and her team are in the early stages of a project called PITH (Process of Incorporating a Transplanted Heart), which employs a qualitative visual methodology to study the effects of transplantation on the recipients. They hope to discover why such a large number of recipients report the experience of "otherness," a disruption of identity, a sense of loss and distress, and even dreams of the donor—not only immediately after the transplant, but well into the "recovered" phase, 3–5 years later. These phenomena cannot easily be explained under the rubric of a positivist, Cartesian biomedical model; consequently, these experiences are usually ignored or psychiatrized. Their research challenges the "spare parts" view of the body that is consonant with a belief in rational autonomy, suggesting instead that an embodied, phenomenological model is more appropriate. They trace the ethical implications of their preliminary findings, responding to conventional bioethics and its insistence on autonomy, confidentiality, and consent; but they also look towards a "postconventional" ethic of intercorporeality drawing on the phenomenology of Maurice Merleau-Ponty.

Roanne Thomas-MacLean's contribution draws on data from the *Visualizing Breast Cancer* project. She offers a reading of several interviews in which Aboriginal women with breast cancer discuss their clinical experience. Focusing on these illness narratives, Thomas-MacLean explores the ways an increased attention to the lived experience of illness—the meaning of which is often taken for granted—might lead to a more ethical and affirming clinical experience. While institutional structures can reinforce and perpetuate a model of healthcare that privileges rational autonomy, she argues that clinicians have a duty to engage with patients in ways that do not reduplicate the dominant ideologies of free choice, autonomy, and paternalism in medicine. Such an approach would serve as an antidote to biomedical orientations and would allow for the recognition of marginalization. Moreover, by turning to the politics and practices of everyday life, she argues that clinicians could better understand how ethical practice emerges from within the intersubjective dimensions of human experience.

Part II, "Biopolitical Interventions," presents chapters that examine the political dimensions of bioscience and its ethical oversight and regulation. While science and technology are frequently presented as apolitical and value-neutral—a move that is often politically strategic—these contributions point to the underlying and hidden powers at play in the governance of life itself. This section opens with a chapter by Ann Robertson, who examines the case of pre-implantation genetic diagnosis (PGD). Robertson defines key biopolitical terms and issues, suggesting that emerging biotechnologies have created a world in which the principle of autonomy can no longer serve as the foundation for governance or for ethics. Based on the Hashmi case in the UK, and using a Foucauldian perspective, her contribution raises some crucial bioethical questions concerning the transformative possibilities of PGD, including the spectre of "saviour siblings" and "designer babies." The ethical implications are discussed further in terms of "biopower" and the notion of "biological citizenship" in the context of a prevailing neoliberal political rationality.

In his chapter, Bradley Bryan discusses the ways that individual subjects—falsely promoted as autonomous—are called into being through biotechnology and biopolitics. Bryan examines how biotechnology arises against the backdrop of an urgent need to manage the conditions that set upon human beings in their very livelihood, including health, illness, and the other vicissitudes of biological existence. Following the insight of French Marxist philosopher Louis Althusser, he argues that "interpellation" or "hailing" is the way the modern subject comes to understand itself as a biological entity. By looking at the preconditions and rhetorical modes of biotechnology, this chapter suggests that individuals recognize themselves as biopolitical subjects in the moment of "being hailed" by biotechnology's (promised) cures.

Stuart J. Murray's chapter invokes the research of Stanley Milgram, the Yale University social psychologist made famous by his experiments on obedience to authority in the early 1960s. Murray argues that an analogous obedience to scientific authority characterizes contemporary Western healthcare, which operates politically according to three interrelated forms of "fascist" ideology: (1) biomedicalization, (2) the political economy of neoliberalism, and (3) biosocial or biocultural discourse. The constellation of these three "fascisms" he terms "biofascism," which is discussed in relation to the phenomenon of genetic screening or "pre-diagnosis." Murray concludes with a discussion on "genetic subjectivity" and offers one way that we might begin to imagine an ethic that would be commensurable with emerging biotechnologies and the kinds of subjects that they foster.

In his chapter, Michael Orsini compares the legal strategies adopted by opposing activist groups in Canada and the USA advancing an autism agenda. One set of groups is appealing to the UN to have people with autism considered a national minority that should be protected from discrimination, while the other is trying to use the law to argue that the state has a duty to cover the costs of applied behavioural therapy, which many parents of autistic children believe can "save" their children from autism. The first group, made up mainly of adult autistics, believes the therapy can be harmful and instead espouses the view that people with autism are "neurodiverse": they are hard-wired differently than the average person. The second group, in contrast, believes that withholding access to this treatment from parents who cannot afford the prohibitive cost is discriminatory. Orsini's contribution deals with the ethical question of who is permitted to speak on behalf of autistic citizens, what treatment(s) should be chosen, and by whom. The debate calls into question what counts as an autonomous person, a person who is presumed to enjoy the right to choose—and to refuse—treatment.

Part III, "Gendered Interventions," takes aim at the ongoing gender bias in biomedical discourse, including the ways the gendered body is represented biomedically and within medico-legal discourse.[1] The gendered body is a site where autonomy claims are played out and fixed, but also troubled and contested. Shelley Wall's contribution is written from the perspective of a biomedical artist. Wall demonstrates that medical illustration in the West shares a long and intimate history with cadaveric dissection, clinical examination, and other medical practices with the body as their object. Her contribution proposes that there is a disconnect between the subjective experiences of patients and the objectifying visual rhetoric of medical and patient education—the clinical gaze. What happens, she asks, when these illustrations function not just as a map, but as a mirror? How do they work to organize the experience of the gendered body? Her discussion takes as its exemplars depictions of sexual anatomy, critiquing them with reference to gender theory, intersex activism, phenomenological accounts of embodiment in healthcare, and the history of medical illustration. It also considers the possibility of alternative—more ethical—visual practices: How can medical illustration rethink the body from the inside out, and better reflect the embodied experience of patients?

Sarah Burgess offers a chapter that reflects on the ways that concepts of autonomy and consent get played out between medicine and the law. Her discussion follows a reading of the UK's Gender Recognition Act (2004). An act that grants rights and a state-issued "gender certificate" to transsexual people according to their "acquired gender," it requires that individuals demonstrate that they have been "living in" a particular gender and plan to do so permanently—a way of being that Parliament refused to clearly define. This chapter explores how this refusal shapes and limits the type of evidence available to subjects who wish to apply for a gender certificate. More specifically, it investigates the effects of removing surgery or other forms of bodily alteration as conditions for a gender certificate. Reading the parliamentary debates and the language of law itself, Burgess argues that this provision introduces a moment to critique how medical evidence is employed (or deployed) in legal and political debates. Such critique is ethically important because it re-defines how a gendered subject is seen and heard within medical contexts.

---

1 For a thorough discussion of gender and postconventional bioethics from a feminist perspective, see Shildrick and Mykitiuk 2005.

Christabelle Sethna and Marion Doull's chapter discusses the ethics of reproductive choice, reporting on a qualitative study of abortion access that tracked the travels of 1,000 women to the Toronto Morgentaler Clinic for the purposes of pregnancy termination in the spring of 2006. The authors demonstrate that access to abortion services has become more difficult since the late 1970s. In light of feminist analyses of reproductive rights, they ask whether the experience of travelling to access pregnancy termination reflects, reifies, and/or exacerbates sociocultural disparities among women. This chapter opens up for discussion bioethical issues of reproductive choice in relation to women's autonomy and women's inequality in Canada. Their data suggest that these women do not experience themselves as autonomous and free.

Part IV, "Cultural Interventions," includes three chapters that variously address medical cultures. Medical discourse has become popular and widespread, informing the terms by which we understand ourselves and others in sickness and in health. The first chapter, by Twyla Gibson, returns to the Hippocratic *Oath*, which has for 24 centuries served as the cornerstone of professional ethics in medicine and the model for all subsequent revisions to ethical codes of conduct. Gibson points out that there has until recently been a significant barrier to new interpretation of this foundational ethical treatise. Applying new findings from the comparative study of ancient literature, she offers an intertextual reading of Hippocrates and Plato in order to bring new meanings to bear on our understanding and interpretation of the *Oath* and the Hippocratic tradition of ethics in medicine. Intertextuality calls into question the autonomy of both author and reader, suggesting that in order to understand ethics, we must turn to the wider communicative, cultural, and historical contexts of our tradition's foundational texts. In so doing, we gain a better understanding of bioethical debates and clinical decision-making today.

Deborah Lynn Steinberg's contribution examines the cultural reception of the gene and genetic science. Steinberg takes as her case study Nancy Kress's popular feminist science fiction novel *Beggars in Spain*, which tells the story of a world in which a class of human beings has been genetically engineered to function without sleep. She reads the work as a parable of emergent values attached to the gene in the late modern era, in particular the uncanny convergence of genetics and neoliberal political economics. Arguably, these are our social values too: a body politics that promises perfect health and beauty, frictionless efficiency, and 24/7 productivity. Attending to the narrative and rhetorical structures of Kress's novel, Steinberg re-visions conventional bioethical discourse with its rigid focus on regulative models and its uncritical affective orientation to scientific progress. She suggests an alternative ethics of ambivalence founded in the "feeling structures" of bodies and knowledge.

Finally, David L. Clark's contribution discusses the world's foremost female Jungian analyst, Marion Woodman, who has long been a vocal critic of conventional biomedical understandings of health and illness. It lies within the power of our respective imaginations, Woodman argues, to make our bodies and minds whole again. Yet Woodman's confidence faced an extraordinary crisis when she was herself diagnosed with and treated for uterine cancer, a process she describes in vivid and moving detail in her memoir, *Bone: Dying into Life* (2000). The triumph of mind over matter that lies at the heart of her health regime threatens at various key points in her autobiographical narrative to devolve into its obscure semblance—namely, an asceticism of the sort that her psychoanalytic project had long railed against. This chapter seeks to show how Woodman's text is haunted by conflicting strata of awareness in which the psychoanalyst's resistance to conventional biomedicine inadvertently quickens a will-to-nothingness that "skeletalizes" the psyche rather than nourishes and enriches it.

It is true that the contributions gathered here do not make an explicit prescriptive ethical claim. But they are not intended to be policy papers. In other words, they do not respond to the crisis in bioethics by offering a moral code or by delineating a set of moral practices or tests. This would render ethics as a piece of positive knowledge, an object within the grasp of an autonomous and free subject, an object to deploy at will. Rather, it is hoped that these contributions will make their claim on the non-autonomous subject, on each of us whose lives are lived alongside—and sometimes for, together with—the lives of others, in sickness and in health. Ethics is not about applying a rule. As Jacques Derrida has said, "There are ethics precisely because … there *is* no rule. There are ethics because I have to *invent* the rule; and there would be no responsibility if I knew the rule … That's where responsibility starts, when I *don't* know what to do" (2003, 31). Ethics is premised, then, on the productive failure of the autonomous "I," beginning where it and its faith in its own knowledge arrive at an impasse, an aporia.

This book hopes to offer more than a consideration of the constitutive social, political, and cultural dimensions of the bioethical field. We hope that readers find in these pages some imaginative possibilities to begin to think and experience bioethics beyond the limits of mainstream bioethical proceduralism—beyond the impasse of liberal voluntarism, autonomy, and rationalism—and toward a critical assessment of the ways that bioethics must respond if it is to meet the complex emerging challenges to healthcare, medicine, the body, and society. More than a critical intervention, then, together these contributions open toward a critical invention—the invention of new modes of ethical relation, new discourses, and a new political ethos that must be forged in virtue of our common and inescapable living-together.

References

Beauchamp, T.L. and Childress, J.F. (2009), *Principles of Biomedical Ethics*, 6th edition (New York and Oxford: Oxford University Press).

Derrida, J. (2003), "Following Theory: Jacques Derrida," in M. Payne and J. Schad (eds), *life.after.theory* (New York and London: Continuum).

McKinnie, M. (2004), "A Sympathy for Art: Sentimental Economies of New Labour Arts Policy," in R. Johnson and D.L. Steinberg (eds), *Blairism and*

the War of Persuasion: Labour's Passive Revolution (London: Lawrence and Wishart).
Murray, S.J. et al. (2008), "Towards and Ethic of Authentic Practice," *Journal of Evaluation in Clinical Practice* 14:5.
Shildrick, M. and Mykitiuk, R. (eds) (2005), *Ethics of the Body: Postconventional Challenges* (Cambridge, MA and London: MIT Press).
Stevens, M.L. Tina (2000), *Bioethics in America: Origins and Cultural Politics* (Baltimore, MD and London: The Johns Hopkins University Press).

PART I
Clinical Interventions

Chapter 1

My Life? My Choice? Ethics, Autonomy, and Evidence-Based Practice in Contemporary Clinical Care

Kim Walker

> We pass our days on the surface of a little star which drifts aimlessly through endless skies, inventing such fictions as we require to make it through the day and persuade ourselves of our significance and meaning. Until at last, weary of its peculiar little local experiment, the cosmos draws another breath and moves on. Then we disappear without a trace. "Knowledge," "obligation," "justice"—these are so many obsolete inventions of the little animals, now useless vapours dissipating in interstellar space. (Caputo 1993, 17)

On Life and Our Lucky Stars

True to form and function, they kept us waiting in the waiting room. Women came and went from the door leading to the clinics behind the receptionist's desk. Time was stalled. At last, Donna was called by a cheery middle-aged woman who had clearly met her before. When we got into the examination room, she asked my sister to disrobe and don the hospital gown, "the surgeon won't be long," she said. We waited, and then waited some more again. The woman, a nurse, it turns out, popped in a couple of times to tell us the surgeon "shouldn't be too much longer." The waiting was excruciating; institutionalized torture masquerading as business as usual. Suddenly, all at once, a trio of women burst into the room. The surgeon looked as if she was on her way to the beach, so casual was her attire; the other two were uniformed in the modern anonymous fashion. Brief introductions all-round; an awkward pause. And then: "I'm afraid it is cancer, Donna." A gush and rush of muted grief and tattered belief as tears welled and Donna grabbed my hand as if to steady herself. Disaster had struck; Donna's guiding star vanished in that ugly, jagged moment and she was cast asunder, bereft.[1] The abyss yawned and invited her into its infinite murk. At once we knew—beyond all doubt—her life was forever to be changed. My sister could no longer indulge the long-held and hard won delusion that she was the main author of her life. The omniscient

1 Disaster, from the Italian, *disastro*, from *disastrato* not having a (lucky) star.

and omnipotent one had snorted with contempt; in this moment He gave Donna a nasty reminder of her precarious mortality, of the sheer contingency of life and, ultimately, the truth for each and every one of us that our being-in-the-world is irretrievably a "Being-towards-death" (Heidegger 1987, 235–67). Donna's self, her sense of herself as invincible and "in control," was no longer something she could happily take "for granted." It was—fleetingly at least—suspended in that truly appalling chasm between faith and fate; being and not-being; presence and absence. And for me, her older brother who had insisted he be there with her for "the moment of truth" and who now sat alongside this suddenly shattered soul, the brute being of Being—our always and only living-in-the-moment—was made mightily all too real. The *evidence* was in (but not the worst of it), *autonomy* was out (my life? my choice?), and *ethics* (the deeply moral dimension posed by what was soon to be re-diagnosed as an incurable cancer) posed its founding questions: What ought she to do? What ought we to do?

And from this *mise-en-scène* of a woman—but not just any woman—struck a terrible blow to my musings. For this once private and personal tale is the same but different from countless many in which every one of you will hear an echo in your own lives. A deep sonority with our shared humanity is what I strive for in this text, so what better way to utter a call to the other but through a tale of the *wounded* other; she whose life has been shipwrecked against desire and need, just when it seemed it could only get better. And I have begun with this tale to open the way for an exploration of a new—or perhaps not so new—mode of ethical comportment in contemporary clinical care, a mode in which the special and local are prioritized over the general and the universal. Most people's lives are parochial in the extreme, and, mostly, their universe is tiny and incestuous, peopled with only a few that really matter, and many more that matter only a little, if at all. This reality underpins much of what follows.

My thinking winds around three premises (none of which are final, all of which can be contested): first, I am against Ethics (or Bioethics, Medical Ethics, Clinical Ethics) as the originary moral ground on which clinicians should, indeed must, stand. Rather, I am for an ethic(s) of care without an E, devoid of its piety and stripped of its philosophical profundity. Because I too share Komesaroff's concern that "there appears to have been no study showing that bioethical theory has produced a beneficial impact on medical decision making, or indeed that it has produced valuable effects in other working ways for doctors (and nurses) or their patients" (1995, 67). With Ramsey I believe that ethics in the clinical field must "deal as competently and exhaustively as possible with the concrete features of actual moral decisions of life and death and medical care" (2002, xxii). And I side with Elliot when he notes that "we have become accustomed to writing and talking in bioethics, where relationships between strangers are in some ways the paradigm for our moral language. The impersonality of conventional bioethics writing also emerges in its (implicit) view of moral agency" (1999, xxix). Feminist writer Shildrick captures neatly for me the central problem: "the field of morality in which biomedicine roots itself has tended to be a fairly restricted one in which the emphasis is on those theories most likely to yield relatively clear guides to action" (1997, 73). Unfortunately, the sorts of actions arising from such theories tend to diminish, rather than elevate, the ontological uniqueness and the exquisite specificity of every individual "patient's" moral condition.

Secondly, I am also against Autonomy as the liberal humanist and political ideal our patients should emulate, and that our health professionals should expect of them (and of themselves). The notion of the human agent as autonomous and sovereign—the liberal individualist—is deeply appealing to modern man and, in fact, defines him (Grosz 1995, 51–2; Johnson 1994, 5–15; Mansfield 2000, 13–24). Instead, I see the subject "as neither sovereign nor autonomous but as always caught up in a network of responsibilities to others" (Elam 1994, 105). I want to run against the grain of much conventional wisdom in healthcare that always positions the patient as endowed with relatively inviolable rights or equally problematically situates the doctor or nurse as a self-defining and regulating professional also endowed with rights. Rather, why can't we move beyond the idea of an autonomous individual and work, instead, with the vulnerable, needy he or she who seeks our help and wants our care? I urge us to recognize the "heteronomic force of the other" (after Caputo 1993) whereby our *obligation* to each other, each palpable, enfleshed, mortal, and fragile other, is something we cannot sequester or abjure in the name of an autonomous, universal, disembodied, "rugged" individualism. I suppose I yearn for times now past, times perhaps no longer possible in our clinical settings beset as they are by rapidity of throughput and diminution of contact, as sheer force of volume and need stretch capacity to its limits. The treadmill that is healthcare today degrades the sense of community and ethos of care that once pervaded even the busiest, largest, and most austere and auspicious of hospitals; the industrialization and commoditization of health has much to atone for.

Thirdly, and finally, I am also against Evidence-Based Practice (EBP) as the governing "episteme" and the shining light for better outcomes in clinical care. Of course these days I am most certainly not alone here as an avalanche of writings has been launched in the last decade, with one journal alone charting over no less than ten editions the rise and rise of EBP and enlisting critique from its antagonists.[2] The scholarly debate in the halls of academe about the place of EBP is fecund indeed; yet it summons barely a flicker of interest amongst most clinicians in the hurly-burly of daily clinical life. Consequently, the idea and practice of EBP suffer from some rhetorical tensions, and in recognizing this I want to play a little deconstructive manoeuvre and reverse the order of its terms (after Rolfe and Watson 2008). Doing this inverts the violent top-down hierarchy—where evidence is imposed on practice—and gives us the idea of practice-based evidence.

2 The editors of *Journal of Evaluation in Clinical Practice* (Blackwell Publishing) have made it their *raison d'être* to engage far-reaching and serial commentary and critique on the state of evidence-based healthcare (1997–2006). It is a fascinating opus and well worth the effort.

While this might seem like mere sleight of hand, it is much more. Both evidence and practice as terms coexist in a mutually binding relationship (like theory and practice and other masterly binaries). But the order in which they appear sets up a tension between them that never quite manages to resolve neatly in terms of letting one have the upper hand because the one without the other is nothing. Prioritizing practice—everyday, ordinary (or extraordinary) clinical practice—as the basis for evidence for future practice opens up a re-appraisal and reinstatement of casuistry: case-based healthcare decision-making.

This approach fully recognizes the ineffable uniqueness of every clinical encounter with each irrepressibly singular human being; it deeply appreciates the unquenchable need each and every one of us has when we are "laid low" to be held in someone else's regard and be offered a "helping hand" out of care—in the Heideggerian (1987, 191–200) sense of concern, solicitude, being-alongside—rather than simply "being nice" (Walker 1997) or just doing our job. Tonelli (2006) and colleagues (Borry et al. 2006; Montgomery Hunter 1989; Mykhalovskiy 2003; Porta 2006; Tannenbaum 2006) call too for a return to casuistry as a response to the limitations of EBP. As Montgomery Hunter reminds us, "the individual case is the touchstone of knowledge in medicine [and I would add nursing and the allied health professions]" (1989, 194). But as she also cautions, "[d]espite an enormous number of reliable, well worn diagnostic and therapeutic paths, there is never enough certitude" (1989, 195).

This "will to certitude" has been the mission of EBP, and it underwrites much of the current obsession in healthcare with risk aversion and containment, as well as the quality and safety agenda and industry both of which consume far more energy and resources than they warrant in my observations. Indeed, they tend to shift clinicians' focus and energies away from care and the ethics of care, much to the detriment of all.

A Disquiet

All this is well and good, you might say to me (even as I say it to myself). But I have misgivings that the intellectual substance of the scholarly debates around each of these weighty words—ethics, evidence, and autonomy—falls mostly on those who have laboured hard to construct the debates in the first instance; they largely fail to reach those who could and should most benefit by them: the clinicians at the sharp and dangerous point of care. I am excruciatingly aware that the vast majority of my colleagues whose quotidian lives are consumed with the busyness of work on the clinic floor will never read this anthology and neither will they care much at all that it has been written. Clinical hospital culture is stained with a perennial anti-intellectualism (Walker 1997; 2000) which disallows substantive analysis and debate about many issues that matter much in clinical care. Such debate is perceived by many clinicians—and perhaps rightly so—not to be oriented around the pragmatic, the mundane, and the everyday. This is something of a shame, both in the sense of our colleagues "missing out," but also in the sense that we ought (those of us who write) to feel shamed if we cannot find ways to better engage our colleagues in such debate. Thus my return to the local in pursuit of the general; a focus on the present-at-hand (Heidegger 1987) at the expense of the "from on high"; a concern with material, contemporary realities, rather than abstract concepts (although clearly the abstract underwrites even the most trivial and concrete instance of the real).

Thus we are headed toward imagining a new form of ethics for contemporary healthcare that, in effect, is a return to an old, if not old-fashioned and even slightly nostalgic notion of "care for and obligation to the other." This concern with obligation arises out of nothing less profound than our being-in-the-world with others (after Heidegger 1987 again); those without whom there would not be a world at all. After all, healthcare is through and through a human service; human beings are both the object and subject of our concerns. In these postmodern times it is salient to remind ourselves that the ethical life is perhaps even harder to define, negotiate, and evaluate than it ever has been, so much have we and our world changed over the last century.

Against Ethics as Merely "Making Things Safe," Toward an Ethos of Obligation as a "Duty of Care to the Other"

As Caputo has suggested:

> Ethics makes safe. It throws a safety net under the judgements we are forced to make, the daily, hourly decisions that make up the texture of our lives. Ethics lays the foundations that force people to be good; it clarifies concepts, secures judgements, provides firm guardrails along the slippery slopes of factical life. It provides principles and criteria and adjudicates hard cases. Ethics is altogether wholesome, constructive work, which is why it enjoys a good name. (1993, 4)

A good name indeed. For to speak against Ethics is perhaps erring too much on the side of the heretic. Leeder suggests similarly (albeit in a very different context to Caputo) that ethics is "soft and warm" (2004, 437). But this Ethics, which Caputo (1993) reminds us is "philosophy," is also tightly and heavily wrapped in piety and profundity, as I suggested at the outset. And this is why it has difficulty resonating with those closest to the ethical fabric of clinical care. There is little that is pious and profound in the day-to-day world of the clinician (in the sense that mostly only superficial regard is given to the religious and deeply humanitarian consequences of being sick in an acute care hospital; there simply isn't time or resources to attend to them any other way). Neither would most clinicians think of their work in these terms; the majority of clinicians are pragmatists with much "work" to be done, and the fact that, without doubt, it is profound work would nevertheless figure little in their imaginations. This is, in part, the reason why we need to cast aside Ethics and consider instead something much more humble, rather less obscure, and certainly much more relevant and meaningful to those at the sharp and potentially dangerous point of care.

Ethics as Institution: The Origins of the Problem

As Borry et al. (2005, 50) remind us, the term, the institution, and traditions of "bioethics" received their canonical status only in the 1970s. So significant has the field of bioethics become that over the last 30 years we have seen the establishment and proliferation of international, transnational, and national bioethics bodies, as well as a World Congress on Bioethics (Dodds and Thomson 2006). A global community of ethics scholars and practitioners of various kinds now generate an enormous body of literature. In fact, as one commentator has observed, "it is perhaps not too much of an exaggeration to say that bioethics now constitutes a substantial academic industry" (Komesaroff 1995, 63). Furthermore, bioethics inserts itself in healthcare policy, procedure, and all manner of protocols and regulations common among which are the all too familiar rituals in hospitals around the gaining of informed consent, the preservation of patients' privacy and confidentiality, discussions about the pros and cons of not-for-resuscitation orders, and similar so-called "ethical dilemmas." Notably, in clinical practice the terms "ethical" and "dilemma" are all but inseparable, and together they frame much of the debate that is conducted in this domain (Komesaroff 1995, 65). McGrath points to a growing critique of a "philosophy based, predominantly abstract, rationalistic, mode of reasoning in bioethics, known as principlism" (1998, 516). As Hunter notes well, "[n]o sure answer is to be found in even the clearest principles … the particularities of human illness … inevitably resist satisfyingly complete abstraction" (1989, 202). Charon (in Frank 1997, 132) and Komesaroff (1995, 64) suggest that this focus on the abstract and principles in clinical ethics is inherently reductive and instrumental.

Why Principlism? Toward a Critique of Autonomy

Beauchamp and Childress's (1994) four founding principles of autonomy, nonmalificence, beneficence, and justice prevail in and underpin most of what passes for ethical discussion in the clinical setting (Borry et al. 2005, 59). But the four principles do not necessarily share equal footing when it comes to clinical and ethical decision making as "[w]e live in the time of the triumph of autonomy in bioethics" (Schneider 1998, xi). Wolpe (1998) and Lupton and Williams (2004) affirm this ascendency. More to the point here, though, the former argues that "autonomy" has become the "default" position when the other principles conflict. This is so, he argues, because "only autonomy is easily codified into a set of rules and regulations pertaining to day-to-day healthcare" (Wolpe 1998, 46–7). Elliot picks up this idea when he suggests the reason for autonomy's pre-eminence is due, in part, to the fact that the "law is the *lingua franca* of bioethics. The language in which bioethics is discussed revolves around quasi-legal notions such as consent, consequence, rights to refuse treatment, to have an abortion" (1999, xxviii). This "codification into rules and regulations" and the legalese through which ethics is presented and discussed in the clinical setting speak to the deep pragmatism that dominates so much of everyday clinical thinking and action. Increasingly, as I hear it in the corridors, the complex philosophical and moral issues surrounding the often very difficult decisions that must be made about treatment options are misrepresented or misconstrued as quasi-legal problems (the patient might sue) or breaches of conduct (the doctor has a conflict of interest).

This over-reliance on the principle of patient autonomy and personal choice has a history. Wolpe (1998, 43–4) argues that the prevailing paternalism of earlier medicine and healthcare was seen as overly repressive and diminished patients' moral rights to make important decisions concerning their health and well being. Tauber, reflecting on his days as a physician, recalls how "[n]ot even the deranged were to be freed from their autonomy. Unless considered dangerous to themselves and others, they were unfettered to roam the streets and fend for themselves as best they could" (1999, 28). Parker, too, is concerned that "[t]o view people solely as individuals and to give priority to individual choice is not, in fact, to empower patients, but rather to emaciate them and to make them vulnerable in new ways" (2001, 88).

For if autonomy were the highest of the principles on which to act ethically in clinical care, then it ought to figure as such in the minds of patients themselves. But, as Schneider notes, "[p]atients want more from doctors than autonomy; they want competence and kindness" (1998, xiii). He concludes that they desire both "more and less than autonomy. From the perspective of the sick, the authority to make medical decisions may not loom so large; but in other ways the sick may want more from doctors—particularly, more personal concern—than doctors have felt called on to give" (1998, xiii). Indeed, he goes so far as to suggest that the current fad with "empowering" patients (through bills of rights and hospital charters and mission statements lauding patient choice, privacy, and confidentiality) may not be at all what patients want or need, and that they may be more in want of complexity, ambiguity, and ambivalence (Schneider 1998). And a more recent study (Joffe et al. 2003) similarly concluded that it is not so much "decision-making" that patients want involvement in, but rather to be treated with respect and dignity and to have confidence and trust in their carers. Remarkably old-fashioned ideas indeed.

Frank, drawing on Bauman's (1992) work, notes well how "[t]he institutional structures of biomedicine too often suppress moral deliberations … modernist medicine works on the rationalisation principle of breaking down problems into smaller and smaller pieces. Illness is broken down into discrete tasks for different specialists" (1997, 144). Elliot (1999) continues this line of thought, discussing the way in which bioethics is framed in the passive voice in the "medical cases" that are presented and discussed (which is arguably more "objective" than the active voice), and in which the agency of the patient is profoundly attenuated if not entirely evacuated.

Ethics (by which I always mean bioethics, clinical ethics, medical ethics) turns on the "case" that is at once singular and multiple. In order for the one to simultaneously encapsulate the many, ethics extinguishes the "proper name" of a real, enfleshed human individual in the name of a de-identified "case" comprising signs and symptoms, pathologies and deviations, dilemmas and perplexities, and ultimately, of course, principles and rules for getting beyond the problems these invoke. But as we know all too well, patients have proper names, and "proper names are so many points on the map of disasters. They are the stuff on which ethics comes to grief and which launches the search for another idiom for disasters" (Caputo 1993, 30). A "case" of advanced breast cancer takes on a very different hue when it is attached to a proper name. As I discovered with my sister Donna, the proper name, when ascribed to her "case," changes everything about it; she is not just another set of signs and symptoms with a prognosis and treatment plan, but my *sister*, her children's *mother*, and my mother's *daughter*. Every seemingly little clinical/ethical decision is heavily invested with significance when the "case" at hand is your own flesh and blood. Generalizations and statistics offer only superficial comfort when one has to walk away from the clinic and live with the consequences of a disaster.

Illness and Moral Agency: Heteronomy as Another Idiom for Disasters

> Clinical ethics is disjunctive from the morality of illness: it does not help people learn who they are. (Frank 1997, 133)

> Health crises confront their victims with something to do and things to decide, but, far more profoundly, such crises assault identity—they force their victims to decide who and how they will be. (May in Ramsey 2002, xxxv)

Frank (1997) advances a theory that the morality of illness has four key dimensions that provide a useful heuristic in helping us to understand better the ways in which autonomy and Ethics are challenged in the context of the acute illness experience and through the effects of acute hospitalization. This heuristic also orients us toward a sharper recognition of the moral force of the "other," and what our response, as healthcare professionals, to this "other" ought to be.

First, the morality of illness is *phenomenological* (after Toombs 1993). The ways people who are ill, such as my sister, are able to construct their inter-subjective relations with others are bound up in intrinsically moral issues concerning the provision of care (who is going to look after me?) and the mutual obligation the provision of care implies (what part do I as the ill person have to play in the reciprocal giving and receiving of care?). The "lived experience" or the phenomenology of illness is exquisitely a dialogical and embodied encounter between carer and cared for, and even in the face of caring for oneself, an inter-subjective element is impossible to exclude in that when we are ill, not all our needs and wants can be met purely by our own means. To be sure, the experience of being ill is precisely as feared as often it is because it amplifies how especially dependent we are on our human and social resources when stripped of our health and well being. The phenomenology of my sister's experience with cancer has invoked a re-consideration for each of her children, her partner, and the rest of our family in terms of how we each interact with our now fatally wounded kin, and what this throws up for each of us by way of obligation and concern.

The morality of illness is inextricably *narrative*, as well in that people live their lives through the stories they tell about those lives (Charon 1994; de Certeau 1984; Ricoeur, 1981; 1984–88). When we are ill, our illness narratives both reflect and construct the meaning illness has for us. Therefore, the morality of illness must also be a *hermeneutic* affair in that our stories of illness require interpretation by others as well as by ourselves. The narrative and hermeneutic dimensions of illness have resonated acutely with Donna and me perhaps more so than with any other of our relatives. Our relationship has been forced to take a radical twist because in my role as a healthcare insider—and her much loved brother—the interpretive work I do with my sister as she finds new narratives to express her changing sense of self and agency, engenders a whole new mode of being for both of us. This mode is very much concerned with an obligation we have to share our anxieties and our hopes and aspirations with each other as we mutually reinforce the life force that still resides in my sister despite the ravages of her treatment and its side effects (which are considerable and considerably depleting of her sense of self and agency).

And of course, the morality of illness is also *sociological* because all ethical choices and decisions are lived within and through the institutional and cultural fields in which we are situated as human agents. Donna's confrontations with the healthcare system and those who people it in New Zealand have indelibly coloured her experiences, given rise to perversely comical and disquieting tales, and left both her and me puzzled and sometimes angry, as well as admiring and grateful at its all too frequent inadequacies, and its small and not nearly frequent enough triumphs.

Each of these dimensions makes apparent how fragile this idea of autonomy really is, and how an Ethics of the ideal ("true" autonomy implies we have no *need* of the other) is always contingent on the politics of the real. No matter how much we might not want to recognize it, we each live far more in "the call of the other" than the ideal of autonomy would or could admit to. Indeed, it is misrecognition of autonomy's precariousness that always gets us into ethical hot water, as it were, and why it is such a limited and limiting concept in the ethico-political domain in healthcare.

We have reached a point where I want to claim, as has Frank, that ethics in clinical practice ought to be considered more as process rather than substance. As he explains it: "Once ethics is endowed with substantive form, it becomes another specialty that *some* people do, and can be left *to them*. This ethics-as-substance can bring some necessary safeguards to clinical work … but imagining ethics this way limits the scope of being ethical" (Frank 2004, 355). Indeed, I would suggest it absolves people from being ethical insofar as they can "pass the (ethical) buck" on to the "expert" to deal with, rather than attempting to deal with it themselves. Horrobin suggests further to this idea of ethics as process that "personhood may be seen to be necessarily a *process*, rather than simply a categorical state" (2006, 290). For him the process of personhood is a melange of our desires and aspirations, our predilections and proclivities, our experiences and all they invoke by way of emotions, memories, and the legacies these create in their wake. Therefore it makes no sense to see ethics and our individual and collective moralities as anything other than another element in the process of personhood, which is "intrinsically open-ended" (Horrobin 2006, 291). This person-as-process is, of course, the postmodernist's rejoinder to the fixed and final, sovereign individual of the Enlightenment, which underscores the notion of autonomy under discussion here.

We need to re-instate the idea of ethics as a practice and not merely as a theory to be "applied" at an appropriate moment for a generic case. We equally need to inculcate in our practitioners a strong sense of what it means to be a moral being in the way that every move we make carries moral implications, not just the "dilemmas" and "quandaries" discussed endlessly in textbooks and arcane journal articles. Unfortunately, ethics is taught mostly, in nursing at least, as a relatively discrete and separate unit from clinical practice and its related subjects, such as bioscience and social theory. It is not positioned as a dynamic and integral, undeniably indispensable aspect of everyday life in healthcare. This, it seems to me, is simply inadequate if we want to nurture a new generation of clinicians who will undoubtedly face even more vexing and complex "ethical dilemmas" than previous generations. But more important still, we need a model of care which will enable such learning by elevating the ethical to a new plane in clinical education and practice.

Against EBP as a "Regime of Truth"; A Return to Casuistry as an Exemplary "Model of Care" in Which the Morality of Illness Can Find Expression

Let us turn now to the ethics of evidence because healthcare is thoroughly an ethical enterprise, and in these evidence-besieged times, it behoves clinicians to turn their thoughts to the morality of clinical decision-making in the midst of more "facts and figures," more treatment options, more potential errors of decision-making and action than ever before. As it has been well-rehearsed by others, the phenomenon of EBP has appeared over the last 15 years as an attempt to help resolve the considerable problem of the burden of evidence that now threatens to crush the very practitioners of the various medical arts under its sheer weight and volume (Feinstein and Horowitz 1997; Gold 2004; Hampton 2002; Harari 2001; Holmes et al. 2008; Jordan and Segrott 2008; Sarasin 1999; Schriger 2000; Tonelli 2001). If ever we lived in times where it was vexing to pose the defining ethical quandary—what are we to do?—these are them.

In medicine specifically and healthcare generally, an enormous quantum of intellectual and political energy and expertise has been invested over the last 15 years in an attempt to shift healthcare culture toward a universal acceptance of the methods of evidence-based practice (Gregson et al. 2002; Kitson 2002; Miles et al. 2003; 2006; and 2007; Rycroft-Malone 2006; Rolfe and Watson 2008). Unfortunately (or perhaps not), universal acceptance, even in the face of such academic and professional profligacy, has failed to materialize (Miles et al. 2003; 2006; and 2007; Williams and Garner 2002). One of the main reasons for this, it seems to me, is that EBP's over-riding concern is the removal of uncertainty by the application of rigorously conducted research evidence that points the way in clinical practice to "what works." But this seems misguided because surely it is a matter not just of the pragmatist's "what works," but what works now, for this particular situation, in this set of circumstances. It is the unrelieved messiness of clinical practice life "in the flux" that renders each and every decision so fraught with potential peril; this is simply a fact of life and will never be erased, no matter how much knowledge we can produce or ever cleverer interventions we can design.

Naylor, speaking of clinical medicine, notes that it seems "to consist of a few things we know, a few things we think we know (but probably don't), and lots of things we don't know at all" (1995, 840). Noting the interval since Naylor made this claim, it is obvious that the more evidence we garner about ever more detailed aspects of the human condition, the more we realize how much there is yet to know (mapping the human genome, for instance, has raised more questions than it has found answers to the mysteries of disease and illness).

In light of this reality, Frank suggests "method [such as EBP] is a procedure for seeking some kind of truth. Method seeks to render analysis, and assertion, trustworthy" (2003, 1414). He continues to add that "[m]ethod, like surgery, aspires to closure; instead, we need witnesses to opening: people who refuse to be either this or that" (2003, 1416). Ultimately, for Frank "the perennial ethical struggle is to get those who invoke the weight of the medical-technological apparatus to listen to the witnesses of the effects of that apparatus" (2003, 1417). This is where I make my case for casuistry as opposed to EBP. For it is in the case-based approach—in which the witness is the patient—that the healthcare provider can enter into dialogue with the other, and the ethical concerns raised by the other's illness experience can best be defined and appropriate action be taken. Parker, too, believes that "[i]ntersubjective discussion and decision is the most reliable procedure for having access to moral truth, since the exchange of ideas and the need to justify oneself before others … broaden one's knowledge and reveal defects in reasoning" (2001, 89).

Montgomery Hunter proffers a definition: "Clinical casuistry … is the comparative analysis of a particular case with all its special circumstances in an effort to relate that case reliably to a system of received principles … [it] is not a matter of theoretical principles but the tested accumulation of generalisations: practical guidelines, clinical dogma, rules of thumb" (1989, 195–6). Clinical casuistry, then, offers itself up as both a process and an outcome. It is a process in the way it is inherently pedagogical; it is designed and required to teach others. All clinicians know and understand all too well how little knowledge the textbooks are really able to impart to them. It is only in the vicissitudes of life "on the wards" that their theoretical knowledge comes alive in the form of individual "cases." Nursing and the allied health sciences also pivot very heavily on this translational process of relating textbook knowledge by way of innumerable encounters with living breathing patients who visibly, viscerally, and vitally embody their diseases (the objective case) and their illness experiences (the subjective case). These days, while officially dead, the apprenticeship model of much clinical learning is, in reality, still very much alive and well for all the health disciplines; it is around the care of discrete, embodied, irregular individuals that most clinical learning takes place, and where the "variables in clinical practice (as elsewhere) approach the infinite: signs shade into the absences of signs" (Montgomery Hunter 1989, 205). This is why casuistry poses such a useful and compelling model, not only for teaching and learning about clinical epistemology, but even more importantly, for ethical decision-making.

But casuistry is equally an outcome. It is an outcome not only in that it produces a tailored and collaborative model of care for each patient, but also in the way it produces in each clinician a degree of humility and wariness of their knowledge and skills, which are vital if healthcare is not to become sclerotic and unable to adapt to new discoveries, new modes of thinking and acting. As Montgomery Hunter puts it, "[s]cepticism in the face of the individual case is the mark of [the medical] profession. With each case they are taught the tentativeness of their knowledge and the uncertainty of their practice" (1989, 200). This is without doubt the most appropriate ethos for grappling with the moral exigencies of clinical care.

Tonelli, a professor of medicine, makes a strong argument for the re-introduction of casuistry as not only a framework for clinical decision-making, but also for ethical decision-making. In doing this he notes that the "major limitations of empirical research evidence relate to the fact that it cannot be directly applied to any particular patient" (2006, 252). Others, too, have decried this shortcoming (Feinstein and Horowitz 1997, 531; Sarasin 1999, 669; Williams and Garner 2002). But Tonelli also recognizes that "reasoning from empirical evidence specifically also represents a form of practical or casuistic reasoning" (2006, 253) because the doctor must decide whether the generalized evidence at hand applies to the specific patient before him or her. As he suggests, "reasoning will be in the form of analogy, with a search for cases, actual or 'average,' that are most similar to the case-at-hand" (Tonelli 2006, 254). Porta concurs, noting that "even if one decides to strictly follow empirical evidence, the very decision of which reported RCT(s), if any, is relevant to a particular case-at-hand remains a process of arbitrary evaluation" (2006, 265). But as Borry et al. caution, "the best choice from an empirical point of view is not necessarily the best from an ethical point of view" (2006, 309). Because ethics is resolutely concerned with values and beliefs, what the case-based approach does allow for, however, and to which I alluded above, is their inclusion not as mere adjuncts to the "real" and important "hard data" of research, but as equal and perhaps even superordinate to such data in certain situations.

We must remember that when evidence-based medicine (EBM) mentions integrating patients' values, "it is writing from the point of view of practitioners. That is, the notion of 'patient values' refers to the fact that people have values, not the actual values themselves" (Gupta 2006, 297). Values held by a patient may not count as evidence for all practitioners, but they certainly count as influences on the types of evidence, empirical or otherwise, that may be allowed to inform a clinical decision that has significant ethical dimensions and consequences for the patient. As Gupta asks, "if casuistry *is* a good model for clinical decision making, does it matter if we classify certain inputs as evidentiary and others as non-evidentiary?" (2006, 298). For me the answer is no, it does not. Practice-based evidence as a form of clinical epistemology is more complex an epistemology to deal with than EBP because it involves acknowledging and working with many variables and highly contingent factors to be incorporated into the decision-making process. But this should not deter us from working with such knowledge if it is best and right for each patient's plan of care.

The case-based approach also restores the moral agency of the patient by returning the health professional to a more humble and less hierarchical position in the order of things. As my sister's experiences with doctors, nurses, and the systems within which they are obliged to work attest, the moral dimensions of her illness experience have frequently been over-ridden by the pressures and demands imposed by hierarchically organized and institutionalized healthcare. This system diminishes a patient's sense of self and agency by reducing them to an attenuated and prefabricated version of a patient (let alone a person).

Of course, this is not to suggest that the majority of healthcare professionals are not inherently caring and concerned individuals. Rather, it is to suggest that over the last several decades, with the rise and rise of ideological and political movements such as EBP and the effects it has had on clinicians, the use of economically driven frameworks, such as diagnostic related groupings and case-mix payments, and the ever present emphasis on the fiscal bottom line, the options available to provide ethical, compassionate, and effective care have become ever more difficult to sustain. And this begs the ethical question once again: What is to be done?

Last Words: From Disaster to Hope

I began this chapter with a lamentation of a disaster where my sister lost her guiding star and simply ran out of luck; life is so much more serendipity than it is strategy, and nothing demonstrated this better to me and to Donna than her diagnosis and subsequent enmeshment in the medico-technological apparatus. All our lives are disasters waiting to happen and all patients are living breathing exemplars of the disastrous made flesh. "Disasters are events of surpassing or irretrievable loss …

a wasting of life, something that cannot be repaired, recompensed, redeemed … You cannot grow another body; you cannot regain wasted years" (Caputo 1993, 29). Taking this as my parting premise, then, as healthcare professionals we must find ways of responding to all the various disasters that present themselves to us and which oblige us, literally *bind* us to the other and make it our task in obligation "to 'begin with' the case—of a disaster, of a damaged life, of an irretrievable loss, of innocent, avoidable suffering" (Caputo 1993, 36). For, as Derrida reminds us, "there is no society without faith, without trust in the other" (in Caputo 1997, 23). As human beings working with other human beings when they are suffering and most in need, clinicians are a privileged group indeed. The care and trust patients both need and want from us extract a considerable energy. But this energy can be restored if we work in intimate collaboration with our patients, always ensuring the evidence is relevant and appropriate for our needs and their hopes and aspirations for the future. Casuistry provides both a pedagogy and a model of care for our uncertain times; it is as relevant as an epistemological and moral framework for clinical practice now as it ever has been. Sometimes what is old is better by far than anything new (and certainly so in the world of human affairs where very little of how we ought to live is unknown to us).

Caputo describes the "heteronomic force of the other" as:

> the feeling that comes over us when others need our help, when they call out for help, or support, or freedom, or whatever they need, a feeling that grows in strength directly in proportion to the desperateness of the situation of the other. The power of obligation varies directly with the powerlessness of the one who calls for help, which is the power of powerlessness. To be sure, the oldest and most honourable work of ethics has been to defend and honour obligation, to make obligation safe. (1993, 5)

But Caputo's deconstruction positions obligation as the point, the moment, the event that makes ethics come unstuck because obligation deals with the here and now, it is always present, it is a condition of "the 'factical life' … as soon as we come to be we find ourselves … enmeshed in obligations. The 'ought' is, in fact, one of the most common features of what 'is,' of what is happening" (Caputo 1993, 7).

If there is to be an ethics of evidence, then, it must be an ethics grounded in this "factical life" (after Heidegger 1987) because that is the only life there is. And if there can be an autonomous individual who is without need, then good luck to him/her, because the evidence before us everywhere suggests quite the obverse. Human beings are inextricably interdependent despite the ruses and follies they perpetrate to convince themselves otherwise. A new form of ethical subjectivity, then, when laid bare and unmasked, stripped of piety and profundity, divested of all historico-political baggage, must, unequivocally and forever, be marked by the call of the other.

References

Bauman, Z. (1992), *Mortality, Immortality, and Other Life Strategies* (Stanford, CA: Stanford University Press).

Beauchamp, T. and Childress, J. (1994), *Principles of Biomedical Ethics*, 4th edition (New York: Oxford University Press).

Borry, P. et al. (2005), "The Birth of the Empirical Turn in Bioethics," *Bioethics* 19:1, 49–71.

Borry, P. et al. (2006), "Evidence-based Medicine and Its Role in Ethical Decision-Making," *Journal of Evaluation in Clinical Practice* 12:3, 306–11.

Caputo, J.D. (1993), *Against Ethics: Contributions to a Poetics of Obligation with Constant Reference to Deconstruction* (Bloomington, IN and Indianapolis, IN: Indiana University Press).

Caputo, J.D. (ed.) (1997), *Deconstruction in a Nutshell: A Conversation with Jacques Derrida* (New York: Fordham University Press).

Charon, R. (1994), "Narrative Contributions to Medical Ethics: Recognition, Formulation, Interpretation, and Validation in the Practice of the Ethicist," in E. DuBose et al. (eds), *A Matter of Principles? Ferment in US Bioethics* (Valley Forge, PA: Trinity Press International).

De Certeau, M. (1984), *The Practice of Everyday Life* (Berkeley, CA: University of California Press).

Dodds, S. and Thompson, C. (2006), "Bioethics and Democracy: Competing Roles of National Bioethics Organisations," *Bioethics* 20:6, 326–38.

Elam, D. (1994), *Feminism and Deconstruction: Ms. En Abyme* (London and New York: Routledge).

Elliot, C. (1999), *A Philosophical Disease: Bioethics, Culture and Identity* (New York and London: Routledge).

Feinstein, R.A. and Horowitz, R.I. (1997), "Problems in the 'Evidence' of 'Evidence-based Medicine,'" *The American Journal of Medicine* 103, 529–35.

Frank, A.W. (1997), "Illness as Moral Occasion: Restoring Agency to Ill People," *Health* 1:2, 131–48.

Frank, A.W. (2003), "Surgical Body Modifications and Altruistic Individualism: A Case for Cyborg Ethics and Methods," *Qualitative Healthcare Research* 13:10, 1407–18.

Frank, A.W (2004), "Ethics as Process and Practice," *Internal Medicine Journal* 34, 355–7.

Gold, M. (2004), "Is Honesty Always the Best Policy? Ethical Aspects of Truth Telling," *Internal Medicine Journal* 34, 578–80.

Gregson, P.R.W. et al. (2002), "Meta-analysis: In the Glass Eye of Evidence-Based Practice?" *Nursing Inquiry* 9:1, 24–30.

Grosz, E. (1995), *Space, Time, and Perversion* (Sydney: Allen and Unwin).

Gupta, M. (2006), "Beyond 'Evidence,' Comment on Tonelli (2006), Integrating Evidence into Clinical Practice: An Alternative to Evidence-Based Approaches," *Journal of Evaluation in Clinical Practice* 12:3, 296–8.

Hampton, J.R. (2002), "Evidence-Based Medicine, Opinion-Based Medicine, and Real-World Medicine," *Perspectives in Biology and Medicine* 45:4, 549–68.
Harari, E. (2001), "Whose Evidence? Lessons from the Philosophy of Science and the Epistemology of Medicine," *Australian and New Zealand Journal of Psychiatry* 35, 724–30.
Heidegger, M. (1987), *Being and Time* (Oxford: Basil Blackwell).
Holmes, D. et al. (2008), "Nursing Best-Practice Guidelines: Reflecting on the Obscene Rise of the Void," *Journal of Nursing Management* 16, 394–403.
Horrobin, S. (2006), "Immortality, Human Nature, the Value of Life and the Value of Life Extension," *Bioethics* 20:6, 279–92.
Joffe, S. et al. (2003), "What do Patients Value in Their Hospital Care? An Empirical Perspective on Autonomy Centred Ethics," *Journal of Medical Ethics* 29, 103–8.
Johnson, P. (1994), *Feminism as Radical Humanism* (Sydney: Allen and Unwin).
Jordan, S. and Segrott, J. (2008), "Evidence-Based Practice: The Debate," *Journal of Nursing Management* 16:4, 385–7.
Kitson, A. (2002), "Recognising Relationships: Reflections on Evidence-Based Practice," *Nursing Inquiry* 9:3, 179–86.
Komesaroff, P. (ed.) (1995), *Troubled Bodies: Critical Perspectives of Postmodernism, Medical Ethics, and the Body* (Melbourne: Melbourne University Press).
Leeder, S.R. (2004), "Ethics and Public Health," *Internal Medicine Journal* 34, 435–9.
Lupton, M.G.F. and Williams, D.J. (2004), "The Ethics of Research on Pregnant Women: Is Maternal Consent Sufficient?" *British Journal of Obstetrics and Gynaecology* 111, 1307–12.
Mansfield, N. (2000), *Subjectivity: Theories of the Self from Freud to Haraway* (Sydney: Allen and Unwin).
McGrath, P. (1998), "Autonomy, Discourse, and Power: A Postmodern Reflection on Principlism and Bioethics," *Journal of Medicine and Philosophy* 23:5, 516–32.
Miles, A. et al. (2003), "Current Thinking in the Evidence-Based Health Care Debate," *Journal of Evaluation in Clinical Practice* 9:2, 95–109.
Miles, A. et al. (2006), "The Evidence-Based Health Care Debate: Where Are We Now?" *Journal of Evaluation in Clinical Practice* 12:3, 239–47.
Miles, A. et al. (2007), "Medicine and Evidence: Knowledge and Action in Clinical Practice," *Journal of Evaluation in Clinical Practice* 13:4, 481–503.
Montgomery Hunter, K. (1989), "A Science of Individuals: Medicine and Casuistry," *The Journal of Medicine and Philosophy* 14, 193–212.
Mykhalovskiy, E. (2003), "Evidence-Based Medicine: Ambivalent Reading and the Clinical Recontextualisation of Science," *Health* 7:3, 331–52.
Naylor, C.D. (1995), "Gray Zones of Clinical Practice: Some Limits to Evidence-Based Medicine," *The Lancet* 345, 840–42.

Parker, M. (2001), "The Ethics of Evidence-Based Patient Choice," *Health Expectations* 4, 87–91.

Porta, M.P. (2006), "Five Warrants for Medical Decision Making: Some Considerations and a Proposal to Better Integrate Evidence-Based Medicine into Everyday Practice. Commentary on Tonelli (2006), Integrating Evidence into Clinical Practice: An Alternative to Evidence-Based Approaches," *Journal of Evaluation in Clinical Practice* 12:3, 265–8.

Ramsey, P. (2002), *The Patient as Person: Exploration in Medical Ethics*, 2nd edition (New Haven, CT and London: Yale University Press).

Ricoeur, P. (1981), *Paul Ricoeur: Hermeneutics and the Social Sciences*, J.B. Thompson (ed. and trans.) (Cambridge: Cambridge University Press).

Ricoeur, P. (1984–88), *Time and Narrative* (vols I–III), K. McLaughlin and D. Pellauer (trans.) (Chicago, IL: University of Chicago Press).

Rolfe, G. and Watson, R. (2008), "Evidence-Based Practice: A Debate," *Journal of Nursing Management* 16, 486–93.

Rycroft-Malone, J. (2006), "The Politics of Evidence-Based Practice Movements," *Journal of Research in Nursing* 11:2, 95–108.

Sarasin, F.P. (1999), "Decision Analysis and the Implementation of Evidence-Based Medicine," *Quarterly Journal of Medicine* 92, 669–71.

Schneider, C.E. (1998), *The Practice of Autonomy: Patients, Doctors, and Medical Decisions* (New York and Oxford: Oxford University Press).

Schriger, D.L. (2000), "One is the Loneliest Number: Be Sceptical of Evidence Summaries Based on Limited Literature," *Annals of Emergency Medicine* 36:5, 517–19.

Shildrick, M. (1997), *Leaky Bodies and Boundaries: Feminism, Postmodernism, and (Bio)ethics* (New York and London: Routledge).

Tannenbaum, S.J. (2006), "Evidence by Any Other Name: Commentary on Tonelli (2006), Integrating Evidence into Clinical Practice: An Alternative to Evidence-Based Approaches," *Journal of Evaluation in Clinical Practice* 12:3, 273–6.

Tauber, A.I. (1999), *Confessions of a Medical Man: An Essay in Popular Philosophy* (Cambridge, MA and London: MIT Press).

Tonelli, M.R. (2001), "The Limits of Evidence-Based Medicine," *Respiratory Care* 46:12, 1435–41.

Tonelli, M.R. (2006), "Integrating Evidence into Clinical Practice: An Alternative to Evidence-Based Approaches," *Journal of Evaluation in Clinical Practice* 12:3, 248–56.

Toombs, S.K. (1993), *The Meaning of Illness: A Phenomenological Account of the Different Perspectives of Physicians and Patient* (Dordrecht: Kluwer).

Walker, K. (1997), "Dangerous Liaisons: Thinking, Doing, Nursing," *The Collegian* 4:2, 4–14.

Walker, K. (2000), "Why Philosophy?: Nursing and the Problem of Truth," in J. Daly et al. (eds), *Contexts of Nursing: An Introduction* (Sydney: McClelland and Petty).

Williams, D.D.R. and Garner, J. (2002), "The Case Against 'The Evidence': A Different Perspective on Evidence-Based Medicine," *The British Journal of Psychiatry* 180, 8–12.

Wolpe, P.R. (1998), "The Triumph of Autonomy in American Bioethics: A Sociological View," in R. DeVries et al. (eds), *Bioethics and Society: Constructing the Ethical Enterprise* (Upper Saddle River, NJ: Prentice Hall).

Chapter 2
"You Might Not Feel Like Yourself": On Heart Transplants, Identity, and Ethics

Jennifer M. Poole, Margrit Shildrick, Patricia McKeever, Susan Abbey, and Heather Ross

Introduction

> A 15 year old girl has received a heart transplant against her wishes in an English hospital … She told her lawyer, "I understand what a heart transplant means—checkups and pills. I am only 15 and don't want a transplant … If I had someone else's heart, I would feel different from anybody else and that's a good reason not to have a transplant, even if it saved my life." The judge ruled that the girl was confused and allowed the operation to proceed … Lawyers have hailed the ruling as humane and just, but medical ethicists have reservations …. (Richmond 1999, 680)

This young woman is not alone in her protests. Since her story appeared in print, anecdotal reports indicate that other patients have refused a heart transplant, defying expectations, denying the extension of life. Some have wanted to give the "gift of life" back after having a transplant operation, maintaining that had they fully known what the process entailed, had they understood the disruption of personal identity and the sense of loss and distress, they would not have given their consent. A few have even tried to undo the procedure themselves, slicing into their own "recovered" bodies because the feelings were too much, the intrusion too great. Yet, seldom do we hear these stories over the din that is the gift-of-life discourse, a chirping chorus about donor heroism and medical miracles. When disquieting instances of resistance, dissent, or suffering make it through the discursive border patrols, such cases are often psychiatrized or dismissed, not reported in the literature or, literally, over-ruled. Yet the troubling talk continues, raising questions around care, consent, and the ethics of transplantation.

According to Cassell, "we must not allow our wonderment over medical technology to cloud our ability to perceive the moral dilemmas that accompany such advancements" (cited in Sharp 1995, 358). Rising to the challenge, in this short chapter we speak to our phenomenologically-informed exploration of heart transplantation and identity. We focus on the dilemmas that accompany what contemporary philosopher and heart transplant recipient Jean-Luc Nancy (2000) calls the "intruding" heart. After a brief tour of the transplantation terrain, we outline our project and its links to the work of Maurice Merleau-Ponty (1989). We then turn to ethics, making clear how the study speaks to both traditional and critical ethicists and suggest some potential ways forward. Although cognizant of the "significant political risks in taking a critical perspective that varies from the progress through medical miracles narrative" (Koenig and Hogel 1995, 396), we end with some of the questions our work has raised, questions that have important implications for researchers, ethicists, professionals, and patients.

On Transplantation

Many know that with cardiac transplantation come medical challenges, such as organ rejection, kidney dysfunction, cancer, and hypertension. Indeed, these challenges are so great that the average life expectancy post transplant is just ten years (Taylor et al. 2008). Relatively little attention tends to be given to the "psychosocial challenges" associated with this kind of life, including poor return-to-work rates as well as high anxiety and distress levels (Dew et al. 2005; Paris and White-Williams 2005; Paris et al. 1993; Taylor et al. 2006). According to Sharp (2006), not only has empirical research about heart transplants historically been "marked by the erasure of the fleshy body" (8), but commentaries about quality of life or suffering have also been rare. However, the tide appears to be turning, with more quality-of-life studies appearing in the literature in recent years. Indeed, one review confirms that issues, such as anxiety, distress, and suffering are not confined to the initial stages of recovery but may appear or be exacerbated at any time (Dew and DiMartini 2005), especially at the three to five year point post transplant. Findings of another study suggest that nearly one third of heart recipients experience substantial, sustained distress over the course of their (post-transplant) lives (Dew et al. 2005).

In the transplant literature, this distress is often psychiatrized, interpreted as depression, anxiety, post-traumatic stress disorder (Stukas et al. 1998), or psychosis (Abbott et al. 2003; Brosig and Woidera 1993; Bunzel et al. 1990; Bunzel et al. 2005; Evangelista et al. 2003; Laederach-Hofman et al. 2002; Salvucci 2004; Triffaux et al. 2002). "Night-time anxiety, feelings of suffocation" (Brosig and Woidera 1993), "delirium" (Triffaux et al. 2002), and "psychosomatic hyperventilation syndrome" (Bunzel et al. 1990) have also been reported. Some psychoanalytically informed researchers have argued these symptoms are linked to mourning, denial, and/or guilt over the donor's death (Bunzel et al. 1992a; Burner 1994; Castelnuevo-Tedesco 1973; Castelnuevo-Tedesco 1978; Goetzmann 2004; Inspector et al. 2004; Kaba et al. 2005; Mai 1986; Rauch and Kneen 1989; Sanner 2003). However, other researchers have posited that these symptoms may be related to recipients' beliefs that they have taken on characteristics of their donors (Brosig and Woidera 1993; Bunzel et al. 1992b; Burner 1994; Inspector et al. 2004; Pearsall 2001; Pearsall et al. 2002; Sanner 2003). For example, an Israeli study of

35 male heart recipients employed five assessment tools to investigate recipients' attitudes toward the graft and the donor. The findings indicated that almost 50 per cent of recipients had an overt or covert notion that they had acquired personality characteristics of the donor along with the heart (Inspector et al. 2004). Another study reported that 21 per cent of respondents said their personality had changed post-operatively, attributing this either to the trauma of nearly dying (15 per cent) or to the grafted heart (6 per cent). The remaining 79 per cent "showed massive defense and denial reactions, mainly by rapidly changing the subject or making the question ridiculous" (Bunzel et al. 1992b).

Importantly, this psychosocial research has made clear that responses, whether reported as denial, distress, depression, or related to the donor, have profound effects on the health and well being of heart recipients (Abbott et al. 2003; Dew and DiMartini 2005). These responses may lead to non-compliance with medications and lifestyle modifications or to harmful or even fatal physical symptoms (Bunzel et al. 1990; Dew and DiMartini 2005; Salvucci 2004).

Intrigued, unsettled, and critical, a handful of scholars in the humanities and social sciences have begun to explore organ transplantation. Speaking to identity disruptions specifically, Waldby (2002; and 2006 with Mitchell) argues that since the "given organ is not a neutral and detachable anatomical component, but rather a fragment that partakes of the identity of the donor" (2002, 248), it follows that recipients sometimes "feel they will be 'invaded' or overwhelmed," overtaken by the "identity associated by the organ" (2002, 248). Similarly, Sharp's (1995; 2006) anthropological research suggests that some recipients actively integrate the donor's personality into their post-transplant identity, despite being chastised by physicians for harbouring such "unscientific" attitudes. Finally, in Nancy's (2000) philosophical account of his own heart transplant, he writes, "never has the strangeness of my own identity … touched me with such acuity," for in "me is the intrus" (10), the new heart. Initially he feels that the "intruder" is twenty years younger than he "is," a "multiple stranger" (11) who unsettles notions of health and sickness, life and death, as well as self and other. This kind of critical writing (see also: Fox and Swazey 1992; Haddow 2005; Hird 2007) raises deeply troubling questions about heart transplantation. However, as contemporary Western medicine still largely endorses a mechanistic, Cartesian, and "replaceable parts" model of the body, such discussions are often devalued or dismissed altogether by most transplant professionals (Sharp 1995; Sylvia and Novak 1997).

Practice, PITH, and Phenomenology

It therefore came as no surprise that at the major Canadian transplant centre where our study is now in the data analysis stage, there is no *official* talk before surgery about possible post-transplant sensations of identity disruption or feelings of otherness. To our knowledge, no potential transplant recipient is informed that s/he may experience a "transformed sense of self" (Koenig and Hogel 1995, 395).

Despite arguments that those who cannot find a way to live with such identity transformations are at much higher risk of immunological rejection (Lock 2002), cancer, and death, no member of the transplant team makes official mention of Sharp's work, of Nancy's experience, or even of the "medical" research articles that indicate that the operation may lead to a life of distress and depression.

At our centre and others, potential recipients typically receive a standard psychosocial evaluation, as well as a manual outlining medical complications, adverse drug reactions, and statistics about life expectancy. If they are conscious (for all are extremely ill when the decision to transplant is made), they are offered a meeting with an approved mentor. Mentors have been through the process and can provide advice on lifestyle modifications, as well as opportunities to discuss "what it's really like" to live with a transplanted heart. Yet, fewer prospective recipients take up the offer than would be expected. Instead, they (and their families) leaf through the manual, make sure their affairs are in order, and with a pager at the ready, assume the "caution and cartwheels" (Trainor and Ezer 2000) position on the all-important waiting list for hours, days, or months.

Wanting to take up these and other issues, to discover whether transplant recipients might not feel like themselves, our interdisciplinary team came together to improve care, as well as consent processes. After designing a study entitled the Process of Incorporating a Transplanted Heart (The PITH Project), we turned away from positivism and the notion of a Cartesian body and turned to the phenomenology of Merleau-Ponty (1989). Merleau-Ponty argued that the self is not a once-and-for-all identity, but a never-ending process of becoming. He also maintained that since we come into the world as bodies, human experience is necessarily embodied, temporal, and spatial. Hence, any modification to the body is a modification to the sense of self (Moss 1989).

Informed by this particular strand of phenomenology, our research project asks how heart transplant recipients perceive their hearts, bodily integrity, and personal identity, and how they imagine and speak about their donors. How do these perceptions, thoughts, and accounts change over time, and is there a relationship between these perceptions and recipients' physical and mental outcomes?

Working with a qualitative visual methodology, we have now interviewed more than 25 heart transplant recipients, videotaped the sessions to capture body language, and are well into the process of data analysis. Sitting through the tapes, we have watched participants speak of identity disruption, distress, depression, dreams of the donor, and a loss so palpable that we have had trouble shifting from our seats at the end of these days. We have been told how patients "should" be prepared, what they wished they would have known, and how some might have done it all differently if given a second "kick" at consent. There have been expressions of gratitude to donors and professionals, as well as caution in these interviews, for some participants seem to want to stay close to official transplant narratives. There have also been disjuncts between what some participants say and how they sound or look, especially when insisting they are "ecstatic" about their gift of life. And yet a detailed report on our findings to date is both entirely premature and outside the remit of this particular chapter. Instead, in the next section, we turn to what our preliminary observations have to say back to the field of ethics.

On the Ethics of Transplantation: Towards Traditional and Critical Possibilities

With respect to heart transplantation, there has always been much ethical hay to be made (Belkin 2003; Bergen 1968; Boniolo 2007; Grande et al. 1998; Halpern et al. 2008; Shildrick 2008; Wright et al. 2005). In 1967, Dr Christiaan Barnard performed the first transplant on a Mr Louis Washkansky, a procedure not only hailed as a medical miracle, but also one that became an international news item. Mr Washkansky lived only 18 days, but those days were spent in the public eye, with complete disregard for the confidentiality and anonymity afforded donors and recipients in Canada today. Akin to the recent case of the French facial transplant (Lafrance 2008), both the recipient and the transplant team were photographed and filmed. The films were aired on television, and various biographical details of the deceased donor were made publicly available.

We argue that for traditional bioethicists, both examples raise issues concerning not just confidentiality and consent (Halpern et al. 2008), but also concerning the status of medical research subjects, the power of medical professionals, and the right to treatment. In addition, reflecting on transplantation generally, dilemmas abound with respect to what limits should be set on the procurement (Kuczewski 2002; Sells 2003), commercialization (Scheper-Hughes 2004; Somerville 2008), and allocation of organs (Childress 1996; Joralemon 1995), the bias of heart transplantation towards male recipients, as well as how to determine when (and if) a donor is really "dead." Indeed, there is much discussion in mainstream ethics circles around brain-stem and cardiac death (Boniolo 2007; Truog and Robinson 2003; Veatch 2000) as the issue of when to transplant for maximum effectiveness is paramount to procedural success and recipient prognosis. However, the boundaries between "alive" and "dead"—between waiting just enough time and too much before procuring the organ—are slippery. On this most debated issue, "bioethicists are asked to establish a binary system of right and wrong, as though a clear distinction between life and death were still possible" (Shildrick 2008, 37).

Although our study is not specifically concerned with the question of when to procure, our findings will raise other dilemmas that are of equal importance for clinical bioethicists. As we have made clear, both the nature and causes of distress in recipients are begging for thorough ethical debate. Similarly, ethicists may need to turn their attention to recipient grief and loss pertaining to the removed heart and/or the new sense of self that is perceived. Most important is the issue of informed consent. Our findings will urge discussion to determine whether, how, and when potential identity disruption and the statistics on depression and distress should be shared with prospective recipients.

At this juncture and for that audience, we will be asked to explore these issues in a "detached and abstract way that cites precedents, applies principles and rules, calculates the numbers, and arrives finally at some determination of the rightness or wrongness of the given procedure" (Shildrick 2008, 36–7). Yet, before that time and task, before we make clear "the myth of rational, free choice based on full disclosure of factual information" (Koenig and Hogel 1995, 395), we want to explore how a critical stance on bioethics begets additional issues and possibilities for heart transplantation.

For us, that critical stance includes feminist challenges to mainstream bioethics, such as the over-reliance on abstract principles, the neglect of context, as well as the meaning of autonomy (Bacchi and Beasley 2005; Nelson 2000; Tong 1997; Tong et al. 2004; Shildrick 2005). And yet, unlike most feminist work, our critical stance also includes recent developments in poststructuralist, postmodern, and phenomenological thought that allow a flexibility and fluidity in bioethics that is always open to the possibility of change (Diprose 2002; Shildrick 1997 and 2005). In the words of PITH team member, philosopher Margrit Shildrick:

> As body theory focuses increasingly on the fragility and vulnerability of embodiment, should we not be prepared to seek out theoretical approaches which reflect that model rather than the autonomous, invulnerable, sovereign subject assumed by traditional bioethics? … It is clear that the boundaries that have previously marked the predictability and uniformity of human form and function are ambiguous and unstable. (2008, 32)

And so, to critically think-through the unstable processes that characterize heart transplantation, we have turned to the "postconventional" practices of Derrida, Foucault, and Merleau-Ponty. These practices eschew laws, absolutes, and universal rules and principles, demanding instead a profound engagement with difficult issues and dilemmas. To engage with heart transplantation in this way is to accept uncertainty. It is also to dispense with the notion of a core self that persists unchanged after the heart "graft."

Following Merleau-Ponty (1989), our critical/postconventional perspective insists that the individual is not an independent, free-standing entity. In place of the rigid and normatively framed autonomous self for whom the body is a possession that gives rise to property rights and questions of alienability, the phenomenological self is inseparable from and only exists in virtue of those who are others. This approach focuses not simply on the abstract interconnections between self and other, but, more fundamentally, on an intercorporeality in which bodies are woven together. As Waldby explains, the "organ recipient is involved in the most direct and literal form of intercorporeality" (2002, 249), and this brings his or her feelings of loss or transference of identity into sharp focus.

Perhaps it may be more ethical to encourage prospective recipients to understand that the graft will never truly be their own, but part of a shared, intercorporeal relationship with the donor. Although transplant professionals may assert that the donor's heart is a neutral "spare part" waiting to be claimed by a recipient, the reality is that each graft comes with DNA that will never lose its separate identity. As this "alien" corporeal matter is always essential to, but never the same as the recipient's body, we suggest that perhaps this otherness should be accepted, integrated into a model of embodiment in transplantation that acknowledges, rather than denies intercorporeality.

Similarly, in the hopes of reducing distress around identity disruption, we maintain that it may be more ethical to teach recipients about postconventional notions of subjectivity in which the self is always "multiple, contradictory and in-process" (Newton 1988, cited in Fook 2002, 74). This understanding could make space for the possibility of other "selves" and identities both during and after the transplant process.

From this follows another argument that it might be more fitting to consider the graft not as a "gift," but as a "guest." Drawing on Derrida's work (1992; 1999; and 2000), we argue that to host such a guest demands an openness, a form of hospitality that does not necessarily come with comfort or clarity. Such a host cannot set limitations on what crosses the threshold of the body but must offer an unconditional welcome, regardless of the outcome.

Finally, our critical stance calls for a recognition of the ways in which prospective and actual heart recipients reject and resist established discourses around productivity, the gift of life, and identity. Recipients may not go back to "work" post-transplant, they may not feel grateful or ecstatic all the time, and they "may not feel like themselves." As Sharp argues, "transplantation is a social act that generates new biographies" (1995, 378), and space must be made for these biographies, many of which will be discursively different. Indeed, we must accept that some "recipients are renegades; defying the rhetoric of transplant personnel, they generate new self-constructions of the (post) industrial body of the late 20th century" (Sharp 1995, 378).

Transforming Transplantation?

We too are renegades. Like the "confused" girl in an English hospital, our study has already received what Holmes et al. (2006) have called the "fascist" responses that come with the insurrection of previously subjugated questions (Foucault 2001). We realize that, if our findings are to be taken up by transplant professionals, our postconventional arguments will demand the kind of elaboration not possible in this short chapter. We realize, too, that our invitations to ethicists both clinical and critical could transform the field of transplantation. On these transformations, we would welcome changes to patient preparation, more elaborate processes of informed consent, and an augmentation of support for those living with (and hosting) the graft. What is more problematic is that our findings and the transformations they might suggest could contribute to a drop in rates of organ donation. Like the elephant in the room, this possibility sits alongside us in our work, asking not to be named (just yet). Indeed, in the words of one patient in our pilot study, most Western societies have "tried to wear blinkers and say, 'there's nothing wrong'" with the process of transplantation as it stands. However, our study, even if it is still in the data analysis stage, suggests otherwise for ethicists, prospective donors, and their future hosts.

References

Abbott, K. et al. (2003), "Hospitalized Psychoses after Renal Transplantation in the United States: Incidence, Risk Factors, and Prognosis," *J Am Soc Nephrol* 14:6, 1628–35.

Bacchi, C. and Beasley, C. (2005), "Reproductive Technology and the Political Limits of Care," in M. Shildrick and R. Mykitiuk (eds), *Ethics of the Body: Postconventional Challenges* (Cambridge, MA: MIT Press).

Belkin, G.S. (2003), "Brain Death and the Historical Understanding of Bioethics," *Journal of the History of Medicine* 58:3, 325–61.

Bergen, R. (1968), "Legal Regulation of Heart Transplants." *Dis Chest* 54:4, 352–5.

Boniolo, G. (2007), "Death and Transplantation: Let's Try to Get Things Methodologically Straight," *Bioethics* 21:1, 32–40.

Brosig, B. and Woidera, R. (1993), "'The Three of Us Must Hold Together': Psychoanalytic Considerations of Experiences of Heart-Lung Transplantation," *Psyche* 47:11 (Nov.), 1063–79.

Bunzel, B. et al. (1990), "The Hyperventilation Syndrome as a Psychosomatic Component of Cardiac Transplantation," [German], *Psychother Psychosom Med Psychol* 40:2, 57–63.

Bunzel, B. et al. (1992a), "Living With a Donor Heart: Feelings and Attitudes of Patients Toward the Donor and the Donor Organ," *J Heart Lung Transplant* 11:6, 1151–5.

Bunzel, B. et al. (1992b), "Does Changing the Heart Mean Changing Personality? A Retrospective Inquiry on 47 Heart Transplant Patients," *Qual Life Res* 1:4, 251–6.

Bunzel, B. et al. (2005), "Posttraumatic Stress Disorder after Implantation of a Mechanical Assist Device Followed by Heart Transplantation: Evaluation of Patients and Partners," *Transplant Proc* 37:2, 1365–8.

Burner, M. (1994), "Organ Transplant: Phantasms of the Receiver and Phantasms of the Donor," [French], *Psychol Med* 26:2, 120–21.

Castelnuevo-Tedesco, P. (1973), "Organ Transplant, Body Image, Psychosis," *Psychoanal Q* 42:3, 349–63.

Castelnuevo-Tedesco, P. (1978), "Ego Vicissitudes in Response to Replacement or Loss of Body Parts: Certain Analogies to Events during Psychoanalytic Treatment," *Psychoanal Q* 47:3, 381–97.

Childress, J. (1996), "Ethics and the Allocation of Organs for Transplantation," *Kennedy Inst Ethics J* 6:4, 397–401.
Derrida, J. (1992), *Given Time: I. Counterfeit Money*. P. Kamuf (trans.) (Chicago, IL: University of Chicago Press).
Derrida, J. (1999), "Hospitality, Justice and Responsibility," in R. Kearney and M. Dooley (eds), *Questioning Ethics: Contemporary Debates in Philosophy* (London: Routledge).
Derrida, J. (2000), *Of Hospitality: Anne Dufourmantelle Invites Jacques Derrida to Respond*, R. Bowlby (trans.) (Stanford, CA: Stanford University Press).
Dew, M. and DiMartini, A.F. (2005), "Psychological Disorders and Distress after Adult Cardiothoracic Transplantation," *J Cardiovasc Nurs* 20:5 (Suppl.), S51–66.
Dew, M. et al. (2005), "Profiles and Predictors of the Course of Psychological Distress across Four Years after Heart Transplantation," *Psychol Med* 35:8, 1215–27.
Diprose, R. (2002), *Corporeal Generosity: On Giving with Nietzsche, Merleau-Ponty, and Levinas* (Albany, NY: SUNY Press).
Evangelista, L. et al. (2003), "Hope, Mood States and Quality of Life in Female Heart Transplant Recipients," *J Heart Lung Transplant* 22:6 (Jun.), 681–6.
Fook, J. (2002), *Social Work: Critical Theory and Practice* (London: Sage).
Foucault, M. (2001), *Fearless Speech* (Los Angeles, CA: Semiotext(e)).
Fox, R.C. and Swazey, J. (1992), *Spare Parts: Organ Replacement in American Society* (London: Oxford University Press).
Goetzmann, L. (2004), "Is It Me, or Isn't It?—Transplanted Organs and Their Donors as Transitional Objects," *Am J Psychoanal* 64:3, 279–89.
Grande, A.M. et al. (1998), "Heart Transplant without Informed Consent: Discussion of a Case," *Intensive Care Medicine* 24:3, 251–4.
Haddow, G. (2005), "The Phenomenology of Death, Embodiment and Organ Transplantation," *Sociol Health Illn* 27:1, 92–113.
Halpern, S.D. et al. (2008), "Informing Candidates for Solid-Organ Transplantation About Donor Risk Factors," *N Engl J Med* 358, 2832.
Hird, M.J. (2007), "The Corporeal Generosity of Maternity," *Body and Society* 13:1, 1–20.
Holmes, D. et al. (2006), "Deconstructing the Evidence-based Discourse in Health Sciences: Truth, Power and *Fascism*," *International Journal of Evidenced-Based Health Care* 4:3, 180–86.
Inspector, Y. et al. (2004), "Another Person's Heart: Magical and Rational Thinking in the Psychological Adaptation to Heart Transplantation," *Isr J Psychiatry Relat Sci* 41:3, 161–73.
Joralemon, D. (1995), "Organ Wars: The Battle for Body Parts," *Med Anthropol Q, New Series* 9:3, 335–56.
Kaba, E. et al. (2005), "Somebody Else's Heart inside Me: A Descriptive Study of Psychological Problems after a Heart Transplantation," *Issues Ment Health Nurs* 25:6, 611–25.

Koenig, B.A. and Hogel, L.F. (1995), "Organ Transplantation (Re)Examined?" *Med Anthropol Q, New Series* 9:3, 393–7.

Kuczewski, M. (2002), "The Gift of Life and Starfish on the Beach: The Ethics of Organ Procurement," *Am J Bioeth* 2:3, 53–6.

Laederach-Hofmann, K. et al. (2002), "Integration Process and Organ-Related Fantasies in Patients Undergoing Organ Transplantation," [German], *Psychother Psychosom Med Psychol* 52:1 (Jan.), 32–40.

Lafrance, M. (2008), "The Gift of Life? Ethics, Subjectivity, Embodiment and Facial Transplant," paper given at the Fourth International Congress on Qualitative Inquiry, University of Illinois at Urbana-Champaign, 14–17 May.

Lock, M. (2002), *Twice Dead: Organ Transplants and the Reinvention of Death* (Berkeley, CA: University of California Press).

Mai, F.M. (1986), "Graft and Donor Denial in Heart Transplant Recipients," *Am J Psychiatry* 143:9 (Sept.), 1159–61.

Merleau-Ponty, M. (1989 [1945]), *Phenomenology of Perception*, C. Smith (trans.) (London: Routledge).

Moss, D. (1989), "Brain, Body, and World: Body Image and the Psychology of the Body," in R.S. Valle and S. Halling (eds), *Existential-Phenomenological Perspectives in Psychology* (New York: Plenum Press), 63–82.

Nancy, J.-L. (2000), *L'Intrus* (Paris: Galilee).

Nelson, H.L. (2000), "Feminist Bioethics: Where We've Been, Where We're Going," *Metaphilosophy* 31:5, 492–508.

Paris, W. and White-Williams, C. (2005), "Social Adaptation after Cardiothoracic Transplantation: A Review of the Literature," *J Cardiovasc Nurs* 20:5, S67(7).

Paris, W. et al. (1993), "Returning to Work after Heart Transplantation," *J Heart Lung Transplant* 12:1 (Pt 1), 46–53; (discussion) 53–4.

Pearsall, P. (2001), "Are Heart Transplant Recipients Receiving Cellular Memories from Their Donated Organ? A Heuristic Study," *Hawaii Med J* 60:11, 282–300.

Pearsall, P. et al. (2002), "Changes in Heart Transplant Recipients That Parallel the Personalities of Their Donors," *Journal of Near-Death Studies* 20:3, 191–206.

Rauch, J.B. and Kneen, K.K. (1989), "Accepting the Gift of Life: Heart Transplant Recipients' Post-Operative Adaptive Tasks," *Soc Work Health Care* 14:1, 47–59.

Richmond, C. (1999), "British Girl Recovering after Forced Heart Transplant," *JAMC* 16:6, 680.

Salvucci, L. (2004), "Solid Organ Transplantation and Post Traumatic Stress Disorder," *Dissertation Abstracts International: Section B: The Sciences and Engineering* 64:8–B, 4061.

Sanner, M. (2003), "Transplant Recipients' Conceptions of Three Key Phenomena in Transplantation: The Organ Donation, the Organ Donor, and the Organ Transplant," *Clin Transplant* 17:4, 391–400.

Savitch, S. et al. (2003), "An Investigation of the Psychological and Psychosocial Challenges Faced by Post-Transplant Organ Recipients," *J Appl Rehabil Counsel* 34:3, 3–9.
Scheper-Hughes, N. (2004), "Parts Unknown: Undercover Ethnography of the Organs-Trafficking Underworld," *Ethnography* 5:1, 29–73.
Sells, R. (2003), "Transplant Ethics: Altruism and Materialism in Organ Donation," *Clin Transpl* 293–305.
Sharp, L.A. (2006), *Strange Harvest: Organ Transplants, Denatured Bodies, and the Transformed Self* (Berkeley, CA: University of California Press).
Sharp, L. (1995), "Organ Transplantation as a Transformative Experience: Anthropological Insights into the Restructuring of the Self," *Med Anthropol Q, New Series*, 9:3, 357–89.
Shildrick, M. (1997), *Leaky Bodies and Boundaries: Feminism, Postmodernism and (Bio)Ethics* (London: Routledge).
Shildrick, M. (2005), "Beyond the Body of Bioethics: Challenging the Conventions," in M. Shildrick and R. Mykitiuk (eds), *Ethics of the Body: Postconventional Challenges* (Cambridge, MA: MIT Press).
Shildrick, M. (2008), "The Critical Turn in Feminist Bioethics: The Case of Heart Transplantation," *International Journal of Feminist Approaches to Bioethics* 1:1, 28–47.
Somerville, M. (2008), "At Heart, It's Slavery by Another Name: All of Us Are Dehumanized If We Treat Body Parts as Merchandise," *The Globe and Mail*, 13 August.
Stukas, A. et al. (1998), "PTSD in Heart Transplant Recipients and Their Primary Caregivers," *Psychosomatics* 40, 212–21.
Sylvia, C. and Novak, W. (1997), *A Change of Heart* (New York: Little, Brown and Co.).
Taylor, D. et al. (2006), "Registry of the International Society for Heart and Lung Transplantation: Twenty-third Official Adult Heart Transplantation Report," *J Heart Lung Transplant* 25, 869–79.
Taylor, D. et al. (2008), "Registry of the International Society for Heart and Lung Transplantation: Twenty-fifth Official Adult Heart Transplant Report," *J Heart Lung Transplant* 27:9, 943.
Tong, R. (1997), *Feminist Approaches to Bioethics: Theoretical Reflections and Practical Applications* (Boulder, CO: Westview Press).
Tong, R. et al. (2004), *Linking Visions: Feminist Bioethics, Human Rights and the Developing World* (Lanham, MD: Rowman and Littlefield).
Trainor, A. and Ezer, H. (2000), "Rebuilding Life: The Experience of Living with AIDS after Facing Imminent Death," *Qualitative Health Research* 10:5, 646–60.
Triffaux, J.M. et al. (2002), "'Take This Heart Away!': From Fear of Rejection to Post-Transplant Delirium," [French], *Rev Med Liege* 57:6 (Jun.), 389–92.

Truog, R. and Robinson, W.M. (2003), "Role of Brain Death and the Dead-donor Rule in the Ethics of Organ Transplantation," *Crit Care Med* 31:9 (Sept.), 239–6.

Veatch, R. (2000), *Transplantation Ethics* (Washington, DC: Georgetown University Press).

Waldby, C. (2002), "Biomedicine, Tissue Transfer and Intercorporeality," *Feminist Theory* 3:3, 239–54.

Waldby, C. and Mitchell, R. (2006) *Tissue Economies: Blood, Organs, and Cell Lines in Late Capitalism* (Durham, NC: Duke University Press), 88–109.

Wright, L. et al. (2005), "The Roles of a Bioethicist on an Organ Transplantation Service," *American Journal of Transplantation* 5, 821–6.

Chapter 3
Embracing the Intersubjective: An Ethics of Care for Chronic Illness

Roanne Thomas-MacLean

> We remain susceptible to oversimplification, of wanting to believe there is one right or good decision to be made, made about life and death, made about bodies … made about research. (Brogden and Patterson 2007, 220)

Introduction

Although many researchers and clinicians have embraced a philosophy of "humane care," it remains that few clinicians are able to address the politics of everyday life and health disparities. This is hardly surprising given the overall structure of national healthcare systems, such as Canada's, yet healthcare professionals are far from immune to the effects of various forms of inequality, such as sexism, racism, and homophobia, and the ways in which these inequities manifest not only in their own lives, but in the lives and illnesses of their patients. While healthcare professionals may grapple with these very inequities in practice, they may also recognize their own inability to address the underlying social constraints that lead to inequities in the first place.

In this chapter, I explore the possibility that if healthcare professionals engage intersubjectively with patients, then connections promoting the recognition of social inequities may be established, potentially influencing social change within the context of ethical healthcare. I begin by looking at conceptualizations of caring, which ultimately leads to considerations of embodiment, narrative, and intersubjectivity. Moreover, the relationships between these theoretical concepts and their applications to qualitative health research will be examined. Next, I outline the ways in which such research may serve as a biomedical antidote, allow for recognition of marginalization, and create opportunities for the acknowledgement of the intersubjective nature of ethical healthcare. This theoretical framework leads to a discussion of the Visualizing Breast Cancer project which involved documenting the experiences of Aboriginal women with breast cancer in Saskatchewan, Canada. Their words illustrate ways in which healthcare may be enhanced through attention to intersubjectivity. I believe their words provide persuasive arguments for the recognition of intersubjectivity as a proponent of more ethical healthcare.

Currently, the Canadian healthcare system functions as a microcosm of broader forms of social inequality, reflecting power imbalances at large. As a contained system with specific objectives, values, and beliefs engrained in biomedical practices, there are few options for patients who seek alternatives to these biomedical orientations. This may be why Quinn asserts that some patients, and healthcare professionals, turn elsewhere: "Patients are looking for caring, healing, wholeness, and spiritual meaning outside of the existing healthcare system because, like nurses, they cannot find it within" (Quinn cited in Mitchell 2004, 129). Mitchell states that for one nursing theorist, Watson, "caring involves a conscious intentional responsibility and 'a moral ideal of nursing'" (2004, 129). While this caring-healing model is laudable, it appears to emphasize choice—i.e., a nurse can choose how to respond in any given situation. The emphasis on the meaning of caring and experiential aspects of illness is important, but "choice" is often (if not always) constrained by countless social factors. How then can a phenomenological sensibility, such as Watson's, be integrated with a more critical or sociological approach that acknowledges the social context of patients' lives? This is potentially unanswerable, yet some possibilities may lie within the interaction itself, by addressing the ways in which micrological practices reflect or resist dominant paradigms.

Engaging with the idea of ethical healthcare and considering what that might look like offers some hope for positive social change. Various scholars have visualized what might serve as theoretical foundations for such an endeavour, drawing upon sophisticated notions of the body. Although such notions rely solely on physical experience, they provide a means to expand understandings of health and illness through attention to the intersections of the physical and the social. Reflections on embodiment are therefore essential for developing intersubjective healthcare. Van Wolputte states that we can trace the emergence of three distinct kinds of bodies in contemporary thought: (1) the "lived" or phenomenological body; (2) the "social body," which refers to the ways in which the body is referenced as a "tool" by which one can understand "social relationships such as gender"; and (3) the "body politic"—the ways in which the body might be disciplined or serve as resistance (2004, 254). All three of these interconnected locations provide points of entry for the establishment of more ethical healthcare. Similarly, Mishler (2005) distinguishes between "micro-ethics" and "macro-ethics," stating that the two must be reconciled. While the former refers to "humane care," the latter refers to "social justice" (Mishler 2005, 432–3). Finally, recent literature suggests that embracing and valuing narratives may provide some direction for understanding the intersections of the personal and the social on a path toward more ethical healthcare. Alone and in isolation, embodiment, micro-ethics, and narratives may not be sufficient for the development of intersubjectivity and ethical healthcare. However, taken together, the three areas provide some sense of the context and imperative for developing intersubjectivity.

Intersubjectivity and Illness Narratives

Illness narratives include references to embodiment and encompass the micro-ethics of which Mishler writes. Mishler notes that in recent decades, many researchers and healthcare practitioners have contributed to a robust body of work about illness narratives, but that this surge of interest has not meant that listening to patients has become a valued "gold standard" (2005, 434). This despite the potential and tremendous impact such listening might have, with respect to the development of intersubjective and ethical healthcare that recognizes the complexity of embodiment. Thus, we find ourselves at a curious paradox—an abundance of storytellers, stories, and researchers, but few corresponding changes to care, beyond minor changes to education and practice. In other words, the "ethic of humane care and its associated line of research on patient-physician communication" has addressed the context of healthcare neither as a system nor as an institution (Mishler 2005, 435). The result is "that health care was defined as if it only included something done by an individual physician to/with her/his patient" (Mishler 2005, 435). Scheurich writes:

> [A]n ethic of caring and support may well entail recognition of factors that reinforce the sick role, such as family reactions or disability payments, but the emphasis is not upon blame or dismissal, but rather upon alliance with the patient and maximization of function and life satisfaction from the patient's perspective. (2000, 465)

To this end, Scheurich advances the possibilities offered by narrative, indicating that stories represent powerful ways to understand the "larger tale" intersubjectively—a task viewed as essential for ethical healthcare (2000, 475).

Intersubjectivity involves recognition that the "self is always dialogically formed" (Swartz 2006, 434). There are opportunities to learn from work that Swartz describes as "African feminist intersubjective therapy," which acknowledges "gender, race, class and power relationships" (2006, 434). Such work, Swartz states, recognizes the impact of colonialism, oppression, and power. Furthermore, this work generates opportunities to create narrative and to recognize intersubjectivity as "essential to change" (Swartz 2006, 434).

One method to gain insight into the intersubjective dimensions of human experience is through qualitative research. Interviews allow for "a unique co-created gestalt to emerge, facilitating the development of new intersubjective thirds" (Snelling 2005, 134). In other words, such dialogue creates a connection transcending both the interviewer and the interviewee. Writing of his own research, Snelling contends that an open approach to interviews "create[s] an intersubjective space in which the emotional or embodied aspects of experience could be privileged," but the "organization, cultural space and the physical environment" (2005, 134–5) determine the extent to which the development of intersubjectivity is possible. To acknowledge and hear the voice of the researcher, and to recognize the possibility of a transcendent connection, runs counter to post-positivistic research imperatives. Similarly, the voice of the patient becomes lost in medicalization (Snelling 2005, 141); nevertheless, to hear such voices may be considered "ethically responsible" (Snelling 2005, 141).

Acknowledging how patients' voices might influence healthcare practices has been the focus of much of my research with women who have experienced breast cancer (Thomas-MacLean 2004a; 2004b; 2005). Most recently, the Visualizing Breast Cancer (VBC) project, with Aboriginal women, provided many possibilities for change and offered ways we might positively influence the healthcare system. The VBC project shows that where "spaces" exist for the creation of genuine and respectful intersubjectivity, so too do opportunities to effect change and to "be ethical" in everyday practices. While I discuss the findings of the VBC project in a subsequent section of this chapter, I draw first upon sections of my Ph.D. dissertation (Thomas-MacLean 2001) which illustrate the potential for qualitative approaches, such as narrative studies, to change the biomedical orientations of medicine. A qualitative exploration of the experiences of women with breast cancer may (1) serve as an antidote to biomedical orientations; (2) allow for recognition of marginalization; and (3) create opportunities for the acknowledgment of the intersubjective nature of ethical healthcare.

An Antidote to Biomedical Orientations

As the nursing scholar Watson (1988) shows, there are elements of illness and caring for the ill that cannot be expressed within traditional medical paradigms. Traditional research is "haunted by the restricted thinking of the medical paradigm that labels, categorizes, manipulates, controls and treats disease; if not disease, patients, if not patients, variables" (17). In contrast, Leder writes, "[t]hrough hearing the patient's *story*, one comes to know in detail of her world as she embodies it .... Only in this broader context will the full significance and etiology of her illness emerge" (1992, 29).

Qualitative studies of the body offer several opportunities for researchers and healthcare professionals to recognize the importance of the role of intersubjectivity in ethical healthcare. For one, orientations toward embodiment in research mean that one may study narratives, or the way illness becomes woven into the fabric of existence. Frank suggests that the "illness narrative is always, at least in part, an oppositional text to this medical inscription" (1993, 50). This emphasis permits an exploration of inequality as it is connected to allopathic paradigms and ideologies of health and illness.

Recognition of Marginalization

Kleinman writes that "[t]he chronically ill live at the margins" (1988, 44). Thus, there is a moral imperative to better understand illness and the body as both medicine and society marginalize "people whose illnesses cannot be cured, whose bodies cannot be restored to perfect shape" (Holmes 1989, 6). Further, Kleinman argues that "cultural meanings mark the sick person, stamping him or her with significance often unwanted and neither easily warded off or coped with. The mark may be either stigma or social death" (1988, 26; see also Frank 1995, 31). Ellis (1998) contributes much to our understanding of stigma, while DeVault states that studies of personal experience "makes excluded voices 'hearable' within a dominant discourse" (1997, 226). Without addressing fundamental inequalities within society and medicine, Kleinman states that medical science cannot "be at all adequate for the needs of patients, their families, and the practitioner" (1988, 29). Studying the meaning of illness may then lead to changes within medical practice. Thus, there is a moral or ethical imperative involved with the qualitative study of illness, particularly given the intersubjective nature of our existence (see Jaggar 2000 for a thorough discussion of feminist ethics).

Intersubjectivity

According to van Manen (1998), illness provides us with an opportunity to study closely the meaning of intersubjectivity: "The phenomenological tradition … maintains that meaning is contextually constructed as an intersubjective phenomenon" (in Anderson 1991, 31). The reading of texts may be thought of as a means to increase the awareness of intersubjectivity. Bell writes that intersubjectivity "acknowledges and even encourages readers' self-conscious engagement with the material" (1991, 247). Denzin states that when "we write about lives, we bring the world of others into our texts" (1989, 82). Kirby and McKenna describe intersubjectivity as "an authentic dialogue … in which all are respected as equally knowing subjects," thereby demonstrating the interconnectedness of marginalization and intersubjectivity (1989, 129).

For Anderson, intersubjectivity involves recognition of the interplay between meaning and social context. She states: "'[m]eaning' is constructed in ongoing relations between people; it is constructed through a dialectical process in everyday interaction" (Anderson 1991, 29). Intersubjectivity is not confined to communication, as it also involves "the whole being," not just the intellect (Barral 1969, 177). For example, Snodgrass (1998) describes her experiences with breast cancer and what the illness has meant for her work as a professor. For her, breast cancer has most significantly changed her "self-perception," but it has also limited her ability to engage with the world in ways she did previously (Snodgrass 1998, 376–7). This means worrying less about time, money, career and valuing more the opportunity to travel, to connect with friends and family, and to facilitate spiritual development (Snodgrass 1998, 376–9). While understanding the role of material resources such as money is important, Snodgrass also suggests that we pay more attention to intangible and intersubjective facets of embodiment as well as their enigmatic aspects.

The VBC Project

Having established some of the theoretical bases for ethical healthcare and the role of intersubjectivity and narrative studies within such a model, I now turn to an exploration of findings from the VBC project and their implications for ethics and healthcare. The VBC project involved the use of "photovoice"—a combination of interviews and photographs taken by the research participants—as a methodology. Twelve Aboriginal women who had experienced breast cancer participated in the VBC project, which was situated in the province of Saskatchewan, Canada. Overall, the data for this study consisted of 24 interview transcripts and over 150 photographs. Details of the research methods, including the ethics approval process, can be found in Thomas-MacLean, Poudrier and Brooks (forthcoming), as well as Brooks, Poudrier and Thomas-MacLean (forthcoming). In this chapter, I focus on interview data pertaining to discussions of healthcare and healthcare professionals. Although healthcare and healthcare professionals figure prominently in the women's narratives, these topics do not easily lend themselves to photographs. As a result, there are few photographs of clinical encounters, likely because the women had finished acute care, though one participant did ask someone to take a photo of her with her physician. That said, the women remembered many details of their interactions with the healthcare system and were eager to describe them.

Two key themes that emerged throughout these discussions relate to the women's experiences of healthcare and their suggestions regarding how healthcare might be more ethical. Both of these themes refer to the importance of healthcare professionals to assume an active and ethical role in the care of patients. This involves: (1) listening, which includes reflecting upon what has been shared; and (2) responding in sensitive and appropriate ways. Essentially, these two themes are connected to the concept of intersubjectivity, the role of narratives, and their implications for ethical healthcare.

Listening and Reflecting

Marion's words illustrate the challenges that might be posed when those who are not valued by society are forced to confront those with privilege. For Marion, her experiences with breast cancer and her encounters with the healthcare system indicate how she might resist the boundaries of power and privilege. She said:

> I used to have a hard time meeting with people, I wouldn't be able to talk … [I would think] 'What am I gonna say? What am I gonna say?' You know like, I was really like, um, I, I just kept to myself, and, after that, after cancer, I realized, 'Okay. Nobody is gonna help me. I gotta try to help myself.' And that's where I learned, I had to just ask any question, even if it sounded stupid. I would just ask.

The broader context of Marion's narrative shows that her interactions with people in positions of authority, like healthcare workers, introduced anxiety about appearing stupid. However, Marion also experienced cancer as empowering; her illness provided her with opportunities to overcome her apprehensions, and enabled her to courageously ask questions, regardless of how she thought they might be interpreted. Nonetheless, Marion's words suggest there are many simple measures healthcare professionals could take that would allow patients to feel more comfortable about asking questions and expressing their feelings of fear and anxiety. Moreover, establishing rapport does not need to involve large -scale political change, nor does it require an increase in funding. Instead, simply by embracing the intersubjective dimensions of healthcare, individuals in positions of authority may help facilitate the ways in which a patient addresses fear and anxiety.

Another example of Marion's dialogue shows how this might occur:

> *Marion*: After the cancer thing like, I always lived with fear. Like, not everyday, hey? But, like for instance, the last time I was with you [interviewer, Carolyn] and my blood pressure was out of control, and I was having the nosebleeds, like that was really scary for me … I was so scared. I thought, 'This cancer came back.' Why was I having nose bleeds so bad? I was so terrified. I, I, I was in total fear. I would just go into my bathroom and cry because I was so scared. And my doctor, he'd keep reassuring me that, it wasn't the cancer.
> *Carolyn*: How did your doctor reassure you, with that?
> *Marion*: He'd sit with me and talk to me … I was telling him, 'I want tests. I want it to stop …. Like it's not normal to have nose bleeds like that.' And he's really easygoing, hey? And he just said, 'Marion, Marion, Marion.' [laughs] And he'd tell me, 'It's your blood pressure ….' He'd say, 'It's not your cancer.' He's more or less like a friend.

As depicted in the preceding quotation, Marion struggled to find words to express her anxiety, yet she was able to communicate her fears about the possible recurrence of cancer. More than any test, it appears that her physician's demeanour and his rapport with her were able to alleviate said fears. Evidently, he listened intently and responded in ways that were reassuring.

However, some healthcare professionals responded in ways that showed that, while they may have listened to what patients were saying, they did not always reflect upon what they heard. Tina's words illustrate how an unwillingness to listen and reflect was conveyed in her interactions with an oncologist:

> In fact, I even told my oncologist, 'I want to go back to work. I need to go back. I need to go back to work because this is, something that is—I need some normalcy in my life and being at work is normal in my life ….' He said, 'Well, I'll keep you at home one more month just to make sure.' Then, I could go back to work.

There is an obvious lack of reflection here. The oncologist responded to what he knew medically, but not to what was being said. He may have been listening, but he was not reflecting. What if finances were an issue, or supporting children? Beyond financial concerns, what meaning or importance is attached to paid work for Tina? Yet, the oncologist's response, which appears to be based solely in a biomedical perspective, does not address these more sociological concerns—an issue which might be avoided by incorporating some degree of reflection upon patients' words and stories.

Furthermore, a lack of reflection may lead to inappropriate responses on the part of the healthcare system. For instance, in an attempt to provide support for Marjorie, one healthcare professional arranged for Marjorie to interact via telephone with another woman who had cancer. In speaking of this experience, Marjorie said:

> I need the emotional support, you know? And that's what like I'd like to see, you know? Someone who's First Nations, someone who can understand, if not necessarily sympathize but you know, if they can even empathize at what the person is going through …. They put me on the phone with some lady that had six months to live, which really set me even back farther because I said, 'Okay, this doctor's not telling me the truth. Why would he get me to talk to somebody that has very little time left, if I'm fine?'

While the type of support arranged for Marjorie is not entirely clear, it is apparent that the person establishing this connection did not reflect upon the type of support Marjorie might need or want. Marjorie wanted to speak to someone who identified as a First Nations woman; instead, she was connected with a volunteer who was dying. This led to Marjorie's questioning of what her physician was telling her. As with Tina, Marjorie experienced a lack of reflective practice.

Responding

An ethical response derives from listening and reflecting. By interpreting a quotation from Shelley, we can recognize that space must be created in order to allow for responses to occur:

> My family doctor was on holidays and she came in to be with me, to be part of the surgery and I thought that was, you know, quite exceptional …. I was so happy that she came, she came to be part of it.

Marion's words are illustrative of a similar type of response that she experienced as positive:

> I actually had a really good oncologist. She'd stay [with me through chemotherapy treatments] …. When I first went to my first treatment I was like a baby. I just cried and cried. I didn't want to go. But she [the oncologist] stayed and she would just be straightforward with me … like I would ask questions, like and,

> I remember this one time when I went this year, I was telling her, 'I'm scared. I know I'm gonna die,' and she said, 'Marion, you're not gonna die.' Like you know, she was just like really, like straightforward she wouldn't, like, treat me like a baby. She would tell me that, 'You have to be a fighter.' She would tell me, 'You have to stand up for yourself, because nobody else is gonna do it. Nobody else is gonna take chemo for you—you gotta do it yourself.' She was just an amazing woman.

Marion's words indicate that her oncologist was aware of what would be reassuring to Marion when she thought she was going to die. The oncologist's response was based on listening to Marion and being aware of how this patient might respond. In contrast, Tina shows what happens when no listening or reflection occurs and clinicians simply respond. Tina was very worried about losing her eyebrows and eyelashes as a result of chemotherapy. She said:

> I went to my room and I said to my heavenly father, 'I know I'm gonna lose my hair, but please don't let me lose my eyebrows and my eyelashes. They've meant so much to me.' I never lost them. My oncologist told me I would. And he told me, 'You're gonna lose them.' And I said, 'No, I am not. I'm going to be fine.' And, when I wore my wig in there, he had no idea that I was losing my hair, or anything. 'Did you lose none of your hair yet?' 'No. It's a wig.' And he said, 'What about your eyelashes?' I said 'No, or my eyebrows. I've never lost them.' I really believe it's because of the faith that I have.

It is unclear whether or not Tina discussed her spirituality with her oncologist, but it is clear that her oncologist did not listen or respond compassionately to the way Tina felt about the possibility of losing her hair. Other women also indicated that they did not share their spiritual experiences with their clinicians. When speaking of Aboriginal healing practices, Mary said:

> Yeah, I didn't think that they [the clinicians] would, um, receive it very well. And so I just didn't bother telling anybody what I was doing. I didn't tell them I went to sweat lodges or anything like that, for fear that they would tell me not to go .... I just didn't tell anybody anything what I was doing. I just went ahead and did it myself.

Mary did not share an integral part of her healing experience because she was uncertain how healthcare professionals would respond. She described clinicians as "cold" and "very hard to talk to." Participants did recognize, however, that responses may be impeded by various factors associated with the structure of the healthcare system. Sandra said:

> I think, you know, it all goes back to the whole system and the lack of money and the lack of doctors and nurses, like they just don't have time. They really

> don't. I mean they can see we're there and people are falling through the cracks. It's just that they can't catch them because they are just trying to catch up. You know when you go into see your doctor you've got five minutes, five minutes! You know, so they diagnose you and rush you out the door.

Discussion

Ethical healthcare involves the integration of listening, critical reflection, and response—actions more frequently associated, perhaps, with sociology and other disciplines, than with biomedicine. De Vries et al. note: "It is no surprise that bioethics and sociology developed an adversarial relationship" (2006, 665). These authors state that reconciliation of these two disciplines means we must face "the challenge of trying to fix in words a dynamic, changing, multi-sited field" (2006, 667). Therefore, contextually speaking, movement toward ethical healthcare will likely entail overcoming traditional biomedical boundaries, even though such restrictions currently reside as ingrained components of professional practice (Mattingly 2005, 458). Figure 3.1 points out various changes that might be considered essential to the dissolution of such boundaries, enabling the emergence of a healthcare system rooted in intersubjectivity and commitment to social justice. The current healthcare system tends to view patients (pts) and healthcare professionals (hcps) as having a somewhat disjointed relationship, depicted by the small circles on the left of the figure.

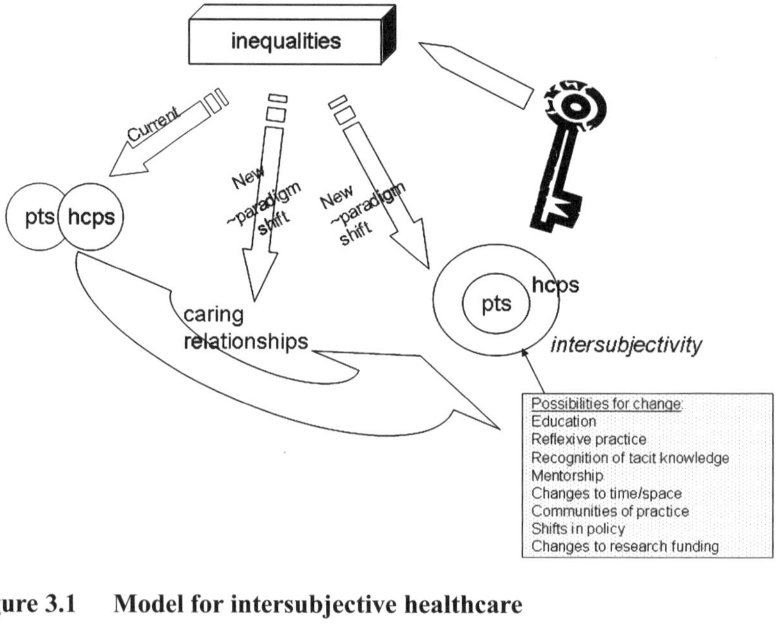

Figure 3.1 Model for intersubjective healthcare

However, through recognition of inequalities and development of caring relationships, a new model of healthcare is proposed, a model with a more direct connection between patients and healthcare professionals. That said, in order to effect such a movement toward ethical healthcare, many dimensions of change, both pragmatic and reflexive, are required; Figure 3.1 lists only a few possibilities. Mattingly states:

> "[T]he good" is not judged by subsuming a particular situation under an abstract ethical rule. Rather, it is judged by locating oneself in a history, or set of histories, that not only point toward a past but toward a future—histories that are still unfolding. While this problem of locating oneself in particular stories one is living out can sound like a purely individual affair, such is not the case. (2005, 465)

By orienting healthcare around the fluid and malleable nature of narrative actions—such as listening, reflecting, and responding—healthcare professionals are provided with the space required for the development of intersubjectivity, thus establishing a relational connection between patient and care provider. And, as the participants in the VBC project have demonstrated, it is through such intersubjective actions that an ethical healthcare system, one that addresses issues of marginalization, can be achieved.

Acknowledgements

The VBC project was supported by a Canadian Breast Cancer Research Alliance (CBCRA) Developmental and Exploratory Research Grant. Additional team members on the VBC project are Dr Jennifer Poudrier and Carolyn Brooks, who contributed greatly to the project's success. I am also exceedingly grateful to our participants for so openly sharing their stories with us. Finally, I would like to thank Paul Spriggs for his assistance with this manuscript and Laurie Schimpf for her help with the list of references.

References

Anderson, J.M. (1991), "The Phenomenological Perspective," in J.M. Morse (ed.), *Qualitative Nursing Research: A Contemporary Dialogue* (Newbury Park, CA: Sage Publications).

Barral, M.R. (1969), "Merleau-Ponty on the Body," *Southern Journal of Philosophy* 7 (Summer), 171–9.

Bell, S.E. (1991), "Commentary on 'Perspectives on Embodiment: The Uses of Narrativity in Ethnographic Writing' by Katharine Young," *Journal of Narrative and Life History* 1:3, 245–54.

Brogden, L. and Patterson, D. (2007), "Nostalgia, Goodness and Ethical Paradox," *Qualitative Research* 7:2, 217–27.

Brooks, C., Poudrier, J. and Thomas-MacLean, R. (forthcoming), "Creating Collaborative Visions with Aboriginal Women: A PhotoVoice Project," in P. Liamputtong (ed.), *Doing Cross-Cultural Research: Ethical and Methodological Perspectives* (Dordrecht: Springer).

Denzin, N.K. (1989), *Interpretive Biography* (Thousand Oaks, CA: Sage Publications).

DeVault, M.L. (1997), "Personal Writing in Social Science: Issues of Production and Interpretation," in R. Hertz (ed.), *Reflexivity and Voice* (Thousand Oaks, CA: Sage Publications).

de Vries, R. et al. (2006), "Social Science and Bioethics: The Way Forward," *Sociology of Health and Illness* 28:6, 665–77.

Ellis, C. (1998), "'I Hate My Voice': Coming to Terms with Minor Bodily Stigmas," *Sociological Quarterly* 39:4, 517–37.

Frank, A.W. (1993), "The Rhetoric of Self-Change: Illness Experience as Narrative," *The Sociological Quarterly* 34:1, 39–52.

Frank, A.W. (1995), *The Wounded Storyteller* (Chicago, IL: University of Chicago Press).

Holmes, H.B. (1989), "A Call to Heal Medicine," *Hypatia* 4:2, 1–8.

Jaggar, A. (2000), "Feminism in Ethics: Moral Justification," in M. Fricker and J. Hornsby (eds), *The Cambridge Companion to Feminism in Philosophy* (Cambridge: Cambridge University Press).

Kirby, S. and McKenna, K. (1989), *Experience Research Social Change* (Toronto: Garamond Press).

Kleinman, A. (1988), *The Illness Narratives: Suffering, Healing and the Human Condition* (New York: Basic Books).

Leder, D. (1992), "Introduction," in D. Leder (ed.), *The Body in Medical Thought and Practice* (Dordrecht: Kluwer).

Mattingly, C. (2005), "Toward Venerable Ethics of Research Practice," *Health: An Interdisciplinary Journal for the Social Study of Health, Illness and Medicine* 9:4, 454–71.

Mishler, E. (2005), "Patient Stories, Narratives of Resistance and the Ethics of Humane Care: à la Recherche du Temps Perdu," *Health: An Interdisciplinary Journal for the Social Study of Health, Illness and Medicine* 9:4, 431–51.

Mitchell, G. (2004), "Advancing the Discipline of Nursing," *Nursing Science Quarterly* 17:2, 128–34.

Robb, M. (2004), "Exploring Fatherhood: Masculinity and Intersubjectivity in the Research Process," *Journal of Social Work Practice* 18:3, 395–406.

Scheurich, N. (2000), "Hysteria and the Medical Narrative," *Perspectives in Biology and Medicine* 43:4, 461–76.

Snelling, E. (2005), "Hungry Researchers: The Tensions and Dilemmas of Developing a Emancipatory Research Project with Members of a Healing Voices Group," *Journal of Social Work Practice* 19:2, 131–47.

Snodgrass, S.E. (1998), "A Personal Account," *Journal of Social Issues* 54:2, 373–80.

Swartz, S. (2006), "The Third Voice: Writing Case-notes," *Feminism and Psychology* 16:4, 427–44.

Thomas-MacLean, R.L. (2001), "Victims, Patients, Survivors, Women: Experiences of Embodiment after Breast Cancer" (Ph.D. dissertation, University of New Brunswick).

Thomas-MacLean, R.L. (2004a), "Memories of Treatment: The Immediacy of Breast Cancer," *Qualitative Health Research* 14:5, 628–43.

Thomas-MacLean, R.L. (2004b), "Understanding Breast Cancer Stories via Frank's Narrative Types," *Social Science and Medicine* 58, 1647–57.

Thomas-MacLean, R.L. (2005), "Beyond Dichotomies of Health and Illness: Life after Breast Cancer," *Nursing Inquiry* 12:3, 200–209.

Thomas-MacLean, R. Poudrier, J. and Brooks, C. (forthcoming), "Envisioning the Future with Young Aboriginal Breast Cancer Survivors," *Atlantis: A Women's Studies Journal*.

van Manen, M. (1998), "Modalities of Body Experience in Illness and Health," *Qualitative Health Research* 8:1, 7–24.

Van Wolputte, S. (2004), "Hang On to Your Self: Of Bodies, Embodiment, and Selves," *Annual Review of Anthropology* 33, 251–69.

Watson, J. (1988), *Nursing: Human Science and Human Care. A Theory of Nursing* (New York: National League for Nursing).

PART II
Biopolitical Interventions

Chapter 4
Biotechnology and the Governance of Life: The Case of Pre-implantation Genetic Diagnosis

Ann Robertson

> I will argue strongly not only for the freedom but also for the *obligation* to pursue human enhancement. (Harris 2007, 9; emphasis added)

Introduction

In a scene from the movie *Gattaca* (1997), a couple meets with a clinical geneticist and discusses the characteristics they desire in their second child.[1] This child will result from the selection (and implantation) of one of several embryos created by *in vitro* fertilization (IVF) using the couple's eggs and sperm. The three discuss such characteristics as height, eye colour, as well as musical and athletic ability.[2]

What this scene illustrates, among other things, is two very powerful and currently prevailing cultural narratives: first, a perennial narrative about human perfectibility, and second, a more recent narrative about "the gene." This chapter is a reflection on how these two narratives weave together to tell a tale—a moral and, arguably, political tale—about biological citizenship in what has been called our "post-genomic" age.

In other words, this chapter is a reflection on the implications of emerging biotechnologies for how we think about fundamental questions about human life: who may live; who should make these determinations; how these decisions should be made; and, finally, questions about the potential social and political consequences of these decisions.

---

1 The movie *Gattaca* is about a society in which there is an elite class of people—the "valids" who are genetically engineered (through IVF and embryo selection)—and an underclass—the "invalids" who are conceived "naturally."

2 In one of the "outtakes" included in the DVD of *Gattaca*, the couple expresses their desire to eventually be grandparents. The clinical geneticist replies, "I've already taken care of that," in a not-so-oblique reference to the "gay gene."

The Enduring Ideal: Biological Mutability/Perfectibility

The idea of human perfectibility, embedded in a larger cultural narrative of biological mutability brought about by the actions of science/technology on Nature, has been a perennial scientific, cultural, and literary theme. The following discussion provides a brief overview of some of the more prominent of these different narratives.

Literary and Cultural Narratives

One of the most well-known stories about the actions of science on Nature in modern Western consciousness is Mary Shelley's *Frankenstein* (2006; originally published in 1818). Many argue that Shelley's story is a morality tale not so much of the failure of the scientist Dr Frankenstein for creating and using his monstrous technology but of his refusal to take any responsibility for the consequences of his technology (Van Dijck 1998).

Likewise, H.G. Wells's book, *The Island of Dr Moreau* (1996; first published in 1894), is a story about a scientist who, attempting to emulate God, is engaged in experiments to perfect the human race by transforming animals into human beings through technological interventions such as skin grafting and transplantation of body parts, among other methods. The moral of this tale follows from the inevitable punishment of the scientist as he ends up being killed by an uprising of his monstrous creations. This compelling cultural motif of an underlying struggle between nature and science is illustrated by the poster for a recent version of the movie *The Island of Dr Moreau* bearing the caption, "where Science breaks the laws of Nature."[3]

And then there is Aldous Huxley's iconic and remarkably prescient *Brave New World* (1967; first published in 1932), a tale of standardized mass production of human beings in a consumer and technologically oriented society. Huxley's imagery of assembly-line produced human workers (the "Gammas") who are kept happily consuming and producing by the ruling classes (the "Alphas") foreshadowed not only our contemporary consumer culture of "getting and spending" but also current re-imaginings of designed human beings.

The idea of human perfectibility/mutability, achieved through the application of modern biotechnologies, continues to be explored in other recent cultural images and icons such as: *The Bionic Woman*; the Borg of *Star Trek: TNG*; and the whole cast of superheroes—from the classic *Superman* and *Batman* to the newer *X-Men* and *Iron Man*—all of which are based on some notion of biological mutability/perfectibility through the work of science/technology on Nature.

As with all literary and cultural narratives, these particular narratives about human perfectibility circulate, in a very general and diffuse way, throughout

3 It has been rumoured that this tale, along with numerous others, is one of the literary inspirations for the popular current TV series, *Lost*.

society becoming part of our collective thinking. At the same time science itself, particularly the "health sciences," has its own narratives about human perfectibility.

Scientific Narratives

More "scientific" notions of human perfectibility/mutability can be found in current health promotion/health education messages about individual "lifestyle" behaviours, such as diet, exercise, substance use, stress reduction, and the like—all strategies for managing one's body, working on one's biology. Indeed, contemporary gyms with their black and chrome decor and soft lighting and music might be viewed as modern-day temples or shrines to the idea of human perfectibility.[4]

With the Human Genome Project's (HGP) successful completion of the project to "map" the human genome, public and scientific imagination has been caught anew by the idea of human perfectibility through the application of technologies that manipulate the genetic material itself, the DNA. These include technologies such as predictive genetic testing, prenatal genetic testing and, more recently, pre-implantation genetic diagnosis (PGD) combined with embryo selection.

The notion of human perfectibility through "selective human breeding" is not a recent idea, as the eugenics movement of the late nineteenth/early twentieth century attests to. A fuller discussion of the history of this movement and its implications for contemporary genomics is beyond the scope of this chapter.[5] However, it is worth noting that the shadow of the eugenics movement's most obscene manifestation in the Nazi notion of racial purity still hangs over anything to do with genetics and genomics.[6]

As briefly outlined above, there are many "stories" about human perfectibility/mutability—scientific, cultural, and literary. In our "post-genomic" age, these stories of human perfectibility mesh seamlessly with contemporary stories about the gene—that is, they can be said to have become, in part, "genetic stories" (Lippman 1991; 2000). These newer genetic stories of human perfectibility underlie the often-triumphal announcements of the "discovery" of certain genes, such as "the Breast Cancer gene" in 1993 or the "gene for aggression" in 2001 (which was "found" on the Y chromosome, the chromosome that determines maleness).[7]

---

4 The "reality TV" series *Extreme Makeover* surely represents one of the most extreme contemporary examples of the enduring power of the notion of human perfectibility.

5 For a comprehensive social history of the eugenics movement, see Paul 1998.

6 See, for example, an exhibit about the Nazi eugenics project mounted by the United States Holocaust Memorial Museum, "Deadly Medicine: Creating the Master Race," http://www.ushmm.org/museum/exhibit/traveling/details/index.php?type=current&content=deadly_medicine.

7 This "discovery" calls to mind the remarkably prescient Philip K. Dick short story *The Minority Report* (2002; first published in 1956)—which was made into a popular movie

The remainder of this chapter considers the implications of a particular genetic technology to explore what it is about "post-genomic" science that seems to promise so much in terms of human perfectibility.

The "New" Genetic Promise

It could be said that what physics was to the twentieth century, biology will be to the twenty-first century. Certainly, the field of molecular genetics reached its current apogee in the HGP's claim that it has successfully "mapped" the human genome—that is, it has located and identified the genes that make up the 23 pairs of chromosomes that carry the genetic information that makes human beings human beings and not toads or toadstools, or even chimpanzees.

Genes have become a dominant cultural icon (Nelkin and Lindee 1995) and have slipped easily into contemporary Western cultural narratives. DNA has been referred to as the "book of life," the code of codes (like the Rosetta stone), a blueprint for life; genes have been referred to as a language, a script, the essence of human life, with the work of the HGP being likened to the mediaeval European legend of the search for the Holy Grail. This has led biologist Evelyn Fox Keller to refer to our current era as the "century of the gene" (Fox Keller 2000). With these powerful metaphoric underpinnings, it is no wonder that stories about genetic possibilities for human perfectibility have claimed a renewed grip on public and scientific imagination. What makes these stories so powerful is that they are simultaneously fascinating, seductive, and disturbing in their implications.

The particular "genetic story" about human perfectibility that I will focus on in this chapter is the genetic technology called pre-implantation genetic diagnosis (PGD). The possibilities for PGD have led not only to a whole host of social, political, and ethical controversies, but also to new terms and metaphors entering the public lexicon, terms such as "designer babies"—as invoked in the scene in *Gattaca* described at the beginning of this chapter—or "saviour siblings"—as illustrated by the landmark Hashmi case in the UK, which is discussed in more detail below.

Pre-implantation Genetic Diagnosis (PGD)

PGD falls into the larger class of genetic screening technologies, which includes pre-natal genetic screening during pregnancy (for, among other things, Down syndrome and cystic fibrosis), newborn genetic screening, and later genetic testing for late onset disease (such as Huntington's or breast cancer).[8] PGD only

in 2002—about genetically altered beings who could "see" future crimes, thereby making it possible for the identification and arrest of *potential* criminals.

8 Currently in Ontario, Canada, all newborns are routinely screened for 29 inherited diseases (See Therell and Adams 2007; see also the Ontario Newborn Screening programme website at: http://www.newbornscreening.on.ca/bins/index.asp).

became possible in the 1980s with the emergence and increasing utilization of new reproductive technologies. In combination with *in vitro* fertilization (IVF), PGD can be thought of as an alternative to prenatal genetic testing and selective abortion, which has already become an acceptable practice for genetic disorders such as Down syndrome. As a genetic screening technology, PGD involves the *in vitro* fertilization of a number of eggs, the testing of the resulting embryos for "undesirable" or "desirable" genetic characteristics for which genetic tests have been developed (e.g., Down syndrome, cystic fibrosis, sex), followed by the selection and the implantation of an embryo without—or with, in the case of selection *for*—the particular genetic "marker." The "excess" embryos are routinely destroyed.

PGD is an extremely controversial genetic technology, raising the highly charged spectres of "designer babies" and "saviour siblings." However, most of the literature on PGD is careful to make the distinction between "embryo selection" and "embryo enhancement." As the UK Human Genetics Commission 2004 Report *Choosing the Future: Genetics and Reproductive Decision-Making* clarifies, embryo *selection* refers to the selection of embryos without a specific serious genetic disorder or chromosomal abnormality. In other words, it is a genetic selection "against" disease. It has also been used for sex selection: to select for female embryos in order to avoid a sex-linked genetic disorder which only affects male children, such as Duchenne muscular dystrophy; for preferential sex selection, a practice which, clearly, has serious implications in terms of gender equity. In some cases, PGD has been used in an attempt to obtain an embryo that is both free of the relevant genetic disorder (beta thalassemia, say) and a tissue match for an existing child with the disease—what has been called the "saviour sibling" phenomenon. Thus, embryo selection, other than preferential sex selection, can be used as a way of preventing, avoiding or treating what are considered to be "genetic diseases."

In contrast, "*embryo enhancement*" refers to techniques to enhance the genetic make-up of a child, either through selection of certain traits, such as beauty or intelligence or musical ability; it also refers to the process of genetic modification to enhance such traits. This taps into the prevailing cultural narratives on human perfectibility discussed earlier. While such a process is not yet technically possible, many observers think it is only a matter of time. Indeed, the recent "discoveries" of the "gay gene" and the "aggression gene" indicate that, clearly, this technique is fraught with all kinds of ethical, social, and political dilemmas (Nuffield Council on Bioethics 2002).

It has been argued that the routinization of pre-natal genetic testing has laid both the clinical and normative groundwork for the public acceptance of PGD (Rapp 1998). Pre-natal genetic testing has such broad public acceptance that not only is it difficult for pregnant women, especially pregnant women over a certain age, to refuse this intervention, many have come to see it as a need or even demand it as a right. It is not inconceivable that the same thing could become true of PGD.

The chapter continues with a discussion, first, of a particular case with respect to embryo selection for a "saviour sibling" and, then, with a discussion of the more hypothetical issue of "designer babies."

"Saviour Siblings": The Hashmi Case

> There is no better reason for having a child than to save the life of another individual. Saviour siblings are therefore not only ethical but also a wonderful, generous and humane decision for parents to make both for the saviour sibling and for the child who will benefit. (Professor John Harris 2005)

The well-known UK case of the Hashmi family's attempt to obtain a "saviour sibling" to help a seriously ill child is a paradigmatic case of many of the ethical, social, and political implications of PGD and is, thus, worth a fuller discussion.[9]

At the time of their initial application to the UK Human Fertilisation and Embryology Authority (HFEA) in 2002, Raj and Shahana Hashmi had a son of six, Zain, who suffered from the blood disorder, beta thalassemia (BT).[10] BT is an inherited condition that occurs relatively frequently in people from the Eastern Mediterranean region (e.g., Cyprus, Sardinia). Since being diagnosed at four months of age, Zain had to undergo regular blood transfusions and was in danger of dying unless a suitable tissue donor could be found for him. Because the best chance of finding such a donor lay in the birth of a compatible sibling, two months after Zain had been diagnosed, Mrs Hashmi conceived naturally in the hope of creating a match for him. The resulting child, Haris, though free of the disease, was not a tissue match for Zain. The Hashmis then launched a worldwide search for a donor but, when that failed, they began to consider alternative options.

The fertility clinic treating the Hashmis applied to the HFEA for permission to carry out not only PGD on embryos created through IVF in order to ensure that the Hashmis would have a child born free of the disease, but also tissue typing to identify which, if any, of the embryos would be a blood match for Zain. A so-called "saviour sibling" could thus be created and umbilical cord blood could be taken and used to treat Zain. The HFEA gave its permission, introducing strict guidelines for the future and noting that future requests would be considered on a case-by-case basis.

Following this decision, the Hashmis produced 14 embryos through IVF but none was a match for Zain. Their efforts to select a saviour sibling were

9 The details of the Hashmi case are taken from the archives of BioNews, a weekly online digest of the top stories in assisted reproduction and human genetics, published by Progress Educational Trust in the UK (http://www.BioNews.org.uk).

10 HFEA is the UK's regulatory body that oversees and rules on the use of new reproductive technologies such as IVF and PGD. For more details, please see http://www.hfea.gov.uk/.

Table 4.1 A chronology of the Hashmi case

October 2001	Hashmis apply to the UK's Human Fertilisation and Embryology Authority (HFEA) for permission to use PGD with tissue typing.
February 2002	HFEA announces decision on Hashmi application, allowing them to go ahead with PGD.
December 2002	CORE challenges HFEA's decision in the High Court which rules that the HFEA had no legal power to authorize the testing of embryos to create "saviour siblings." Hashmis are ordered to stop treatment.
April 2003	HFEA launches appeal to High Court decision. Court of Appeal overturns High Court decision.
May 2003	Court of Appeal publishes detailed reasons for its decision. Hashmis begin third IVF attempt.
January 2004	CORE launches a further legal challenge to Court of Appeal decision.
July 2004	The Hashmis stop treatment after six unsuccessful attempts.
July 2004	HFEA changes its policy to allow PGD with tissue typing to create "donor siblings."
April 2005	The Law Lords rule that the decision taken by the HFEA on the Hashmi case was lawful.

then brought to a halt by a legal challenge from the pro-life pressure group, Comment on Reproductive Ethics (CORE). CORE argued that in granting the Hashmis permission to proceed, the HFEA had exceeded the bounds of the authority accorded it under the Human Fertilisation and Embryology Act of 1990. Specifically, CORE's argument in the House of Lords was that HFEA's authority over licensing tissue-typing was specifically "designed to determine whether embryos are suitable [to be placed in a woman]" and that "suitable" in this context must mean *only* capable of becoming a healthy child who is free of abnormalities. Any broader construction of "suitable," such as taking account of the wishes of the Hashmis as to a future child's particular characteristics, CORE argued, would pave the way for the creation of "designer babies" chosen on the basis of non-health characteristics, such as hair and eye colour; in other words, the proverbial—and, therefore, singularly unhelpful—"slippery slope" challenge.

The HFEA subsequently brought a counter suit arguing for a broader understanding of "suitable," suggesting that the Hashmis would be entitled to regard an embryo as "unsuitable" unless it was *both* free of abnormality *and* a perfect match for Zain. While the judge in the High Court found for CORE and a narrow interpretation of "suitable," eventually, after a long legal battle (see Table 4.1 "A Chronology of the Hashmi Case"), both the Court of Appeal and House of Lords found unanimously that the HFEA had acted originally within its powers in allowing the Hashmis to go ahead with IVF combined with PGD to obtain an embryo who was a tissue match for Zain. When the House of Lords announced its ruling in 2005, Shahana Hashmi made the following statement to the press:

> It's nice to know that society has now embraced the technology to cure the sick and take away the pain. It has been a long and hard battle for all the family and

> we have finally heard the news we wanted to hear. *We feel this ruling marks a new era* and we are happy to move forwards now. We hope and pray that we get what we need for Zain. (Harris 2005; emphasis added)

Precisely what this "new era" consists of is not clear. As of 2007, the Hashmis have not been successful in creating a "saviour sibling" for Zain.

Questions Raised by the Hashmi Case

The Hashmi case provoked a storm of media interest and widespread questions regarding the ethics of the deliberate creation of so-called "saviour siblings," including:

- Do these procedures violate a core Kantian principle by creating a child as a means to some other end, albeit a benevolent one?
- Do such actions take adequate account of the welfare of the child who is to be born as a "saviour sibling"? Is this truly in their "best interests"?
- Do parents have a more general right to pre-determine the genetic characteristics of their own children?
- Does allowing the selection of "saviour siblings" place us on a slippery slope towards allowing full-scale "designer babies"?

The issue of "saviour siblings" also raises questions at a more social and political level, including:

- Who should make these decisions and how should they be made?
- Should the sorts of issues raised in the Hashmi case be left to the conscience of individual parents and the professional discretion of clinicians, avoiding the need to parade the private tragedy of a family through committees, courts, and the media?
- Is it better that these decisions should be located in the hands of a body like the HFEA with its ability to draw on medical, legal, ethical experts, and lay members?
- Or, rather, are the ethical issues raised by these kinds of "private decisions" of such fundamental public importance that they would be more appropriately determined by a public body? And if yes, then what sort of public body—a legal court, parliament, a publicly constituted ethics commission?

These are all questions that, clearly, have no easy answers. They are all questions of fundamental importance about the nature and parameters of human life: about what is life, who may live, who makes those determinations, and how.

While the issue of "saviour siblings" has been a prominent "genetic story," particularly in light of the Hashmi case, it is the issue of "designer babies" that most clearly weaves into the cultural narrative about human perfectibility.

"Designer Babies": Why Not the Best?

> It may be possible to produce great benefits for individuals and even for society as a whole through some kinds of enhancement .... (Buchanan et al. 2000, 195)

Is there a difference (social/ethical/political) between using PGD for therapeutic embryo selection against certain genetic diseases, or even for "saviour siblings," and using PGD for "preferential" embryo selection? This selection could be either *for* certain characteristics—such as sex, athletic ability, or IQ—or *against* certain behavioural characteristics like "shyness" or "aggression," all of which are either technically possible now (sex) or within the foreseeable future (IQ).

In their book, *From Chance to Choice: Genetics and Justice* (2000), Buchanan and his colleagues ask, "What could be more natural than parents seeking the best children?" Indeed, they argue that parents have an explicit obligation not only to protect their children from harm but also to produce the best children they can, not only in the interests of those future children but of society in general.

> If genetic techniques gave parents a way to enhance the resistance of their children to certain diseases ... should parents be free, *or even required* in some instances, to use them? (Buchanan et al. 2000, 157; emphasis added)

Buchanan et al. go on to make the point that parents do everything they can to provide the best for their children, from immunization, music lessons, orthodontics, to private tutoring.[11] They argue, by somewhat specious analogy, that genetic selection and even genetic enhancement (if and when this becomes technically possible) could be seen to be a natural and logical extension of these sorts of parental efforts and choices.

A fuller discussion of the range of social, political, and ethical questions that are raised by the possibility of "designer babies" is not possible here but one question that stands above all is the question: "is this eugenics?"[12]

From Eugenics to Genomics?

Is there a straight line from eugenics to genomics (Kerr and Shakespeare 2002)? Does the issue of "designer babies" represent nothing more—and nothing less—than the old eugenics in the new clothing of biotechnology? A eugenics that is cleaned up, white-coated, with the aura of science surrounding it? Many people have argued that what is different about the new genomic technologies, such

11 Buchanan and his colleagues are clearly referring to middle-class, privileged parents and their children.

12 For fuller discussions of these issues see, for example: Chadwick 1999; Chadwick et al. 2005; Evans 2002; Harris 2007; Kamm 2005; Sandel 2004 and 2007; Verlinsky 2007; Wilkinson 2005.

as PGD, is that, because they are couched in the language of individual choice and improved quality of life (for some, that is), their eugenic potential is hidden. This has led Troy Duster to refer to the new genomic technologies as "backdoor eugenics" (Duster 2003).

As Alan Petersen (1998; 1999) argues, this "user friendly" eugenics—unlike the old eugenics, which was more about species or racial improvement—is driven primarily by market forces and individual consumer desire. The desire is, in part, for healthy, beautiful, intelligent, talented children; in other words, for human perfectibility. This raises fundamental ethical questions about the "given-ness" of human life, what Michael Sandel refers to as the "unbidden":

> the deepest moral objection to enhancement lies less in the perfection it seeks than in the human disposition it expresses and promotes.. *The problem lies in the hubris of the designing parents*, in their drive to master the mystery of birth … [which] would … deprive the parent of the humility and enlarged human sympathies that an openness to the unbidden can cultivate. (Sandel 2004, 5; emphasis added)

It has been argued that genomic technologies, like PGD and more conventional pre-natal testing, are inherently discriminatory towards persons with disabilities, and directs attention away from providing appropriate supports for such persons and their families (Lippman 1991; 1999; and 2000; Peterson 1998; 1999).

Jeremy Rifkin (1998) argues that genetic engineering tools are *by definition* eugenics instruments. Along these lines, biologist Richard Lewontin makes a critical distinction when he reminds us that "to conflate … the prevention of *disease* with the prevention of *lives* that will involve disease is to traduce completely the meaning of preventive medicine" (Lewontin 1997, 5; emphasis in original).

Well-known British sociologist and disability rights activist, Tom Shakespeare, has weighed into this particular debate in his recent controversial book, *Disability Rights and Wrongs* (2006). Shakespeare argues, in part (see Chapter 6), that pre-natal testing and termination does not necessarily express disrespect or discrimination against people with disabilities, as has been argued by many disability rights groups.[13] Both sides of this particular debate are eloquently expressed by this "lay" member of the UK Human Genetics Commission who, himself, has an inherited disability:

> I believe that parents should be allowed to give their children the best possible chance to live a healthy and successful life. *On the other hand, I would not have been born ….* (UK Human Genetics Commission 2004, 26; emphasis added)

The issues relating to "saviour siblings" and "designer babies" raise further issues about what Nikolas Rose (2001; 2007) has called "the politics of life itself."

13 For an extended discussion of the debate raised by Shakespeare's book, see *Journal of Medical Ethics* 34 (2008).

PGD and the Governance of Life

In the remainder of this chapter, I will consider what contribution social theory might make to our understanding of new and emerging biotechnologies, like PGD, in terms of the broader social and political context within which these technologies have emerged and are located: that is, Western society characterized by a neoliberal political rationality, a capitalist mode of production, and a consumer culture.

Specifically, I will discuss three interrelated concepts based on the work of French philosopher, Michel Foucault, that not only shed light on these issues but also open up space for further discussion, namely: (1) biopower, (2) neoliberalism and governmentality, and (3) biological citizenship.

The brief overview that follows is intended to demonstrate the utility of these concepts for examining PGD, in particular, and genomic technologies, in general.

Biopower

In comparison to earlier sovereign forms of government, Foucault contended that modern programmes of governance in the West, which he argues emerged in the seventeenth and eighteenth centuries, have come to rely less on repressive, juridical modes of power, and to operate primarily through "biopower" or power exercised through a precise and calculated management of life itself (Foucault 1977; 1978; and 1984a). According to Foucault, biopower operates in relation to two interconnected poles:

> 1. the first pole, the *anatomo-politics of the individual human body*, aims to usefully train and discipline the individual body-as-machine and distributes bodies in time and space by rendering the body as an object of knowledge and surveillance;
> 2. the second pole of biopower, the *bio-politics of the population*, focuses on the species body and aims to develop knowledge about the mechanics of life and biological processes of the population as a whole—e.g., birth rates, death rates. (Foucault 1984a)

Foucault argues further that it was during the shift from juridical forms of rule to biopolitical modes of governance in the seventeenth and eighteenth centuries that a range of disciplines emerged, including demography, public health and hygiene, and so on, all of which took "population" as an object of knowledge and surveillance and as a target for practical intervention (Foucault 1984b and 1991). As a result, a "technology of population" came into being that operated more in terms of norms that classified individuals according to scientific, statistical distributions (Castel 1991; Ewald 1991). Statistics emerged as one of a number of strategies for states to gain information about populations in order to manage them.[14] Indeed, several statisticians of the late nineteenth/early twentieth centuries, like Galton and Pearson, were enthusiastic supporters of the eugenics movement.

According to Foucault, modern forms of governance operate not by oppressing or suppressing people, but rather by inciting or eliciting certain desires: for example, through prevailing cultural messages about the kinds of persons we should be, the kinds of bodies we should have, the kinds of thoughts, beliefs, attitudes we should have, and so on. Foucault was interested in how we come to think of ourselves as certain kinds of people, or subjects, and in the practices that we take on and in which we engage in order to make ourselves certain kinds of subjects.[15] Foucault referred to these practices as "technologies of the self," which "permit individuals to effect by their own means, or with the help of others, a certain number of operations on their own bodies and souls, thoughts, conduct, and way of being, *so as to transform themselves* …" (Foucault 1994, 225; emphasis added).

Foucault argued further that these practices—the ways in which subjects freely "transform themselves"—do not originate *sui generis* from within the subject, nor are they universal, transhistorical, or transcultural. Rather they are generally prevailing and circulating in the culture and thus are, always, historically and culturally contingent and constituted:

> *these practices [of the self] are nevertheless not something invented by the individual himself* [*sic*]. They are models that he finds in his culture and are proposed, suggested, imposed upon him by his culture, his society, and his social group. (Foucault 1994, 291; emphasis added)

From this perspective, it could be argued that, with the coming together of the narrative of human perfectibility and the narrative of the gene in the late twentieth/early twenty-first centuries, we have become constituted as "genetic subjects." Indeed, *Gattaca*'s main character (an "invalid") says at one point, "My real resume is in my cells"—in other words, in his DNA.

Neoliberalism and Governmentality

Foucault used the term "governmentality" to refer to this shift in the strategies of governance toward those that increasingly spread beyond the domain of the state itself and permeate the social body through such apparatuses as the media, popular culture and entertainment, the consumer marketplace, education, health

14 It is interesting to note here the etymological relationship between the words "statistics" and "state," both from the Latin *status*, meaning "manner of standing, position, condition." Statistics is, then, an essential tool of statecraft, that is, of governing.

15 As Foucault explains: "There are two meanings to the word *subject*: subject to someone else by control and dependence, and tied to his own identity by a conscience or self-knowledge. Both meanings suggest a form of power which subjugates and makes subject to" (1983, 212).

and social services, and so on. Many scholars have written about the particular form that governmentality takes on in the contemporary neoliberal context (see, for example: Barry et al. 1996; Burchell et al. 1991).

Briefly, "neoliberalism" is the term used by many scholars to refer to the political rationality that emerged in the West in the late 1970s/early 1980s with the election of the politically and fiscally conservative governments of Margaret Thatcher in the UK and Ronald Reagan in the USA, marking the end of post-Second World War welfare state development in Western industrialized nations.

This political rationality, which replaced an older one and which persists today, rests on underlying principles of classical liberalism such as: the dominance of a "free market" ethos; a minimal role for government; and, an emphasis on individual freedom and choice along with responsibility and self-reliance. This focus on "individual responsibility" was captured in Margaret Thatcher's (in)famous statement shortly after she was first elected in 1980: "There is no such thing as Society. There are individual men and women, and there are families"—the notion of "family" being a decidedly narrow one.[16]

Neoliberalism, or "advanced liberalism," is distinguished by Nikolas Rose (1996) from classical liberalism in terms of three characteristic shifts:

1. *A new relation between expertise and politics*—in which individuals and society are to be rendered manageable (invoking Foucault's two poles of biopower) by new domains of professional expertise that operate at a distance from formal centres of state power through social apparatuses such as schools, hospitals, genetic testing clinics; as such, the role of experts becomes central to the exercise of power;[17]
2. *A new pluralization of "social" technologies*—which reconfigures the earlier political relationship between social citizens and their common society as a relationship between the responsible individual and their self-governing community;
3. *A new specification of the subject of government*—from citizen to consumer—of health services, of education, of social services, of genetic testing; the citizens of neoliberalism are individuals actively engaged in the "enterprise of themselves" (Petersen 1997) in order to maximize their individual quality of life—and that of their children—through exercising free choice in a marketplace of consumer commodities, which might include new biotechnologies such as PGD.

According to Deborah Lupton (1999) a crucial aspect of governmentality as it is expressed in neoliberal states is that the regulation and disciplining of citizens is directed at the autonomous self-regulated individual:

16 Quotation from: http://womenshistory.about.com/od/quotes/a/m_thatcher.htm.

17 For a further discussion of the role of expertise in relation to health see, for example: Petersen 1997; Petersen and Lupton 1996; Polzer 2005.

> the strategies of governmentality, expressed in neo-liberal states that emerged in the west in late modernity, include both direct, coercive strategies to regulate populations, but also, and most importantly, less direct *strategies that rely on individuals' voluntary compliance with the interests and needs of the state.* (Lupton 1999, 87; emphasis added)

Within older forms of governance, individuals were primarily regulated by agents of the state whereas within neoliberal forms of governance individuals regulate or police *themselves*; that is, they exercise power *upon* themselves as normalized subjects who are in pursuit of their own best interests and freedoms, who are interested in self-improvement, seeking happiness and healthiness (Burchell 1996). In other words, we are governed *through* our freedom (Rose 1990; 1996).[18]

The problem of governance (that is, all of the "governing" institutions and forces in society, not just the formally constituted elected governments), then, is to find the means by which individuals may be made responsible for themselves through their individual choices, through their own shaping of a lifestyle according to practices that are widely disseminated throughout the culture. These practices include, among other things: the uptake of all of the strategies for self-surveillance and self-management that we have come to take for granted, such as diet, exercise, dress, body adornment (piercings and tattoos, for example); the cultivation of certain kinds of tastes in food, clothing, music, etc.; in other words, all of those body/self projects that we take on to make of ourselves certain kinds of people. To these governmental practices we can now add genomic technologies such as PGD.

The social or political implications of increasingly thinking of ourselves as "genetic subjects" can be captured, in part, by considering the notion of "biological citizenship."

Biological Citizenship

The term "biological citizenship" has been used to refer to the multiple ways in which, at any given historical moment, beliefs about the biological existence of human beings—as individuals, as embodied members of families, communities, populations, races, a species—are linked to particular notions of citizenship (Polzer 2006; Rose and Novas 2005).

It has been argued that in the present historical moment, characterized by a neoliberal political rationality, the notion of biological citizenship—as, primarily,

---

18 It is important to note here Foucault's argument that "we need to see things not in terms of the replacement of a society of sovereignty by a disciplinary society and the subsequent replacement of a disciplinary society by a society of government; in reality one has a triangle, sovereignty-discipline-government, which has as its primary target the population ..." (1991, 102). (For further discussions of this point, see also: Dean 1999; Hindess 2001; Valverde 1996.)

"genetic citizenship"—facilitates the engagement of active subjects in particular practices such as genetic testing/screening and PGD (Bunton and Peterson 2005; Petersen 1999; Polzer 2006). These practices tie personal life trajectories into broader political imperatives in which individuals have a right to genetic health. In addition, within this political rationality, the case has been made (as discussed above) that parents have not only a right but also a positive duty—to their children and to society—to ensure the "genetic health" of the population.

This increasing tendency to "geneticize" health and disease is occurring in a context of a major shift in world view: the commitment to social welfare institutions that focus on the support, training, and rehabilitation of the ill and disabled appears to be declining in favour of a new technologically-driven imperative towards genetic prevention and genetic intervention (Lippman 1991; 1999; Petersen 1998). By further individualizing social approaches and responses to health and disease, this trend contributes to an ongoing "desocialization" and "depoliticization" of health and disease.

Conclusion

This chapter has introduced some of the social, ethical, and political issues that are raised by emerging genomic technologies. To be sure, some of these technologies will have some beneficial applications that will surely reduce human suffering, none of which I have discussed here.

As indicated earlier, it has been said that what atomic physics was to the twentieth century, biology, in particular molecular genetics, will be to the twenty-first century. But do we know where we are going on this particular journey, or more to the point, do we know where we *want* to go? Is the case of PGD simply a matter of responsible and good genomic science—that is, getting the science "right"—and then applying that science to reducing the burden of disease? But, history teaches us that, like Mary Shelley's monster, every technology developed through human ingenuity, however seemingly beneficial, carries hidden dangers. It remains to be seen what form the "fallout" from genomic technologies, like PGD, may take.

This chapter is not intended as a neo-Luddite, anti-science/technology argument against emerging biotechnologies, in general, or genomic technologies, in particular. However, I would argue that, as social scientists and bioethicists, our first responsibility is always to question the powerful and seductive cultural and scientific narratives that surround us, including the enduring narrative on human perfectibility in its current genomic version. For as Foucault reminds us:

> The … point is not that everything is bad, but that everything is dangerous … If everything is dangerous, then we always have something to do. (Foucault 1984c, 343)

References

Barry, A. et al. (eds) (1996), *Foucault and Political Reason: Liberalism, Neo-liberalism and Rationalities of Government* (Chicago, IL: University of Chicago Press).

Buchanan, A. et al. (2000), *From Chance to Choice: Genetics and Justice* (Cambridge: Cambridge University Press).

Bunton, R. and Petersen, A. (eds) (2005), *Genetic Governance: Health, Risk and Ethics in the Biotech Era* (London: Routledge).

Burchell, G. (1996), "Liberal Government and Techniques of the Self," in A. Barry et al. (eds).

Burchell, G. et al. (eds) (1991), *The Foucault Effect: Studies in Governmentality* (London: Harvester/Wheatsheaf).

Castel, R. (1991), "From Dangerousness to Risk," in G. Burchell et al. (eds).

Chadwick, R. (1999), "Genetics, Choice and Responsibility," *Health, Risk and Society* 1:3, 293–300.

Chadwick, R. et al. (2005), "Discussion (day 1, session 2): Designer Babies," *Reproductive Biomedicine Online* 10, 40–42.

Dean, M. (1999), *Governmentality: Power and Rule in Modern Society* (London: Sage Publications).

Dick, P.K. (2002), *The Minority Report* (New York: Pantheon Books).

Duster, T. (2003), *Backdoor to Eugenics*, 2nd edition (New York: Routledge).

Evans, J.H. (2002), *Playing God?: Human Genetic Engineering and the Rationalization of Public Bioethical Debate* (Chicago, IL: University of Chicago Press).

Ewald, F. (1991), "Insurance and Risk," in G. Burchell et al. (eds).

Foucault, M. (1977), *Discipline and Punish: The Birth of the Prison* (New York: Random House).

Foucault, M. (1978), *The History of Sexuality, Volume I: An Introduction* (New York: Random House).

Foucault, M. (1983), "The Subject and Power," in H. Dreyfus and P. Rabinow (eds), *Michel Foucault: Beyond Structuralism and Hermeneutics* (Chicago, IL: University of Chicago Press).

Foucault, M. (1984a), "Right of Death and Power over Life," in P. Rabinow (ed.), *The Foucault Reader* (New York: Pantheon Books).

Foucault, M. (1984b), "The Politics of Health in the Eighteenth Century," in P. Rabinow (ed.), *The Foucault Reader* (New York: Pantheon Books).

Foucault, M. (1984c), "On the Genealogy of Ethics: An Overview of a Work in Progress," in P. Rabinow (ed.), *The Foucault Reader* (New York: Pantheon Books).

Foucault, M. (1991), "Governmentality," in G. Burchell et al. (eds).

Foucault, M. (1994), "Technologies of the Self," in P. Rabinow (ed.), *Michel Foucault: Ethics, Subjectivity and Truth* (New York: Pantheon Books).

Fox Keller, E. (2000), *The Century of the Gene* (Cambridge, MA: Harvard University Press).

Gattaca (1997), Film. Directed by A. Niccol. Produced by Columbia Pictures, USA.

Harris, J. (2005), "Press Release," *Science Media Centre* [website], <www.sciencemediacentre.org/press_releases/05-04-28_HashmiRuling.htm>.

Harris, J. (2007), *Enhancing Evolution: The Ethical Case for Making People Better* (Princeton, NJ: Princeton University Press).

Hindess, B. (2001), "The Liberal Government of Unfreedom," *Alternatives* 26:1, 93–111.

Holm, S. (2008), "The Expressivist Objection to Prenatal Diagnosis: Can It Be Laid to Rest?" *Journal of Medical Ethics* 34:1, 24–5.

Huxley, A. (1967), *Brave New World* (Harmondsworth: Penguin).

Kamm, F.M. (2005), "Is There a Problem with Enhancement?" *American Journal of Bioethics* 5:3, 5–14.

Kerr, A. and Shakespeare, T. (2002), *Genetic Politics: From Eugenics to Genome* (Cheltenham: New Clarion Press).

Lewontin, R. (1997), "Science and the 'Demon-haunted World': An Exchange," *The New York Review of Books* 34:4 [website], (published online 6 March 1997) <http://www.nybooks.com/articles/1246>, accessed 6 March 2007.

Lippman, A. (1991), "Prenatal Genetic Testing and Screening: Constructing Needs and Reinforcing Inequities," *American Journal of Law and Medicine* 17:1–2, 15–50.

Lippman, A. (1999), "Prenatal Genetic Testing and Screening: Constructing Needs and Reinforcing Inequities," in D.E. Beauchamp and B. Steinbock (eds), *New Ethics for the Public's Health* (New York: Oxford University Press).

Lippman, A. (2000), "Geneticization and the Canadian Biotechnology Strategy: The Marketing of Women's Health," paper presented at The Gender of Genetic Futures: Canadian Biotechnology, Women, and Health, York University, Toronto, 11–12. February 2000.

Lupton, D. (1999), *Risk* (London: Routledge).

Nelkin, D. and Lindee, S. (1995), *The DNA Mystique: The Gene as Cultural Icon* (New York: Freeman).

Nuffield Council on Bioethics (2002), *Genetics and Human Behaviour: The Ethical Context* (London: Nuffield Council on Bioethics).

Paul, D.B. (1998), *Controlling Human Heredity: 1865 to the Present* (Amherst, NY: Humanity Books).

Petersen, A. (1997), "Risk, Governance and the New Public Health," in A. Petersen and R. Bunton (eds), *Foucault, Health and Medicine* (London: Routledge).

Petersen, A. (1998), "The New Genetics and the Politics of Public Health," *Critical Public Health* 8:1, 59–71.

Petersen, A. (1999), "Public Health, the New Genetics and Subjectivity," in A. Petersen et al. (eds), *Poststructuralism, Citizenship and Social Policy* (London: Routledge).

Petersen, A. and Lupton, D. (1996), *The New Public Health: Health and Self in the Age of Risk* (London: Sage).

Polzer, J. (2005), "Choice as Responsibility: Genetic Testing as Citizenship Through Familial Obligation and the Management of Risk," in R. Bunton and A. Petersen (eds).

Polzer, J. (2006), "Genetic(optim)ization, Risk and the Neoliberal Biological Citizen," paper presented at the Annual Conference of the British Sociological Association, Medical Sociology Group, Edinburgh, 16 September 2006.

Rapp, R. (1998), "Refusing Prenatal Diagnosis: The Uneven Meanings of Bioscience in a Multicultural World," in R. Davis-Floyd and J. Dumit (eds), *Cyborg Babies: From Techno-Sex to Techno-Tots* (London: Routledge).

Rifkin, J. (1998), *The Biotech Century: Harnessing the Gene and Remaking the World* (New York: Jeremy P. Tarcher/Putnam).

Rose, N. (1990), *Governing the Soul: The Shaping of the Private Self* (London: Routledge).

Rose, N. (1996), "Governing 'Advanced' Liberal Democracies," in A. Barry et al. (eds).

Rose, N. (2001), "The Politics of Life Itself," *Theory, Culture and Society* 18:6, 1–30.

Rose, N.S. (2007), *The Politics of Life Itself: Biomedicine, Power, and Subjectivity in the Twenty-first Century* (Princeton, NJ: Princeton University Press).

Rose, N. and Novas, C. (2005), "Biological Citizenship," in A. Ong and S.J. Collier (eds), *Global Assemblages: Technology, Politics, and Ethics as Anthropological Problems* (Malden, MA: Blackwell Publishing).

Sandel, M. (2004), "What's Wrong with Designer Children, Bionic Athletes, and Genetic Engineering," *The Atlantic Monthly* [website], (published online April 2004) <http://www.theatlantic.com/doc/print/200404/sandel>.

Sandel, M. (2007), "Designer Babies: The Problem with Genetic Engineering," *Tikkun* 22:5, 40–43, 84–5.

Shakespeare, T. (2006), *Disability Rights and Wrongs* (New York: Routledge).

Shelley, Mary Wollstonecraft (2006), *Frankenstein* (London: Bloomsbury).

Therrell, B. and Adams, J. (2007), "Newborn Screening in North America," *Journal of Inherited Metabolic Disease* 30:4, 447–65.

UK Human Genetics Commission (2004), *Choosing the Future: Genetics and Reproductive Decision-Making* (Commission Report, UK Department of Health).

Valverde, M. (1996), "'Despotism' and Ethical Liberal Governance," *Economy and Society* 25:3, 357–72.

Van Dijck, J. (1998), *Imagenation: Popular Images of Genetics* (New York: New York University Press).

Verlinsky, Y. (2007), "Ethics of Preimplantation Genetic Diagnosis," *Reproductive Biomedicine Online* 14, 102–3.

Wells, H.G. (1996), *The Island of Dr Moreau* (New York: Modern Library).

Wilkinson, S. (2005), "'Designer Babies,' Instrumentalisation and the Child's Right to an Open Future," in N. Athanassoulis (ed.), *Philosophical Reflections on Medical Ethics* (New York: Palgrave Macmillan).

Chapter 5
"Hail the Cure!": Althusser, Biotechnology, and Biopolitics

Bradley Bryan

Orienting Remarks: Confronting Biotechnology's Cures

When struck by illness, it is more than tempting to turn to a cure. "More than tempting" because it is not a question of "resisting" whether to think of our illness in terms of a cure. The notion of a cure is implied from the outset, it is an intrinsic part of thinking in terms of an illness, along with all the hope it carries in rescuing us from a death that has already been made present. Today biotechnology offers a wildly wide range of "cures" to conditions and situations that had not previously been thought of as illnesses: ageing, being overweight, forgetfulness. The idea of a cure rescues us from our frailties. When we begin to see ourselves in terms of a cure, we are also provided the critical opportunity to pay close attention to how we have come to be swayed by the hopeful promise of a cure. Who are we that we have come to think of ourselves in this way? One particular way that has been advanced to assist with interpreting our own self-interpretation is the French philosopher Louis Althusser's notion of interpellation (1971). The following is an attempt to show the usefulness of interpellation for thinking through biotechnology's cures, with the added proviso that we cease to think simply in terms of ideology and the subject, as we do with Althusser, and rather think of biopolitics and the "subject" of biotechnology. In other words, this contribution investigates the manner in which biotechnology and biopolitics increasingly provide the terms by which the subject is subjected—the powerful terms in which subjects are spoken and rendered politically coherent and meaningful.

One of the more fruitful interpretations of Althusser's notion of interpellation has demonstrated how "subjects" come to understand themselves as the kind of subjects they in fact are; however, one of the limits of interpellation has been the totalizing nature of ideology it seems to presume. Faithful to Marx, Althusser defined ideology as a "system of ideas and representations which dominate the mind of a man or a social group" (1971, 158). In what follows I try to navigate a course between the fruitful orientation of interpellation and the idea that one's "subject position" is somehow either totally ideological or, in reprieve, at least always already given. Through a reading of biotechnology, I will show that interpellation should be thought in terms other than of "subject formation," according to ideology, or even within "discourse." By locating biotechnological discourses (always plural) within the sphere of biopolitics and thereby thinking of "subjects" as self-interpreting accordingly, interpellation can be rearticulated in terms of the way the human is recruited as the kind of being it ostensibly is, in the kind of world that it ostensibly is in. And more specifically, when we look at biotechnology and its biopolitical modes and histories, we see that the kind of being that one comes to be is as a "subject" that exists over and against a world of "objects" in the strict sense: the interpellation of beings in a world of sciences presumes the "subject/object" divide. As Althusser remarks, an account of interpellation must be clear about what "a subject" actually is. In articulating what it is to be a biotechnological subject, we cannot rush straight to them, but must instead travel along the routes of their interpellation, i.e., along the routes that biotechnology takes in articulating the conditions of subjectivity itself.

Biotechnology's Cautious Subjects

Jeremy Rifkin (1998) has written extensively on the "inherent dangers" of biotechnology, and he has also worked tirelessly in Washington, DC, and around the world to influence and write policy to regulate biotechnology. Reading Rifkin, one feels as though one is witnessing an individual traumatized by the knowledge of what biotechnology could represent. The same is true of William Leiss. Leiss is a major figure in the debates over biotechnology in Canada and around the world, and is, as he readily admits, also traumatized by what he has seen and sees coming. "Researchers in biotechnology have surpassed every milestone they have set in a much shorter time frame than imagined possible. Should we be concerned about the promises and perils of biotechnology? You bet we should. Believe me, they're coming and they'll be here sooner than you think" (Leiss 2005). Hailed as one of Herbert Marcuse's most promising students, Leiss claims that his own confrontation of science with policy is "Hegelian" and that it is the Hegelian dialectic that drives him to attempt to face technology—a fact not to be lost on those who would wonder why he thinks of "subjects" and "objects" of knowledge. And with the vocabulary of Hegel, Leiss thereby suggests a deep historical and philosophical urgency to confront the desire to dominate nature that inheres in biotechnology (Leiss 1972).

Rifkin and Leiss typify debates over biotechnology by presenting this sense of urgency, inviting each of us to take up a position that would stand against it. Leiss demands that we start thinking about possible responses, adding that "the future is here" and it is time to "do something." He says that when we are called upon to accept or reject a particular aspect (read: product) of biotechnology, we will be asked, "what else would you like us to do today…," as though the seeming plasticity of our existence will be offered up for our design. Leiss denies that our seeming omnipotence is only a giddy moment at a genetic supermarket where body parts are fetishized commodities. Rather, for Leiss and others, this apparent power could result in the complete destruction of everything human as we know it. This commodification of life and the domination and destruction it supposedly represents is what unites policymakers like Rifkin and Leiss with poststructural Marxists like Finn Bowring and Slavoj Žižek, and with Neo-Conservative political theorists like Francis Fukuyama; and they have all set their sights on opposing what they take to be the dehumanizing elements of it (see, for instance: Bowring 2002; Fukuyama 2002; Žižek 2003). From Rifkin to Žižek, we are being asked to imagine ourselves in two specific but different registers when confronting and being confronted by biotechnology: what one would do when confronted with a specific example of biotechnology, and what one would do about biotechnology in general or on the whole?

In the first register, notice the variety of places in which we can imagine ourselves confronted by biotechnological innovations: in the supermarket as a customer, in the office of a physician as a patient, in a government as a policymaker, in a lecture hall as an expert. In each of these locations there are parameters set on what a "confrontation" with biotechnology might be. In a supermarket, "confronting" biotechnology might take the form of refusing to purchase foods with genetically modified ingredients in them. In a physician's office it may mean refusing to undergo or accept treatment that involves medicinal products procured through biotechnological processes. Notice also that what is "confronted" in each instance is discrete; missing this detail has us running the risk of thinking that we have somehow confronted biotechnology itself (i.e., on the whole) in each of these instances (which in some sense we have, but biotechnology is not thwarted by such refusals or acceptances). As there are two registers in Leiss's specific invitation to confront biotechnology, there are (at least) two different kinds of moments of decision posed—but what is to be decided remains unstated and out of view. Those who would claim that we need to come to a decision about biotechnology on the whole are asking, begging, that we figure out a *way* to think of biotechnology beyond its particular examples—*assuming we could find a method or procedure to guide us in confronting biotechnology in its particular manifestations*. While we might imagine a discrete decision about a particular innovation in biotechnology as involving values and conceptualizations of risk whilst we shop or decide as officials or researchers, a decision or method for deciding about biotechnology *in toto* demands attention to the relation of the human *to* biotechnology—as though these two registers were separable, and as though the human could stand against biotechnology in the specific mode of *decision on the whole or in general*.

Consider the following two analogies that show the practical impossibility of achieving a relation of decision with respect to biotechnology. Over the past 20 years there has been a transformation in the kind of gear worn by the average hockey player. Where it was once the norm to play without helmets or facemasks or extensive padding, it is no longer possible: ice arenas will not allow players without helmets (as their insurance would be void), and those playing without visors or masks are not individually insured, as such conduct shows a voluntary assumption of the risks. And of course it makes complete sense to wear protective equipment. But as many an elderly hockey player will attest, the advent of better equipment has meant more careless play, more "raised sticks," and a new kind of cavalier attitude. While the equipment is an obvious way to reduce the number of injuries associated with hockey, it also allows a new type of play that does not pay heed to the same kinds of practices that were formerly necessary. So too with biotechnology. Particular technical innovations rise to meet a plethora of daily needs, concerns, and ailments—and to such a degree that it becomes hard to imagine how we would live without them, even though we know that we once did.

A second analogy can be found in the procedure of having one's stomach stapled to a much smaller size in order to avoid eating too much. The difficulty with regulating one's intake of food is that it is contingent on one's ability simply to refuse to eat more despite the desire (or habit) to continue. Stomach stapling makes overeating very difficult, since the sensation of "being full" comes much sooner during a meal than it otherwise would. In some sense, then, it is a perfect solution, for it avoids the difficulty of having to pay attention to one's eating habits—which would require the inculcation of another habit, something the various meanderings of daily life and nutrition make increasingly difficult. Protective gear in hockey and stomach stapling operations solve the problem of *a systematic lack of care*.

These two analogies focus on the way technical solutions work to solve immediate problems arising out of a certain set of practices. The solutions issue from a troublesome decision about these practices: a decision to design either a product or procedure that solves some situation too difficult for individuals to continue to manage on their own. These solutions are perfect *precisely because* they sidestep human willing in a moment of design. The technical, present in moments of human planning, delivers the human from its frailty. Even though technicity is both systemic (insofar as it belongs to the notion of system itself) and systematic (insofar as its deployment follows a logic), the operation and proliferation of technical solutions are *systematic* (rather than systemic) insofar as they purposefully subvert and avoid human decision, according to the logic that such subversion renders behaviour more regular. Why on earth might anyone argue against protective gear or devices preventing unhealthy behaviour, let alone other technical advances like seatbelts, air traffic safety checklists, or medicinal products? Arguing against these devices seems wantonly irresponsible, or, perhaps more troublesome, seems to traffic in the language of "bearing up" and "taking responsibility," something the technical addresses precisely because "responsibility" either consistently fails or is not really an issue where simple seatbelts are the concern.[1] More importantly, particular resistance to facemasks or stomach stapling will do nothing about hockey or eating on the whole. This is a contradiction entailed in "resistance" itself: "speaking truth to power" is not simply making oneself heard before authorities. "Addressing" or "confronting" biotechnology, like confronting dangerous play in hockey or confronting over-eating, is perhaps nothing more than to think about who we take ourselves to be in

1 On the specific way that safety equipment displaces the "ethics" of responsibility, see Simon 2002, 177–208.

the fears we have and the utterances we make.[2] In doing so we demand of ourselves that we try to understand why and how we have come to be in the world as we are. In an age of biotechnology, we have come to understand the living beings of this world as somehow available for us to think about in their materiality, and we think we can approach this materiality *in principle* to solve particular problems with our bodies. This ordinary way of grasping biotechnology's mundane task is present in the everyday way biotechnology circulates as a way of thinking about living beings. In accepting that biotechnology involves how we come to grasp living beings in the way we do, we avoid assuming that biotechnology is merely a set of practices in which we engage; we must acknowledge that we are implicated in biotechnology in the very way we speak and act today.

Biotechnology and Interpellation

The kind of critical thinking advocated here does not seek to be for or against biotechnology or biopolitics, nor does it attempt to solve the problems with biotechnology's technicity, nor does it present biopolitics as a discourse of solutions, as though the question of the subjectivity of biotechnology were a problem of knowledge. Rather, the kind of critique advanced here attempts to think through what we are doing when we "come into contact" with biotechnology, and of the kind of human being we are taken to be in speaking of it in the way we do. Many prominent contemporary accounts of biotechnology invite us to see biotechnology as involving various issues on which we can take a stand, and according to these accounts the kind of critique of biotechnology advanced here might be thought irresponsible for not addressing biotechnology's apparent challenge. What does it mean to "challenge" biotechnology? "Where" is biotechnology that we might challenge it? Why does biotechnology present a challenge that makes many (of us) think (to ourselves) "something must be done"? Do we stand in a relation to these kinds of practices or activities such that we could pronounce upon them? The point of asking these questions is not to answer them, but to point us toward the question of how we come to be situated to ask the kinds of questions about biotechnology that we do, i.e., "what should we do about biotechnology?" To ask the question of our situatedness is to intervene in biotechnology while sidestepping any normative claim about it. To see that we are somehow *involved* with biotechnology as the political venture that it is, i.e., that facts appear by virtue of our understanding of our own finitude, is not to say that we cannot achieve some kind of orientation (perhaps even *an*—as opposed to *the*—appropriate orientation) for thinking about it. Acknowledging our involvement in biotechnology implies that we recognize that the drive to stand outside, over, and against biotechnology is conditioned by biotechnology itself, and hence is fraught with the perils of attempting to be "objective" about it.

2 Though hardly seeming to be a "method," I take this way of phrasing my approach from Hannah Arendt (see Arendt 1958, 6).

In order to understand the way that biopolitics underlies the at once obvious and desirable features of modern society while also presenting an abhorrent authoritarianism, we need to see how any one of us comes to be positioned as subjects of biopolitics *by way of* the discourses of biotechnology. The conditions of this positioning are betrayed in the "moment" in which we come to identify ourselves as biopolitical subjects, a "moment" that is not an actual moment but an accretion of many. This "moment" is helpfully elucidated by Louis Althusser's notion of *interpellation* or "hailing" (1971, 159–65), which I will situate in the context of biopolitics as part of the problematic of how we come to be framed by biotechnology's frames of reference.

In what way are we involved with biotechnology in our everyday existence? At its most basic, it can be said that during daily life one finds it difficult to think of his or her body as not composed of matter, as not responsive to pills or poisons, as not "producing oneself" in the very act of responding to the various calls for attention to our present biological situation. The singling-out and identification of the subject as a biological entity vulnerable to the commands of its genes, for instance, is carried out by biotechnology, and it takes place upon the invitation to see our bodies "scientifically," in some sense. Althusser referred to this manner of "being identified" by something external as "interpellation." The initial articulation of the subject as "hailed" created a stir in Marxist circles because of the way Althusser used this notion in the attempt to solve the problem of the false consciousness of the worker: how does the worker come to identify *with* capitalist ideology? He understood "interpellation" as the way the capitalist system "hailed" the worker to understand herself in the very terms of capitalist ideology itself. "Ideological state apparatuses," such as educational and healthcare institutions, function to identify the individual as a particular kind of productive subject, and encourage her to (self-)identify as such. But rather than provide a psychological account of the formation of "beliefs," Althusser was concerned to show that ideology itself was at work in a particular "moment" in which the worker self-identifies as a worker.

The example Althusser used to explain how interpellation works to produce the self-identification of subjects through ideology was of a police officer calling out: "hey, you there!" (1971, 162–3). In the moment of being hailed by the police officer one is also identified as someone in relation to the police officer, i.e., as a suspect, such that all the background understandings that make sense of the statement also serve to identify oneself in relation to the police officer and police authority—a relation to sovereign power. This relation is instantiated at the moment the hail is issued. We can also say that the police officer's "hey you!" is a performative utterance, but one that does more than "doing by saying"; the police officer's "hey you!" constructs an identity in the very moment it is deployed—there is, in effect, no identity prior to it.[3] Analogously, biotechnology is an instance of biopolitics, and as such "interpellates" or hails the liberal subject as

3 This is perhaps akin to the way something is "done" or "performed" in the saying rather than represented or expressed (see, for instance, Austin 1975, 8–11).

a biological entity—threatened as that subject is by the vicissitudes of biological existence. The biopolitical subject is not hailed by biotechnology *on the whole* but by a particular instance or innovation that speaks to an aspect of one's finite existence. Biotechnology is not "total" in the sense that Althusserian ideology is, but it is akin to ideology insofar as it is not possible to stand outside its frame as it calls the biopolitical subject forth.

Biotechnology hails us in terms of biopolitics. It promises to remedy deficiencies long thought endemic to the human condition, and now reveals them as politically manageable. We are hailed as biologically constituted entities, hailed through urgent promises and invitations to see ourselves as constructed of elemental matter configured to "produce" who we are and who we take ourselves to be. "Who we take ourselves to be" occurs to us when asked if we will participate in moments of biotechnological rallying like the "Run for the Cure" for breast cancer research. In these moments we are not asked if we would like to give time, money, or research opportunities to very large pharmaceutical companies to pursue clinical trials of any number of drugs or forms of therapy—gene therapy among them. We are asked instead if we would like to help support the cure for cancer, or rather, if we would like to *help fight the battle* against cancer. *And of course we do—how could we not?* In that moment we take ourselves to be concerned with the suffering that accompanies cancer, and we accept the invitation to solidarity and the concomitant challenge to somehow mediate that kind of suffering. To respond to this way of being "interpellated" or "hailed" by biotechnology does not require my participation in the actual "Run for the Cure," it simply requires that I am set upon or "recruited" as one who can get cancer or know someone who can or did. Althusser describes the interpellation of the subject by ideology in that it "'acts' or 'functions' in such a way that it 'recruits' subjects among the individuals (it recruits them all), or 'transforms' the individuals into subjects (it transforms them all)" (1971, 162–3). Biotechnology hails us in the moment that it draws attention both to and away from our finitude. Once I have become a biopolitical citizen in such a moment, from then on any discussion that tries to bring the cure into question will not just seem foolhardy to me, it will seem almost incomprehensible. The promises of biotechnology work to produce a particular sense of how one stands with respect to one's own finitude. When interpellated this way, we "recognize" ourselves as having genes, as being subject to molecular forces at work in our bodies and brains, and as vulnerable in a way we do not wish to be. Because biotechnological innovations are presented to solve real problems, we take seriously the plans and systems for managing and distributing these innovations despite the way it turns our existence into an object of knowledge.

No "Outside": A (Re)Vision of Althusser

The "subject" of biotechnology is the one who is subjected to its call, and the one who is made to think of him- or herself (as him- or herself) in terms of biotechnology's "facts." There is no particular subject or self "there" other than the kind of being that is called forth to stand there by the hailing of biotechnological discourses. Now, it is clear that there are many ways in which beings and individuals are called forth and reckoned with, placed and named and identified. In order for a being to be made sense of, it hearkens to a world. The "world" that presents itself by way of the named being is made present through language; language, however, does not exist in a straightforward or obvious or thing-like way. As Wittgenstein (1958) and Heidegger (1971) both say, language's heterodoxy is irreducible to any particular sense (and hence has no intrinsic "meaning" or "value"). But we can see and say that what comes to us by way of words allows us to see ourselves in light of the way what is said claims us. To be told that a cure for cancer of a certain kind exists not only allows me but compels me to think of myself in terms of the kind of being it makes sense to imagine as one who is at the whim of cancer. If it is prostate cancer, I am well on my way to grasping how I have already been recruited as the kind of biological subject I would have to be in order to become a subject of that kind of cancer, and for that kind of possible cure.

The way such words come is not in a haphazard way, but nor is it necessarily in the totalizing onslaught of ideology. That is, the way I am claimed by a world is not in the singular way that Althusser suggests, but in variegated ways that are themselves contingent. My so-called subject position is necessarily untenable as any kind of necessary or *a priori* subject; so too, then, is it untenable to think of a subject that somehow exists apart from these, or even of the kernel "on" which any kind of subject must attach;[4] so too, then, is it untenable to hold fast to the "individual" as ontologically preceding the subject. We can dispense with it as a ghost of false necessity. While Althusser noted that *all* individuals are recruited as subjects, and that we are always already subjects, he held to the notion of the individual as an epistemological necessity for explaining both ideology's presence and its force. But without the individual, and *a fortiori* without the "subject," we are led to see not simply the way a biotechnological "subject" is recruited, but rather the way we can see ourselves as already within the fold of a biopolitical discourse. It is not to say that all "subjects" are captured by discourses, nor that all discourses are biopolitical. Rather, it is to invite reflection on what it means to think of ourselves as subject to the kind of power that reigns when sovereign power has been displaced—namely, biopower (see Foucault 1978). Biopolitics is the kind of politics that encourages us to think of ourselves as *subject to biological necessity*, and hence beholden to the power of a cure. The sovereign's pardon has become biotechnology's curative.

---

4 As seems to be the case with two particular critiques of Althusser: is there a "kernel" of consciousness to which the subject position must attach? (See Butler 1997, 106–31; Dolar 1993.)

From Ideology to Discourse: Biotechnology and Biopolitics

Biotechnology belongs to the urgent management characteristic of modern societies, witnessed in everything from pension plans to healthcare schemes to traffic to labour relations. It integrates scientific knowledge into the productive force of the economy by promising to revolutionize medicine, agriculture, material production, as well as environmental remediation; it mobilizes resources for need. But the rise to prominence of biotechnology happens against the backdrop of a way of understanding what it is to be a human being in the world, a way often called "biopolitics." Biopolitics characterizes the rise of a specific form of political subjectivity in modernity, one defined by this seemingly urgent need to manage the conditions that set upon human beings in their very livelihood.

Initially coined by Michel Foucault, "biopolitics" designates the way modern politics takes its rationale from an ability to organize and control the "conditions of life." "By ['biopolitics'] I meant the endeavor, begun in the eighteenth century, to rationalize the problems presented to governmental practice by the phenomena characteristic of a group of living human beings constituted as a population: health, sanitation, birthrate, longevity, race" (Foucault 2003, 202). These criteria for tracking and measuring allow the state to assert the contours of the body politic, specifying that the human being exists as a member of an organized and regularized population, and hence as an object of disciplinary study (also see: Foucault 1978, 139). The human's objective status is identified in relation to other members of a population according to certain non-arbitrary features. This is normalization. It should be noted that even among those who think critically about what has come to be called biopolitics, the term suffers from a kind of rich ambiguity, an ambiguity that is fruitful so long as it is maintained (Brown 2001, 100–104). While there is something obvious about the existence of the human as a member of a populace, it is not obvious that this way of characterizing existence is a hypothetical postulate used to foster a loose, anonymous grasp of the people of an area for managing the consequences that befall them. While early activities of organizing and inspecting behaviour aimed at the disciplining of a subject with productive habits, the widespread organization and inspection of a population's conditions of livelihood itself was termed "biopower" by Foucault—and it is this biopower, this bringing of life into the explicit calculations and techniques of statecraft as its *raison d'être* (Foucault 1978, 143), that differentiates the austere conditions of the disciplinary mechanisms of bureaucracy and the threshold of modern life manifest by way of biotechnology.

The provocation embedded here is that biotechnology only makes sense because it occurs in a time and place of *biopolitics*, and not just of a bioethics *applied to* things like biotechnology. This provocation also implies a differentiation, but of a different sort than the first one. "Biopolitics" refers to modern state institutions that have an obvious necessity to them, obvious in the sense of managing an aspect of our lives in need of being managed by statecraft of one kind or another. And yet biopolitics also seems to threaten us precisely because it manages, organizes, and orders us into populations that provide data for our further management, organization, and ordering. The institutions of state that typify biopolitics are at once obvious in their necessity, and yet abhorrent in the way they discipline the subject.

Biotechnology exhibits biopolitics (without being an example of it) by virtue of the way it manifests these two distinct aspects: its innovations seem somehow obvious and necessary, and yet are carried out in ways that, when characterized in terms of biopolitics, set upon individuals and their "parts" as objects of biological study and mobilization inimical to freedom. Notwithstanding that biotechnology must proceed on the basis of biological explanations thought ultimately to condition human existence by underlying it, the grounding of human existence implicit in such explanations is undercut by the humane needs biotechnology openly seeks to address.

It is unmistakable that modern society *requires* intense management. We "need" institutional arrangements such as emergency response teams tied through telephone systems (i.e., dialling 911). Are we not "thinking" when we adopt such systems? Am I blinded by the biopolitical here, because it seems so very reasonable and obvious to me? But it is equally unmistakable that bureaucratic management reaches a threshold when it sets upon "the biological conditions of a population"—and such a threshold is a condition of rationalized, bureaucratic management. At once completely obvious, institutional arrangements nevertheless threaten us in their very institutional form. Biopolitics is in this sense an amplification of bureaucratic management, moving from conditions of sovereignty to conditions of "life and livelihood." Biopolitics mobilizes each of us as members of various populations (for we can at once be members of very different kinds of populations), and it mobilizes us by flocking our "biological markers" through statistical analyses thought to safeguard collective livelihood. It is indeed through the intense "depersonalization" of statistical analysis that biopolitics projects a possibly horrible face on the body of bureaucracy. However, while Weber's characterization of bureaucracy's "iron cage of reason" seems to present an inevitable historical logic of sovereignty, the unfolding of biopolitics is less clear. Part of the difficulty of reducing the ambiguity of biopolitics stems from the seeming obviousness and naturalness of a state pursuing conditions that guarantee the living standards of its population, whether or not these are territorially or otherwise defined. "Politics" today is about the authorized exercise of power over a population for the welfare and benefit of that population, and even the "right" to take life is justified insofar as it safeguards the life of others. As Foucault notes, "the power to expose the whole population to death is the underside of the power to guarantee an individual's continued existence" (Foucault 1978, 137). By dealing with the characteristics of a population, the state is enabled to organize and manage the well-being of the population through the very biological characteristics the state has identified.[5] The

5 This powerful observation was first made by Hannah Arendt regarding the way the "masses" were "shaped" by totalitarian propaganda in *The Origins of Totalitarianism* (1951, 362–4). Arendt added to this insight later, remarking that the rise of "mass society"

logic of bureaucratic management moves according to the dictates of the biological health of the population because the "facts" of biological existence appear by way of the very apparatuses that sanction their use. And it is in this exact way that biotechnology occurs as an example of the biopolitical: it exists not just in the drive, promise, and warranty to repair or improve the conditions attendant to the so-called biological status of being a human being, but in the very conditions that allow the facts of manipulable biological existence to come into view in a way that makes them seem *a priori*.

That biotechnology does not proceed from an official enactment or as a specific project of the state does not mean it is not an example of biopolitics. Rather, biopolitics is manifest in the descriptions put forth in biotechnology's circles, and these descriptions cannot themselves be reduced to specific institutions or legislative acts, just as bureaucracy itself cannot be reduced to the specific instance of institutional regulation. While biotechnology designates a set of practices through which biopolitics goes to work on the populace, it too is somehow not quite reducible to these practices. If biotechnology (and practices like it) were reducible to specific institutional mobilizations, then one could say that biopolitics is nothing more than a specific kind of institution defined by its purpose, i.e., one that includes safeguarding living conditions. Because biotechnology is not reducible in this way, however, we can see that its practices are manifest in the way we speak of them; that is, when we speak of biotechnology, we name its specific instantiations as well as the way it exists beyond these.[6] Instead, biotechnology exists as an example of biopolitics because biotechnology participates in the ambiguous way that we come to think of ourselves as biologically constrained subjects.

The Interpellating Embrace of Biopolitics

Biopolitics presents an embrace, inviting *us* to embrace *it*. There can be little doubt that broad and bountiful data about various factors of the "health" of a given population, given nuance and specificity, will allow a state to rationalize and regulate that "health" extremely effectively—indeed, more effectively than any other presently known scheme. The moment of embrace comes not when we endorse such institutions but prior. It comes when we find ourselves believing in "things" that address our "health," in the straightforward effectiveness of pills, in the existence of effective medical technologies. For it seems that it is true that pills like ibuprofen work as molecules released into my own bodily system, one that reacts to such molecules—how can it be denied? But this hits the (not ironic) crux of why and how biotechnology is "not mysterious," in Max Weber's sense:

becomes possible only when differences are absorbed and individuals are atomized (see Arendt 1958, 38–40).

6 A distinction first drawn by Plato in *The Republic*, Bk VI, 507b (see Plato 1961, 742).

"principally there are no mysterious incalculable forces that come into play, but rather that one can, in principle, master all things by calculation" (Weber 1948, 139). We speak of biopolitics as somehow strange and abhorrent while reaching for the ibuprofen, and it is in this gesture that we reach with a healthy dose of irony—an irony that somehow does not relieve symptoms of tension. We embrace a language of codes as though it were inscribed beneath and beyond words because we have been robbed of any other way of bringing our embodied life to words than by a calculative pursuit of codification. Because biotechnology threatens us in our very words, we desperately try to seek *better words* to describe and abstract from the circumstances that biotechnology presents. We seek such words in ethics committees and policy proposals to keep intact the illusion of control—an illusion that belongs centrally to biotechnology.

Part of the sway of biopolitics is in the illusion of control it provides, an illusion with much force in "bioethics." What is most challenging about the way biotechnology recruits us as biopolitical subjects is the way recruitment is hidden in the very way we come to recognize "truths" and "truthfulness" in biotechnology unmistakably. The challenge that frames this chapter, then, is not simply to imagine the conditions under which such recruitment is possible (which would require a treatise on interpellation and psychology), but on the conditions of the recruitment itself. These "conditions" are the ones we take to be true, and include the various ways that "truths" about biotechnology are put forth. We cannot step "outside" of these conditions to assess them, but can only see the way they are put forth implicitly in the actual claims and practices of biotechnology. *This way of being situated by the terms of biopolitics—by being interpellated by biotechnology—ushers in a way that calls each of us to be concerned about the health and safety of others: it is the vocation of the biopolitical citizen.* I say "each one of us" because there is no way to avoid the sensation that draws us to be concerned to find technical solutions to the systematic absence that haunts our ways of engaging each other. With biopolitics, each one of us unavoidably enters an unchosen arrangement "with the system," as opposed to the one who claims to remain "outside" or "beyond" its corruption. We "turn up" as biopolitical agents because we cannot choose the conditions of biopolitics as the conditions of contemporary subjectivity, even though we may claim to be aware of them.

That is to say, we all occupy this position with respect to biotechnology, whether or not we recognize our "complicity" with it. We are utterly implicated with biotechnology, such that any attempt to challenge it or "think outside" is not possible simply because there is no way to think of human subjectivity apart from the condition of the biopolitics that renders biotechnology legible and cognizable at all. This is the position occupied by the interpellated subject, one who wishes to understand the conditions of her own subjectivity, and yet cannot step outside of them. If biotechnology is somehow implicated in the very way that we characterize and think of living beings, is there any *other* way for us to properly "get biotechnology in hand"? It is because I wonder about the possibility of establishing a moment of clarity about biotechnology that I am suspicious of the drive to "debate" biotechnology or to offer up ways of confronting the "values" that are at stake "in" biotechnology. I wonder, then, how it might be possible for us to gain clarity about what is at stake in biotechnology if it is the case that the "worldview" or, better, frame of reference, is in some sense at the edges of our vision, so to speak.

Concluding Remarks

This chapter purposefully does not enter debates over biotechnology even though it does speak to them; instead, I hope to have unearthed the interpretive background that animates our understanding. To unearth the interpretive background requires throwing light on some of the descriptors that resonate there: to grasp why it is so difficult to understand how we are drawn into biotechnology's particular ways of casting the "truths" of biological existence. *The hailing of a cure does not recruit us; the hailing of a cure shows us that we are always already recruited as the kind of "subject" that is in need of something like a cure.* The foregoing has taken some steps towards the characterization of the moment of interpellation, of *seeing as*,[7] where and when we come to see ourselves through the interpretive lens of biotechnology.

We are not out to get "the whole picture" of how biotechnology proceeds, nor are we proceeding simply to turn the cultural assumptions of biotechnology into "objective knowledge" (as this would be carrying on in the same fashion as biotechnology itself—treating biotechnology as a problem of knowledge). This is because attempts to do so lose sight of the specifically historical grounding of the event of biotechnology, since "only that which has no history can be defined" (Nietzsche 1967, II:13). Thus, we need to pay heed to the historical elements that can direct our attention to the events that render the occlusiveness particular to biotechnology. "*Understanding proves to be an event*, and the task of hermeneutics, seen philosophically, consists in asking what kind of understanding, what kind of science it is, that is itself advanced by historical change. We are quite aware that we are asking something unusual of the self-understanding of modern science" (Gadamer 1989, 309). In some ways, Gadamer is advancing a common claim about science, i.e., that it is historically conditioned. But that insight *alone* does not help us to see the way we are at stake in biotechnology, the way we are hailed by it, nor the particularly pressing kind of experience we undergo in being hailed by biotechnology, a hailing that puts ourselves at issue through a confrontation with our own finitude. For even if we can blandly say that our finitude is contained in the experience of our continual and original interpellation as biotechnological subjects, we have not yet seen ourselves at stake because we have only given a

7 This refers to Wittgenstein's description of the problem involved in describing what it means to see something "as" something, such as a rabbit or a duck (see Wittgenstein 1958, 90ff.).

formally abstract account of our subjectivity without seeing our particularities: the offer of a cure is always directed particularly at any one of us. Where Althusser wants to set out the ideological bases of the moment of interpellation, finitude is expressed only in the precise *and differing* ways truths are put forth to capture and situate us through our particularities.

References

Althusser, L. (1971), "Ideology and Ideological State Apparatuses," in *Lenin and Philosophy and Other Essays*, B. Brewster (trans.) (London: New Left Books), 159–65.

Arendt, H. (1951), *The Origins of Totalitarianism* (New York: Harcourt Brace Jovanovich).

Arendt, H. (1958), *The Human Condition* (New York: Anchor).

Austin, J.L. (1975), *How to Do Things with Words*, J.O. Urmson and M. Sbisà (trans.) (Cambridge, MA: Harvard University Press).

Bowring, F. (2002), *From Seeds to Cyborgs: Biotechnology and the Appropriation of Life* (London: Verso).

Brown, W. (2001), *Politics Out of History* (Princeton, NJ: Princeton University Press).

Butler, J. (1997), "'Conscience Doth Make Subjects of Us All': Althusser's Subjection," in *The Psychic Life of Power: Theories in Subjection* (Stanford, CA: Stanford University Press).

Dolar, M. (1993), "Beyond Interpellation," *Qui Parle* 6:2 (summer).

Foucault, M. (1978), *The History of Sexuality, Volume I: An Introduction*, Robert Hurley (trans.) (New York: Vintage).

Foucault, M. (2003), "The Birth of Biopolitics," in *The Essential Foucault*, P. Rabinow and N. Rose (eds) (New York: New Press).

Fukuyama, F. (2002), *Our Posthuman Future: The Consequences of the Biotechnology Revolution* (New York: Farrar, Straus & Giroux).

Gadamer, H.-G. (1989), *Truth and Method*, 2nd edition, J. Weinsheimer and D.G. Marshall (trans.) (New York: Continuum).

Heidegger, M. (1971), *On the Way to Language*, P.D. Hertz (trans.) (New York: Harper and Row).

Leiss, W. (1972), *The Domination of Nature* (New York: G. Brazilier).

Leiss, W. (2005) "Biotechnology, Religion and the Body," Lecture, Pacific Centre for Technology and Culture, Victoria, BC, 25 Jan. 2005, <http://www.pactac.net/pactacweb/web-content/video11.html>.

Nietzsche, F. (1967), *On the Genealogy of Morals*, W. Kaufmann (trans.) (New York: Vintage).

Plato (1961), *The Republic*, in *The Collected Dialogues*, E. Hamilton and H. Cairns (eds) (Princeton, NJ: Princeton University Press).

Rifkin, J. (1998), *Biotech Century: Harnessing the Gene and Remaking the World* (New York: Putnam).
Simon, J. (2002), "Taking Risks: Extreme Sports and the Embrace of Risk in Advanced Liberal Societies," in T. Baker and J. Simon (eds), *Embracing Risk: The Changing Culture of Insurance and Responsibility* (Chicago, IL: University of Chicago Press), 177–208.
Weber, M. (1948), "Science as a Vocation," in *Max Weber: Essays in Sociology*, H.H. Gerth and C.W. Mills (trans. and eds) (London: Routledge and Kegan Paul).
Wittgenstein, L. (1958), *Philosophical Investigations*, G.E.M. Anscombe (trans.) (Oxford: Basil Blackwell).
Žižek, S. (2003), "Bring Me My Philips Mental Jacket," *London Review of Books* 25:10 [website], (updated 22 May 2003) http://www.lrb.co.uk/v25/n10/zize01_.html.

Chapter 6
The Perils of Scientific Obedience: Bioethics under the Spectre of Biofascism

Stuart J. Murray

Introduction

This chapter invokes the research of Stanley Milgram, the Yale University social psychologist made famous by his experiments on obedience to authority in the early 1960s. I argue for the relevance of Milgram's insights in the context of modern Western healthcare, claiming that the rhetoric of healthcare demands a perilous obedience to scientific authority. This argument extends beyond medicine's proverbial paternalism; indeed, the rhetoric of healthcare has become internalized as a worldview, and has come to authorize and regulate a limited set of normative terms—a language—in and through which individuals relate to the social world, to themselves, to their bodies, and even to their own genetic material. In other words, healthcare discourses extend seamlessly beyond the medical sphere to touch every aspect of human life and death, increasingly underpinning modern subjectivity and identity—effectively spelling the end of the rational, autonomous subject in the traditional sense of the term. Taking an ethical and political perspective, this chapter draws on the implications of Milgram's eponymous experiments to support the stark claim that emerging healthcare discourses tend toward totalitarian or fascist modes of (self-)governance. I limit my analysis of healthcare rhetoric to three interrelated instances of "fascist" ideology in play: (1) biomedicalization, (2) the political economy of neoliberalism, and (3) popular biocultural discourses. The constellation of these three "fascisms" I call "biofascism," and I turn to the phenomenon of genetic screening or "pre-diagnosis" as an illustrative example that cuts across all three. Given that we are subject to biotechnologies and healthcare discourses that clearly exceed our understanding and control, the challenge will be to imagine an ethic that is not fettered to an obsolete principle of autonomy. I conclude with a discussion on "genetic subjectivity" to suggest how we might begin to imagine subjects who are not "autonomous," but who are nevertheless responsible to understand—and to resist—the perilous political and moral authority of healthcare rhetoric and practice.

It is no coincidence that Milgram's well-known experiments at Yale University began just a few short months after the beginning of the Adolf Eichmann trial in Jerusalem. A high-ranking Nazi officer charged with war crimes and crimes against humanity, Eichmann claimed that he was innocent because he was merely "following orders," obeying the authority of the *Führerprinzip*. In a nutshell, then, the Milgram experiments engaged the terms of Eichmann's defence, and set out to test the extent to which ordinary citizens could be prompted by an authority figure to act against their own political and moral conscience. I begin here because the Eichmann case dramatizes for us, as it did for Milgram, the conflict between individual autonomy and collective responsibility. On the one hand, we demand that Eichmann be held responsible for his crimes; on the other, however, we acknowledge that he formed part of a fascist, ideological "machine," and therefore cannot be considered to be "autonomous," *sensu stricto*. There is no contradiction here. Indeed, I shall conclude below that ethical responsibility ought to be re-conceived in broader terms, and need not presume—or shore up the fiction of—the autonomous subject. If traditional bioethics continues to insist on founding itself in autonomy, it will grow increasingly irrelevant in the face of burgeoning biotechnologies that evacuate that autonomy, as I argue below.

It is worthwhile recalling the main experiment. Research subjects were recruited from the general public and told they would be participating in an experiment that tested the effects of punishment on learning. Two subjects drew lots to determine who would be the "teacher" and who would be the "learner"; in reality, the roles were fixed. The learner was played by an actor whose lines were scripted, while all subjects were cast in the teacher role. The learner/actor was strapped into what resembles an electric chair, and electrodes were attached to his body. The teacher/subject was then led into an adjoining room and seated in front of an elaborate machine with switches ranging from "Slight Shock" and "Moderate Shock" through to "Extreme Intensity Shock" and "Danger: Severe Shock." Two switches beyond these bore the obscene label, "XXX." The "shock generator" was clearly marked with a voltage output from 15 to 450 volts. The teacher/subject was asked to read simple word pairs to the learner through a microphone and then test the learner's ability to remember and repeat the words correctly. For an incorrect answer, the teacher/subject was instructed by the experimenter to "shock" the learner, beginning at 15 volts and increasing each shock by 15 volts for each incorrect response. Despite scripted screams of pain from the learner, the outcome of the experiment was that most subjects were fully compliant, administering the maximum, lethal shock of 450 volts. Only a few participants refused to comply—but these did not refuse until reaching or surpassing the 300 volt level.

Much like Hannah Arendt (1963) had depicted Eichmann, Milgram held that his research participants were "ordinary" or even "good" people, neither monstrous nor innately sadistic:

> After witnessing hundreds of ordinary persons submit to the authority in our experiments, I must conclude that Arendt's conception of the banality of evil comes closer to the truth than one might dare imagine. The ordinary person who shocked the victim did so out of a sense of obligation and impression of his [or her] duties as a subject—and not from any peculiarly aggressive tendencies. (Milgram 1973, 75)

There is an ordinariness, then, to our obligation to authority, just as there are ordinary social pleasures that attend our sense of duty, of discipline, and loyalty to what we might call a dominant symbolic order, to fulfil socially mandated roles. "Morality does not disappear," Milgram suggests, "it acquires a radically different focus: the subordinate person feels shame or pride depending on how adequately he [or she] has performed the actions called for by authority" (1973, 77). In this view, morality becomes reconfigured as social compliance. If Milgram's work has had a tremendous afterlife and is invoked to help make sense of such phenomena as US torture at Abu Ghraib and Guantánamo (see, for instance: Fiske et al. 2004; Packer 2008), it is because the individual's place in contemporary society is increasingly mediated by command hierarchies, a sociopolitical machinery of obedience. And while they might appear to be "banal," as Arendt would say, our increasingly militarized and corporatized structures of governance divide human labour and diffuse individual responsibility. In our submission to authority, we come to displace our personal responsibility onto that authority. Again, if we consider the murders and other US crimes in Iraq, Afghanistan, and so on, we find ourselves directed toward a vague and amorphous hierarchy, to the point where one wonders if anyone at all is responsible. This was Eichmann's defence. There is always potential displacement, (im)plausible deniability, the shadows and shadow-men of extralegal bureaucracy. Milgram concludes: "The person who assumes responsibility has evaporated. Perhaps this is the most common characteristic of socially organized evil in modern society" (1973, 77).

This chapter will reflect on the kinds of sociopolitical structures that prompted Milgram's bleak comment on "socially organized evil." Below, I apply Milgram's insights to the rhetoric of healthcare, asking, what is left of personal responsibility if there is no person, no autonomous subject, in the traditional sense of the term? Milgram writes: "The most far-reaching consequence is that the person feels responsible *to* the authority directing him [or her] but feels no responsibility *for* the content of the actions that the authority prescribes" (1973, 77). But Milgram's explicit distinction between "responsibility to …" and "responsibility for …" must be pushed further still. We are not just responsible for the "content" of our actions, including those prescribed by authorities, symbolic or otherwise: in a civil society we are also responsible for those structures of authority themselves, for the system of rewards, right down to the conditions of possibility by which we experience duty, loyalty, and discipline. In other words, being "responsible for …" surpasses the question of obedience to pose the question of consent, which is often tacit. Discussing the Nazi collaborators, Arendt writes: "the question addressed to those who participated and obeyed orders should never be, 'Why did you obey?' but 'Why did you *support*?'" (2003, 48). To be sure, whether or not to consent, condone, support, or otherwise authorize wider cultural systems of governance and meaning-making is much more complex outside the experimental situation where there are few clear authority figures and where social roles are less well-defined. Milgram's more speculative statements bear this out: "when … they are asked to carry out actions incompatible with fundamental standards of morality, *relatively few people have the resources needed to resist authority*" (1973, 76; emphasis added). What would these resources look like? And what could they mean, particularly when that authority is nearly total, an immersive environment, where authority is disembodied, and social roles poorly defined or differentiated?

The work of social psychologists, such as Milgram, offers a common way to map "evil" and our ethical responses to it. In another case, Philip Zimbardo's 1971 prison experiment at Stanford University draws similar conclusions (see, most recently: Zimbardo 2007). These experiments claim to provide insight into "how good people turn evil." Such work is described as a "situationalist" ethics because it seeks recourse to the situation or social context, rather than to principles, such as autonomy or nonmaleficence. In Zimbardo's experiment, wholesome young university boys became cruel, authoritarian, and sadistic when they were cast in the role of prison guards, meting out such frightening punishment on the boys who were "prisoners" that the experiment had to be cut short. Zimbardo explains that these boys were not predisposed to adopt a "guard mentality," but that their behaviour can be explained by the social roles and expectations that encourage, condone, or authorize it. In short, the social situation turns them bad, a "Lucifer effect." Unsurprisingly, Zimbardo appears frequently in the media as an expert on "prison abuse," brought in to explain the situational "causes" of the abuse, arguably undermining the moral gravity of these crimes, exonerating the criminals. Rejecting Zimbardo's conclusion, however, need not return us to an ethics based on personal responsibility and autonomy, as I discuss below.

Three Fascisms: Socially Organized Evil in the Rhetoric of Healthcare

Here I would like to consider "socially organized evil" within the specific context of the healthcare industry. While we may not be persuaded by their conclusions, Milgram and Zimbardo lay out the problem rather well: Is ethics a matter of personal responsibility and autonomy—a "responsibility to …"? Or must we take account of something inherently more social and political, a question of collective responsibility—a "responsibility for …"? This conflict arrives at a crisis in all manner of "total institutions" (Goffman 1961)—whether this is in the laboratory, the prison, the medical clinic, or society at large where these institutions authorize and regulate a limited set of normative terms in and through which individuals are (self-)governed. Below I discuss the case of genetic screening or "pre-diagnosis." Before doing so, however, I would like to build on earlier work (Holmes et al. 2006) in the politics of healthcare to sketch three closely related political ideologies—or "microfascisms"—at play in the way that healthcare, increasingly, is deployed rhetorically.

Biomedicalization

The first microfacism is in the seemingly inexorable "biomedicalization" of healthcare management and delivery. As my colleagues and I have argued (Murray et al. 2007), the healthcare industry is a mind-boggling nexus, a tangled web that includes Big Pharma, innumerable government lobbies, government agencies and public policymakers, academia and its research sponsors, the convergence of research and business with its multiple public and private "stakeholders," and the insurance industry, to name just a few. For the person who is (potentially) ill, this complex system can be barely navigable, and it is not farfetched to imagine the apparently autonomous individual disappearing into this apparatus, subject to the "disciplining" (Foucault 1977) frenzy of best-practice guidelines, evidence-based medicine (EBM), bureaucratic proceduralism, and the like. What I point to here is not simply the expansion of medical authority and practices into new realms; rather, it is the emergent paradigm by which we are coming to understand the relation between medicine, health, and life itself. I follow Adele Clarke and her colleagues who characterize biomedicalization as a number of interrelated phenomena, including the new political economic valences of biomedicine, the rise of risk factors and risk surveillance, and the emergence of biomedical or technoscientific identities, to name just a few (Clarke et al. 2003).

While it is undoubtedly a polemical position, it is nevertheless worthwhile to consider obedience to this new scientific authority in Milgram's terms and to trace how it operates as a pervasive ideology, politically, as a form of fascism. Milgram himself refers to the political writings of Arendt and considers at length the social and political implications of his findings (see Milgram 1974)—whether there could be ethics after Auschwitz, we might say. Dave Holmes and his colleagues have more recently turned to the work of Michel Foucault and Gilles Deleuze to demonstrate the *microfascism* of current medical practices, examining in particular the narrow ideologies and methodologies that govern evidence-based medicine (EBM). Following Foucault and Deleuze, they:

> understand such fascist logic as a desire to order, hierarchise, control, repress, direct and impose limits. *Fascism* is one of the many faces of totalitarianism—the total subjection of humanity to the political imperatives of systems whose concerns are their own production. (Holmes et al. 2006, 184)

EBM, as one instance of biomedicalization, is a totalizing logic because it privileges the randomized controlled trial (RCT) above all else, foreclosing upon other possible ways of knowing. Holmes and his colleagues argue that evidence-based practitioners, much like Milgram's subjects, reap institutional rewards and the pleasure of "a job well done," dutifully capitulating to a scientific authority that is authoritative merely because it has the institutional imprimatur of Science. Patients, too, are interpellated into this regime through the promise of "better outcomes"; they are not told that their own narratives are ranked as "low evidence" according to the Cochrane Hierarchy. "Evidence" is arranged hierarchically: RCTs are on top, while clinician experience is typically located somewhere near the bottom, and patient narratives rarely appear at all. The hierarchy works authoritatively to pre-judge the relative value of "evidence," determining in advance what—and who—will be authoritative.

The Political Economy of Neoliberalism

What is more, the totalizing impulse of biomedicalization maps neatly onto the political economy of neoliberalism, arguably the reigning ideology of contemporary Western democracies. Here healthcare is aligned with what I am calling a second "fascism," where neoliberal political economic discourses supplement and feed on biomedicalization. Each demands greater efficiency and greater economy in the face of dwindling financial resources and soaring healthcare costs. Biomedicalization, from EBM to self-surveillance and risk-management, is enabled by the neoliberal ideology that expresses an almost evangelical faith in free market capitalism (see, for instance: Barry et al. 1996; Bunton and Petersen 1997; Rose 1996b; Rouvroy 2008). And *vice versa*. From academe and its research granting bodies to hospital ethics review boards and the medical insurance industry, the dominant discourse is borrowed from the corporate sphere: client-based (also known as a patient-centred mantra), key performance indicators (KPIs), outcomes, best-practice guidelines (BPGs), knowledge mobilization and transfer (also known as scientific transfer), capacity building, operationalization, commercialization, and so on. "Client" patients are encouraged to conceive of themselves in "entrepreneurial" terms, which means relating to their own bodies and to their genetic material instrumentally and economically, as "biocapital" (see, for instance: Sunder Rajan 2006). The phenomenon of private "biobanking"—storing one's umbilical cord blood, eggs, semen, or other stem cells for later use, should the need arise—is one instance where the economic relation to oneself is literalized through one's own body (see, for instance: Waldby 2006).

In Michel Foucault's terms, the neoliberal subject is "an entrepreneur and an entrepreneur of him- or herself" (Foucault 2004, 232; translation mine). In this form of its self-relation, the subject is not just a consumer but is doubled: "The consumer, in so far as he or she consumes, is a producer" (ibid.). It is a closed economy where the subject herself is imagined to produce the satisfactory health and wellbeing that she will enjoy and "consume"; she repays her own debt. It is a model of self-sufficiency, a circuit that is closed by responsibilization and the politics of risk—"technologies of the self." Under neoliberalism, the subject's own self-improvement is internalized as a moral duty. Many healthcare models are based on the self-care ideology (see, for instance, Orem's nursing conceptual model). In the case of illness, she is expected herself to compensate for the deficits imposed by her disease, and this relation is marked as both a responsibility to one's own body and to the population as a whole. Within a market economy, the person who is ill accrues a kind of social debt which must be redeemed by locating herself within compensatory discourses that are both social and corporeal—that is, they must be performed publicly and they must be done to the body, whether something is cut from or added to that body. If this sounds like "autonomy," it is an extreme and reductive form in which the terms of self-relation must obey a narrow econometrics.

Popular Biocultural Discourses

Biomedical and bioeconomic discourses work in tandem to inform wider cultural perceptions of health and the individual's relation to his or her body and to the healthcare system and industry in general. Here I identify a third "fascism" that is sociocultural. It has less to do with biomedical facts or with bioeconomic imperatives and their measures, but with shifting perceptions—with the dominant popular terms that circulate and with the ways that these terms shape our self-understanding in the quotidian. This is best illustrated through an example. Consider the ways that the gene has entered popular discourse and has come to inform how we understand human life and the body, the individual's relation to history, and to health and illness more generally. In his speech on the occasion of the mapping of the Human Genome, former US President Bill Clinton typifies the kind of thinking that has entered the mainstream:

> With this profound new knowledge, humankind is on the verge of gaining immense, new power to heal. Genome science will have a real impact on all our lives—and even more, on the lives of our children. It will revolutionize the diagnosis, prevention and treatment of most, if not all, human diseases. In coming years, doctors increasingly will be able to cure diseases like Alzheimer's, Parkinson's, diabetes and cancer by attacking their genetic roots. (Clinton 2000)

The metaphor of the "map" complements popular conceptions of genetic "blueprints" and the gene as the "book of life" (Fox Keller 2002). What emerges is a social and cultural science fiction of the gene, a popular discourse that increasingly informs our understanding of kinship relations, health, and medicine in the post-genomic age. This authority and "knowledge" is internalized. And, true to the logic of the gene, the "internalization" is both figurative and quite literal. While the gene has become a dominant rhetorical figure for individuality and identity, the "matter" of genes is of paramount importance because they are considered to be the most elementary particles of the body, the very authors of who we are, from eye colour to personality.

The "genetic" discourse is compelling. In a world of disenchantment, where transcendent truths are increasingly unfashionable, genomics fulfils a deep cultural desire for Truth. As Nelkin and Lindee argue, in popular culture DNA is not just a dominant trope for individual identity, in many respects DNA also functions as a secular equivalent of the Christian soul. Seemingly independent of the body, DNA appears to be immortal; it extends indefinitely into the past and, if one has children, it stretches indefinitely into the future. DNA has become fundamental to identity, charged with the tremendous power to explain individual differences, moral order, and human fate. Incapable of deceiving, genes seem to be the locus of the "true self" (Nelkin and Lindee 1995, 2; also see Nelkin 2001). The gene thus operates as a cultural science fiction, offering what is at times a deeply moralistic vocabulary that masquerades as Science and Truth. But the meaning of DNA is culturally mediated, conveyed through particular social and historical contexts that are nevertheless contingent. When genes are raised to the level of Truth, the inherent danger is that cultural values become "naturalized," no longer subject to discussion and interpretation. Bill Clinton continues:

> Today's announcement represents more than just an epic-making triumph of science and reason. After all, when Galileo discovered he could use the tools of mathematics and mechanics to understand the motion of celestial bodies, he felt, in the words of one eminent researcher, "that he had learned the language in which God created the universe." Today, we are learning the language in which God created life. We are gaining ever more awe for the complexity, the beauty, the wonder of God's most divine and sacred gift. (Clinton 2000)

This rhetorical excess is politically dangerous; it casts the scientist as God, and marks scientific knowledge with divine—and hence, indisputable—authority.

The Birth of "Biofascism"

I use the term "biofascism" to point to the constellation of the biomedicalized, bioeconomic, and biocultural microfascisms that I have sketched above. In other words, biofascism invites, if it does not demand, a totalitarian obedience to scientific authority, to the ideological political economic coordinates of neoliberalism, and to the cultural science fiction of genetic "truth." These spheres overlap; they are mutually implicated in complex ways. Together, they form a totalizing ideology that governs life itself—whether "life" is located in the most microscopic biological terms, or whether it is deployed in the widest possible sense, as something sacred and inviolable. No matter; the governing structures are nimble enough to be applied across a range of social spheres in the project of biopolitical governance (Foucault 2004).

I would like to explain my use of the term "fascism" and to argue for the value of provoking an ethical and political reflection on the emerging crisis in healthcare rhetoric and practice. What kind of totalitarianism is biofascism? Slavoj Žižek argues that historically there are two totalitarianisms, the first, which is aligned with Hitler and National Socialism, and the second, which is properly Stalinist. As Žižek writes, "In the Stalinist ideological imaginary, universal reason is objectivised in the guise of the inexorable laws of historical progress, and we are all its servants, the leader included" (2005). Stalinism conceived of itself as following Enlightenment principles, hence the famous show trials where individuals "confessed" and, as so-called rational subjects, were held responsible for their "crimes." As Žižek points out, for the Nazis there was no such pretence: a Jew was guilty by virtue of his genetic makeup alone. But what if we imagine a kind of synthesis of the Nazi and Stalinist ideologies: where, for example, the Jew is *de facto* guilty, thanks to his genes, but is now made to confess publicly, to be responsible for, and to wholeheartedly believe and to adopt the ostensibly rational and enlightened perspective according to which he will demand his own execution in the name of hygiene, History, Science, Progress, and Nature? It is not difficult to imagine a totalitarianism, an ideology of "life," obedient in the first instance to scientific authority. While Arendt famously writes that totalitarianism "is quite prepared to sacrifice everybody's vital immediate interests to the execution of what it assume[s] to be the law of History or the law of Nature" (2004, 461–2), here the term "sacrifice" becomes nonsensical because the programme is implemented in the very name of "vital immediate interests," in the name of life. We might call this a vital self-subjectivation, where the individual concedes to the Truth of his being, and the ideology is internalized so completely that he demands this knowledge, makes it public, and even yearns for it. Ironically, it appears that such a system preserves the liberal, rational subject—and perhaps even vouchsafes a perverse "ethics" based on the enlightened principles of "freedom" and "autonomy." And yet, it fosters such a subjectivity only to have it delight in its own self-annihilation.

There is a distinct parallel here with the way that traditional bioethics fetishizes the liberal, autonomous subject, preserving it at the cost of that subject itself. Even mainstream bioethics tends to embrace biomedicalizing, bioeconomic, and biocultural discourses because they *appear* to shore up patient autonomy, giving individual patient-clients the tools for self-knowledge, self-surveillance, and self-regulation, so that they can become entrepreneurial managers of their own healthcare regimens. In reality, however, the subject is increasingly tied to expert advice and a cadre of medical authorities, increasingly inculcated into a regime that ultimately hijacks the liberal, autonomous subject in the guise of freeing it (Novas and Rose 2000; Rose 1996a; Rose 2001). And as the two examples below suggest, genomic medicine itself renders the notion of a unified, rational, and autonomous subject practically obsolete.

Two Examples: Genetic "Pre-Diagnosis"

The scientific authoritative constellation I call "biofascism" can be demonstrated through the phenomenon of genetic screening, or what I call genetic "pre-diagnosis." The first case is a relatively rare condition in which an individual is genetically pre-disposed to develop stomach cancer. Hereditary Diffuse Gastric Cancer (HDGC) is associated with the *CDH1* gene and a particular encoding of the protein E-cadherin (Gayther et al. 1998). The genetic predisposition can now be detected by a blood test. Women with this genetic condition have a 70 per cent chance of developing stomach cancer; for men, the numbers are somewhat lower. With HDGC, women also carry a 50 per cent chance of developing lobular breast cancer. Because the stomach cancer is virtually undetectable with scopes or biopsies, and thus regular screening is not likely to detect it, the recommended treatment is a prophylactic gastrectomy—removing the stomach and attaching the oesophagus directly to the small intestine. The operation has a high potential for morbidity and mortality; risks and long-term complications are legion, including extreme weight loss, infection, anastomotic leaks (where the oesophagus joins the small intestine), blood clots in the lung(s), spleen, or liver, and sometimes death. Roughly half of those who test positive opt to have the surgery—surely an unthinkable and terrifying decision.

The second case is much more well-known. By screening for the BRCA1 and BRCA2 genes, geneticists can predict the likelihood that a woman will develop breast cancer in her lifetime. Based on epidemiological statistics, she is assigned a risk factor. Perhaps she learns that she has a 29 per cent chance of developing breast cancer. She must now decide whether or not to undergo a prophylactic bilateral mastectomy. Whether or not she opts for the surgery, she will be forced to weigh her 29 per cent risk in "real" terms. The number, I would suggest, is a maddeningly unreal artefact; the discourse on risk is alien, it belongs to the insurance industry, to epidemiology, to mathematics. But it is on this terrain that she must find the normative terms by which she will be compelled to relate to herself, to her body, and to her future. The numbers are probabilities, uncertainties. While she may be cancer-free at the moment of the test, with a positive test result she will be inducted into the strange temporality of medical surveillance; she will be expected to take responsibility for a spectral disease that may or may not affect her at some indeterminate point of time. She will be expected to avail herself of expert service-providers while calculating the value of a life she has not yet lived. She will be expected to calculate and weigh the costs and the benefits of various treatment options. She will be summoned to think like a "health economist," rationally plotting her "Quality Adjusted Life Years" (QALY)—the number of years that would be added by the medical intervention, each year ranked from 0 through 1, with 1 representing perfect health and 0 representing death. She will be railroaded into an impossible temporal and epistemological relation with herself: she must account for a future-self and must do so in terms that may have little phenomenological relevance to her bodily and psychic life.

Discussion: An Autoimmunity Response

The cases above draw on and contribute to a "genetic" worldview; however, despite the appeal to scientific authority, this world is not necessarily rendered more navigable. I suspect that for the client-patient this "geneticized" network of healthcare services and their attendant structures can invoke a kind of "autoimmunity" response—a condition where the organism fails, as it were, to recognize its own constituent parts as part of itself, and therefore attacks them in a perverse form of "self-defence." I borrow the metaphor of "autoimmunity" from Jacques Derrida. Giovanna Borradori describes it as follows: "Autoimmune conditions consist in the spontaneous suicide of the very defensive mechanism supposed to protect the organism from external aggression" (in Habermas et al. 2003, 150). Thus, the organism succeeds in destroying its own defence mechanisms, "immunizing" itself, paradoxically, against its own immunity. "One function of the concept of autoimmunity," Borradori continues, "is to act as a third term between the classical opposition of friend and foe" (151). "Friend" and "foe" here must be understood metaphorically, but just barely: with genetic "pre-diagnosis," the classic political binary between friend and foe soon breaks down. If the threat comes from my genes, are my genes then the enemy? Or are they not also "me," my body, my self? In Milgram's terms, are we "responsible to ..." our genes, "responsible for ..." them, or some strange hybrid of the two? And how are we either constituted by or free to relate to the "geneticized" network of healthcare services and their attendant structures? After all, they authorize and regulate a limited set of normative terms in which to locate oneself. Not only have I been subjectivated by these terms, the strange indefinite futurity of the "pre-diagnosis" binds me to a potentially open-ended and fluctuating set of terms and practices as I am inducted into the imaginary futures of medicine. While we are accustomed to speak of the ongoing "war" on diseases such as cancer, with genetic "pre-diagnosis" there is no certain infection, no invasion, no attack on the body. Rather, we imagine the body poised to attack itself or as leaving itself open to attack because of defective defences—both autoimmunity responses.

Borrowing his metaphor from medicine, Derrida discusses autoimmunity in relation to terrorism and the War on Terror, where the enemy is imagined as anyone who could be anywhere, and the Western coalition might properly be said to be waging war against itself, ostensibly, in its own rational self-defence. I see this as akin to the sinister combination of the two totalitarianisms from Žižek, discussed above, where the subject's biological self-subjectivation becomes biopolitical as well, ostensibly obedient to an Enlightenment political rationality. For Derrida, autoimmunity is a deconstructive "third term," meant to upset the problematic binary between friend and foe, us and them. With genetic "pre-diagnosis," however, friend and foe are already unstable categories: self and other are radically uncertain when we seek to locate "genetic selfhood" and "genetic alterity." Moreover, the "we" who "seek" in this formulation is itself without stable ground, ethically and epistemically: is it an inquiry on behalf of "me," "my kin," "DNA," or some "stakeholder" in the biomedical-industrial complex? The information from a genetic "pre-diagnosis" raises the terror of the spectral disease to a new level, inscribing my potential illness in terms that can be spoken and claimed by no one. Not only are the subject and her body seemingly at odds, not only will she be at pains to locate her subjectivity and her body spatiotemporally, not only will she founder when she wonders who speaks in her name when she seeks the meaning of her genes, but all of this occurs as she navigates between the authority of and obedience to biomedicalizing, bioeconomizing, and biocultural discourses. She will now be forced—unable to refuse—to consent to these terms; she will be forced—unable to refuse—to choose whether or not to act with a pre-emptive medical strike. Once she is armed with this genetic information, she is unfree not to choose. Patients frequently describe their DNA as a "ticking bomb," borrowing from a military vocabulary and a logic that authorizes "pre-emptive strikes" and even torture. It is this self-sacrifice that must be made, the paradoxical and impossible demand of autoimmunity, in the name of life itself.

Conclusion: The Address of the Gene

Where are genes located? No place, no physical address, inside and outside. In biomedical terms, they introduce a strange temporality into a subject's self-understanding. While they have no physical address, we are addressed by genes. We are called into being genetically, through biomedicalizing, bioeconomizing, and biocultural addresses. And we are at pains to formulate an appropriate, ethical response that would be commensurable with the new forms of subjectivity that arise in tandem with burgeoning biotechnologies. From the foregoing, it should be clear that the total situation is more complicated than any "genetic essentialism" that might characterize the materialist position. Regardless of the ontological underpinnings of the gene, however, when it faces the complexity of genetic discourses, bioethics will be forced to admit that the modern liberal principles of freedom, autonomy, and reason are rather shaky foundations, indeed. Attempting to reinstall the liberal subject through the structures of biomedicine, a political economy of neoliberalism, or through the naturalizing manipulation of our wider cultural conceptions, ultimately robs the subject of freedom, autonomy, and reason—telling a lie in order to induct the subject into a biopolitics under the spectre of biofascism, where the terms of the subject's self-understanding and the meaning of life itself are too narrowly prescribed.

If the traditional foundations of bioethics have become obsolete, does this mean that we cannot have an ethic? In reply, we might gesture toward a poststructuralist response and ask, as Judith Butler does, "which foundations have come under criticism, and how is it—through what means—did we come to understand foundations to be a kind of *sine qua non* of ethics in the first place?" (Murray and Butler 2007, 419). Butler mobilizes the terms, understands them to be in relation. This is one way to think about the address of the gene, neither as a fixed abode nor as a command that I, the subject, receive in any stable fashion, for I, too, am of no fixed address, and the command calls or entreats me, demanding a response rather than obedience. "This self is distributed in its relational, social, and historical dimensions," Butler says,

> But this fact does not destroy the idea of responsibility; all it does is to relocate responsibility as a problem of my relationality, of the fact that I am constituted fundamentally in a relationship with others, and that that constitution does decenter me; it both decenters me and provides the condition of a certain kind of responsibility. (Murray and Butler 2007, 419–20)

This relocates ethics from its presumptive foundations into a "scene of address" (see Butler 2005). Thus, we might begin to understand ethics as a responsibility for the scene of address itself, for the myriad conditions in and by which an address or claim will be made, in and by which the terms of our relation to ourselves and to others will make sense and will circulate socially, politically, and biomedically.

How shall we account for the "genetic" scene of address, and to what—and whose—terms shall we be obedient? In the early pages of *The Human Condition*, Arendt claims that "speech is what makes man a political being," and she warns against biotechnological modes of relationality: "the 'truths' of the modern scientific world view, though they can be demonstrated in mathematical formulas and proved technologically, will no longer lend themselves to normal expression in speech and thought" (1998, 3). Here Arendt distinguishes technological know-how from thought and speech. She writes further:

> If we would follow the advice, so frequently urged upon us, to adjust our cultural attitudes to the present status of scientific achievement, we would in all earnest adopt a way of life in which speech is no longer meaningful. (1998, 3–4)

In other words, our relations are in danger of becoming meaningless if they are obedient to a technoscientific vocabulary. Within the coordinates of biofascism, these terms have a powerful normative authority, constraining the subject and installing her within a particular discourse that limits her freedom by regulating and prescribing the available terms in which her "free choice" might be exercised. If she refuses these terms she risks appearing unrecognizable, inhuman, since the discourse has already defined the human ontologically, as genetic, and epistemically and ethically as embodying a particular normative relation to one's own genetic material. This sets out in advance what will be permissible and impermissible expressions of the human, recognizable and unrecognizable life. The word "fascism" is therefore warranted, and perhaps not even scandalous enough. It is at this basic level of signification, of meaning-making, that we might begin to intervene.

I began this chapter with Milgram and Zimbardo because they raise the problem of obedience to authority in concrete terms; however, their analyses are limited because they continue to represent the "commonsense" view that responsibility is no more than a rational self-relation, posing questions to oneself in a particular way, and of drawing on one's own personal resources to muster the courage simply to refuse or consent. This view continues to dominate popular impressions of what responsibility is: the domain of the self. But this is to bypass or to downplay the power relations—in part, political and biomedical—through which the subject came into being in the first place. And it is to deny the ethical implications of these relations both as conditions for the emergence of a meaningful subject and, equally importantly, as that for which the subject is also in part responsible by taking account of those conditions that set any scene of address.

Milgram begins his essay, "The Perils of Obedience," with the assumption that "Obedience is as basic an element in the structure of social life as one can point to" (1973, 62). He claims that "Some system of authority is a requirement of all communal living" (ibid.). When asked about this claim, Butler responds as follows:

> It may well be that authority is necessary for social life, its regulation and control. But it may also be that the means for a critical contestation of authority in the name of justice is equally important for social life, or any number of other political matters. (Murray and Butler 2007, 441)

The task might be to resituate obedience and authority within a critique that locates justice as the basic element of communal living. Here we might begin by asking: What is community? What is life? In her discussion, Butler contests Zimbardo's work as an apologist for US murder and torture at Abu Ghraib. Were these men good soldiers and good patriots, as Zimbardo claims? Rather than ask the question of obedience—"Why did you obey?"—she takes an Arendtian tack and points to the conditions under which the prison guards supported, consented, condoned:

> these experimental scenarios … cannot actually look at the generation of political, social, and cultural norms—in particular, those that valorize lawless violence in the name of the nation, in the context of a war effort—and see how they actually enter into the individual actions of prison guards … But what if torture has become the very sign of patriotism within the lexicon and normative culture of this war? (Murray and Butler 2007, 442)

Butler demonstrates that patriotism and goodness—terms that are ostensibly self-evident—are themselves contestable because they are part of a wider normative discourse. So too are the crimes that are committed in their name.

This critique maps onto the broader political, social, and cultural norms of healthcare rhetoric. Just because norms are operating, just because there is a command hierarchy, it does not mean that nobody is responsible. However, nor does it mean we must return to a principle of autonomy in order to ground responsibility. Responsibility opens onto the scene of address, a scene in which we are all players—each of us, whose responsibility extends beyond the limits of our skin, spatially, and out into a world beyond the immediate effects of our individual actions, temporally. This is a different view on subjectivity. Here, responsibility is not simply a "response" to the given scene in which we find ourselves: it is a creative, forward-looking endeavour. We must create possibilities to refuse the terms, to rearrange them, to set them into different scenes, to imagine counter-scenes, and to critically intervene in order to expose vested powers and interests. To say that we are responsible for the scene of address does not imply that we "know" it and hold it before our mind's eye; instead, it might mean that we feel it, that we "try on" another scene, that we are "in" it but not "of" it. Here we can begin to respond to Milgram when he claims that his subjects lacked the "resources" to refuse to obey: "there would have to be other cultural norms and other cultural resources and other legal traditions to which one could turn in order to draw upon the resources that one needs to make the claims of justice," Butler suggests.

> This is because we do not have access to some Platonic idea of justice and we do not have access to a natural right. Instead, we have a set of texts, cultural traditions, various kinds of philosophical and social movements and institutions that have been articulating justice and producing it as a cultural resource precisely for these moments. (Murray and Butler 2007, 443)

It is incumbent upon us, theorists and practitioners alike, to foster these philosophical and social movements and institutions, to safeguard the texts and traditions that will serve as valuable resources when we need them. We must struggle together against the collapse of meaning, to make speech and thought possible, and to claim responsibility for those scenes of address in which life itself might emerge from under the spectre of biofascism. Here we might begin to imagine, together, the renovation of bioethics through relations that neither return us to the unreconstructed authority of personal autonomy, reason, and liberalism, nor force a capitulation to the biomedicalized, bioeconomic, and biocultural discourses that now hold us in their grip.

References

Arendt, H. (1963), *Eichmann in Jerusalem: A Report on the Banality of Evil*, 1st edition (New York: Viking Press).

Arendt, H. (1998), *The Human Condition*, 2nd edition (Chicago, IL: University of Chicago Press).

Arendt, H. (2003), *Responsibility and Judgment* (New York: Schocken Books).

Arendt, H. (2004), *The Origins of Totalitarianism* (New York: Schocken Books).

Barry, A. et al. (eds) (1996), *Foucault and Political Reason: Liberalism, Neo-Liberalism, and Rationalities of Government* (Chicago, IL: University of Chicago Press).

Bunton, R. and Petersen, A.R. (eds) (1997), *Foucault, Health and Medicine* (New York: Routledge).

Butler, J. (2005), *Giving an Account of Oneself* (New York: Fordham University Press).

Clarke, A.E. et al. (2003), "Biomedicalization: Technoscientific Transformations of Health, Illness, and US Biomedicine," *American Sociological Review* 68:2, 161–94.

Clinton, W. (2000), "Remarks by the President, Prime Minister Tony Blair of England (via satellite), Dr. Francis Collins, Director of the National Human Genome Research Institute, and Dr. Craig Venter, President and Chief Scientific Officer, Celera Genomics Corporation, on the Completion of the First Survey of the Entire Human Genome Project," *The White House, Office of the Press Secretary* [website], (updated 26 June 2000) <http://www.clintonpresidentialcenter.org/legacy/062600-speech-by-president-on-completion-of-first-survey-of-entire-human-genome.htm>, accessed 18 May 2008.

Fiske, S.T. et al. (2004), "Why Ordinary People Torture Enemy Prisoners," *Science* 306:5701, 1482–3.

Foucault, M. (1977), *Discipline and Punish: The Birth of the Prison* (New York: Pantheon).

Foucault, M. (2004), *Naissance de la biopolitique: cours au Collège de France, 1978–1979* (Paris: Gallimard/Seuil).

Fox Keller, E. (2002), *Making Sense of Life: Explaining Biological Development with Models, Metaphors, and Machines* (Cambridge, MA: Harvard University Press).

Gayther, S.A. et al. (1998), "Identification of Germ-Line E-Cadherin Mutations in Gastric Cancer Families of European Origin," *Cancer Research* 58:18, 4086–9.

Goffman, E. (1961), *Asylums: Essays on the Social Situation of Mental Patients and Other Inmates* (New York: Anchor).

Habermas, J. et al. (2003), *Philosophy in a Time of Terror: Dialogues with Jürgen Habermas and Jacques Derrida* (Chicago, IL: University of Chicago Press).

Holmes, D. et al. (2006), "Deconstructing the Evidence-Based Discourse in Health Sciences: Truth, Power and *Fascism*," *International Journal of Evidence-Based Healthcare* 4:3, 180–86.

Milgram, S. (1973), "The Perils of Obedience," *Harper's* (December), 62–77.

Milgram, S. (1974), *Obedience to Authority: An Experimental View*, 1st edition (New York: Harper and Row).

Murray, S.J. and Butler, J. (2007), "Ethics at the Scene of Address: A Conversation with Judith Butler," *Symposium: Review of the Canadian Journal for Continental Philosophy* 11:2, 415–45.

Murray, S.J. et al. (2007), "No Exit? Intellectual Integrity Under the Regime of 'Evidence' and 'Best-practices'," *Journal of Evaluation in Clinical Practice* 13:4, 512–16.

Nelkin, D. (2001), "Molecular Metaphors: The Gene in Popular Discourse," *Nature Reviews: Genetics* 2:7, 555–9.

Nelkin, D. and Lindee, M.S. (1995), *The DNA Mystique: The Gene as a Cultural Icon* (New York: Freeman).

Novas, C. and Rose, N. (2000), "Genetic Risk and the Birth of the Somatic Individual," *Economy and Society* 29:4, 485–513.

Packer, D.J. (2008), "Identifying Systematic Disobedience in Milgram's Obedience Experiments: A Meta-Analytic Review," *Perspectives on Psychological Science* 3:4, 301–4.

Rose, N. (1996a), "Governing 'Advanced' Liberal Democracies," in A. Barry et al. (eds), 37–64.

Rose, N. (1996b), *Inventing Our Selves: Psychology, Power, and Personhood* (New York: Cambridge University Press).

Rose, N. (2001), "The Politics of Life Itself," *Theory, Culture & Society* 18:6, 1–30.

Rouvroy, A. (2008), *Human Genes and Neoliberal Governance: A Foucauldian Critique* (Abingdon, UK: Routledge-Cavendish).
Sunder Rajan, K. (2006), *Biocapital: The Constitution of Postgenomic Life* (Durham, NC: Duke University Press).
Waldby, C. (2006), "Umbilical Cord Blood: From Social Gift to Venture Capital," *BioSocieties* 1:1, 55–70.
Zimbardo, P.G. (2007), *The Lucifer Effect: Understanding How Good People Turn Evil* (New York: Random House).
Žižek, S. (2005), "The Two Totalitarianisms," *London Review of Books* [website], (published online 17 March 2005) <http://www.lrb.co.uk/v27/n06/zize01_.html>, accessed 18 May 2008.

Chapter 7
Contesting the Autistic Subject: Biological Citizenship and the Autism/Autistic Movement

Michael Orsini

Introduction

This chapter explores the constitution of subjectivity in the so called "autism wars," which have pitted parents of autistic children seeking access to treatment/therapy against those who are more interested in advancing a notion of autism that frees it from the straitjacket of being viewed as a crippling disability. I argue that the ways in which the autistic subject is framed has important implication for the types of activist strategies advanced by the key actors in the autism and autistic movements. I use the term "autism movement" to distinguish activists or advocates more interested in pressing for policy change around the treatment for autism and concern with its causes, versus the term "autistic movement," which normally refers to the efforts of activists to create a positive identity for autistic people using, albeit not exclusively, a disability rights frame. Of course, the autistic movement is not made up entirely of autistic individuals; non-autistic parents of autistic children who support the goals of this fledgling movement take part, as well. In general, members of the autistic or autistic rights movement decry the focus on and language of "curing" autistics. In an entry on her blog, "The Autism Crisis," Michelle Dawson, a prolific Canadian autistic advocate and researcher, is more direct: autism advocacy "is the widespread effort to make the world as free of autism—of autistic people—as possible" (Dawson 2007). Some of the most influential autism "experts" have spoken of the need to treat children who are undergoing treatment as a blank slate; that one needs to start from scratch in developing the personality of autistic children.[1] Others speculate that the three common symptoms experienced by autistic children—abnormal social development, problems with communication, and the lack of pretend play—may

1 Ivar Lovaas, a leading proponent of this theory, says: "You see, you start pretty much from scratch when you work with an autistic child. You have a person in the physical sense—they have hair, a nose and a mouth—but they are not people in the psychological sense. One way to look at the job of helping autistic kids is to see it as a matter of constructing a person. You have the raw materials, but you have to build the person" (quoted in Dawson 2005).

be related to the autistic person's poor mindreading ability (Baron-Cohen 1997, 63). Lacking a "theory of mind," Baron-Cohen contends, autistic people suffer from "mindblindness," or the inability to read behaviour.

The first section of this chapter situates autism in some politico-legal context, drawing on a 2004 Supreme Court of Canada decision (*Auton v. British Columbia*) as a springboard to discuss the constitution and framing of autistic subjectivity. The second section analyses autistic and autism activism through the prism of "biological citizenship," a notion first developed in Adriana Petryna's *Life Exposed* (2002) and expanded upon by Nikolas Rose and Carlos Novas (2005) and Rose (2006). The idea of biological citizenship is useful, albeit somewhat problematic, when considering the subjectivity of children; indeed, it reveals the Janus-faced character of biological citizenship and autistic subjectivity. The sharing of aspects of one's biological identity can be a potent force for collective mobilization, bringing together groups of otherwise disparate individuals in what Rabinow (1996) has termed "biosocial collectivities." It also has the potential, however, to isolate autistic individuals from non-autistics (or neurotypicals, as some refer to them), and to essentialize the differences between autistic and non-autistic people (see Nadesan 2005).

Autism in Politico-Legal Context

> There are parents that are forced to put kids in schools that are completely overcrowded and 12 kids and 1 teacher. And the—the kids don't make progress. But I remember that was a very scary moment for me when I realized that I had sat in the car for about 15 minutes and actually contemplated putting Jodie in the car and driving off the George Washington Bridge and that that would be preferable to having to put her in one of these schools. And it's only because of Lauren, the fact that I have another child (who is not autistic) that I probably didn't do it. (Alison Tepper Singer, mother of Jodie, an autistic child, speaking in the controversial documentary, *Autism Every Day* [2006], produced by US organization, Autism Speaks)

> When parents say, "I wish my child did not have autism," what they're really saying is, "I wish the autistic child I have did not exist, and I had a different (non-autistic) child instead." This is what we hear when you pray for a cure. This is what we know, when you tell us of your fondest hopes and dreams for us: that your greatest wish is that one day we will cease to be, and strangers you can love will move in behind our faces. (Autistic activist Jim Sinclair, co-ordinator of Autism Network International, a US self-advocacy organization run by autistic people; see Sinclair 1993)

The first quotation, taken from an interview with the mother of an autistic child, sparked an outcry among autistic activists who reject the vision that autism must be cured, and that autistic people need to be fixed, lest they be a financial, emotional, and psychological burden on their families and on society (see Standing Senate Committee on Social Affairs, Science, and Technology 2007). Nothing seems to anger autistic activists more than hearing about the crushing economic burden of autism, as if to say that autistic people are nothing but a drain on their families and on society. The claim, by the father of an autistic son who appeared before the Canadian Senate Committee hearings, that "autism is worse than cancer in many ways, because the person with autism has a normal lifespan," stood out among some autistic activists as particularly egregious (Standing Senate Committee on Social Affairs, Science, and Technology Proceedings 2003, 9:12).

In defending the use of the candid interview material in their documentary, *Autism Every Day*, the filmmakers said they wanted to present an honest portrait of life as the parent of an autistic child, and to show, albeit in dramatic fashion, the toll autism takes on families, especially mothers. Critics of the documentary pointed out, on blogs and in internet chat rooms, that what was even more repulsive than expressing the thought of murdering your own daughter was the fact that the mother in question made this statement within earshot of her non-autistic daughter (see Don't Speak for Me).

It would be an understatement to suggest that there are deep divisions or disagreements in the autism and autistic communities. The advocacy promoted by mainstream organizations such as Autism Speaks (the prominent US organization that produced the above documentary), Families for Early Autism Treatment (FEAT), and Cure Autism Now, is generally centred on the benefits of treatment/therapy for autistic children. There is some disagreement, however, in the autism community with respect to the etiology of autism, with some activists pointing the accusatory finger at childhood vaccines, while others are more interested in advancing genetic research. A recent article in the *New York Times* revealed a particularly bitter rift in the large autism charity, Autism Speaks, which was founded by a former television executive whose grandson was diagnosed with autism. The founder's daughter has criticized her parents for not lending enough support to the claim that autism has environmental causes (Gross and Strom 2007). As proof of these advocacy groups' considerable political clout, the US Senate and Congress passed the Combating Autism Act in late 2006, which committed more than $900 million to autism spending over a five-year period. (Not surprisingly, perhaps, Canadian activists have been pressing government to fund a similar strategy.) In a relatively short period, autism has attracted significant media attention and scores of celebrity supporters, including comedian Bill Cosby and R&B singer Toni Braxton in the US and comedian Eugene Levy in Canada, to become the celebrity *cause du jour*.

Some autistic self-advocates vehemently reject as unproven and, worse, potentially harmful, treatments such as Applied Behavioural Analysis (ABA), which was pioneered by Karl Lovaas in the 1960s and was at the centre of a landmark Supreme Court of Canada ruling in 2004. Intensive, costly, and time consuming, ABA is a form of behaviour modification that claims to help autistic children by teaching them to unlearn "dysfunctional" behaviours and replace them with adaptive ones (Nadesan 2005, 102). Adopting what disability studies scholars term "a social model of disability," autistic advocates argue that the real injustice lies in the way non-autistics treat people with autism. A term often used by some activists to describe autistic people is "neurodiverse": autistic people's brains are simply "hard wired" differently. Just as we embrace other forms of difference based on race, gender, or sexuality, citizens should accept and accommodate the needs of those who are neurologically diverse. "Curing" them would amount to destroying their personalities.

Autistic adults often speak out against the silencing of autistic people in mainstream autistic organizations. Michelle Dawson, for instance, operates a website, provocatively titled "No Autistics Allowed," in which she rails against the exclusion of autistic individuals in the everyday practices of the organizations that purport to speak for autistic people. When autistic people like herself do speak out, they are attacked for not being autistic enough, almost asked to prove that they are authentic representatives for autistic individuals. If they are too articulate, appear to be too "normal," their autistic identity is immediately called into question. Dawson's case is particularly intriguing as she blurs the line separating scientific and lay forms of knowledge. The former postal worker's own experiential knowledge of life as an autistic individual deeply informs her online activities, and she has recently been collaborating on academic research with Laurent Mottron, a noted psychiatry professor and autism expert in Montreal. The two have been dubbed the "odd couple" of autism research (Picard 2006). Their work has been published in a number of leading scientific journals, and has been presented at scientific conferences. The main thrust of their current research is that researchers have underestimated the intelligence of autistic people because they have been using the wrong measurement tools.

In order to support a thriving autistic culture, activists have organized gatherings of autistics such as Autreat, a yearly meeting organized mainly by Jim Sinclair of Autism Network International. Autreat "focuses on positive living with autism, NOT on causes, cures, or ways to make us more normal" (Sinclair 2005).[2] Autistic activists such as Sinclair and Dawson are also quick to point out that the lion's share of advocacy in the name of autism and autistic people today does not necessarily advance their interests or validate their authentic autistic selves. Autism advocacy, they claim, is bent on erasing the autistic subject. The primary spokespeople for autism, they argue, are non-autistic parents of autistic children who believe strongly in the benefits of interventions such as ABA. As noted earlier, autism activists who support ABA treatment are generally parents of autistic children (namely mothers), although it is important to stress that not all parents who advocate for their autistic children support ABA. Nonetheless, parent-led activism does raise some interesting questions about agency as these

2 The information provided to potential participants at Autreat describes some of the ground rules at the meeting, including information for those who wish to attend but prefer to limit their social interaction. Participants can signal their chosen form of interaction by wearing a colour-coded badge.

advocates claim to speak for their "voiceless" children. The fact that mothers are in the forefront of such activism is also significant since they were originally blamed for causing their child's condition in the first place. Once dubbed "refrigerator mothers," it was suggested that their cold, distant parenting forced children to retreat into their own world. Bruno Bettelheim's book, *The Empty Fortress: Infantile Autism and the Birth of the Self* (1967), provides one of the better-known accounts of this theory, which is rooted in psychoanalytic thought. Bettelheim argued that autism was linked to a form of psychopathology in mothers, which led them to react inappropriately to normal aspects of their child's development, such as an initial withdrawal from their environment (Nadesan 2005; Schreibman 2005). Unlike most mothers who react to this in positive ways with increased "mothering acts," some mothers "respond with extreme negative feelings, rejection, and even counterwithdrawal" (Schreibman 2005, 79). The behaviours often characterized as autistic, such as self-stimulation or echolalia, are simply defensive responses to what they perceive as a "threatening and hostile reality."

Although Bettelheim's theory has been roundly condemned and discounted, one of the unfortunate consequences of this is that the "ghost of the refrigerator mother" still haunts the autism research community (Nadesan 2005). It stands in the way of promising research that would examine the influence of the social environment on autism for fear that it may somehow reproduce similar blame-the-parent type theories (Nadesan 2005, 176). At the very least, it is remarkable that mothers, who were initially the scapegoats, have become central figures in autism advocacy over the last few decades.

Traditional autism advocates adopt a liberal agenda advancing the notion that the welfare state has a moral duty to cover the costs of this "medically necessary" treatment, which some parents believe can "save" their children from the damaging effects of autism. Withholding access to this treatment to parents who are unable to cover the prohibitive cost, it is argued, is unjustly discriminatory. Canadian autism advocates made this argument, albeit unsuccessfully, in Canadian courts, suggesting that it violated the principles of the Canada Health Act as well as the equality rights enshrined in the Canadian Charter of Rights and Freedoms.

The heated debates surrounding funding for autism treatment reached a peak in 2004 in Canada when the nation's top court heard an appeal regarding the responsibility of the state to pay for the treatment, which can run to upwards of C$60,000 per year per child. As noted earlier, ABA is an intensive one-on-one treatment that typically requires a commitment of 40 hours per week. Supporters of the Lovaas technique, to which it is sometimes referred to distinguish it from generic ABA treatment, claim that if the therapy is to be effective, it must begin as early as a child is diagnosed, preferably by age two. Although the intricacies of this case have received some attention within legal circles, and among health policy scholars interested in the nexus between constitutional law and health (see Greschner and Lewis 2003; Jackman n.d.; Manfredi and Maioni 2005), this chapter focuses instead on the constitution of the autistic subject in these unfolding discourses. The project of making the autistic subject is, of course, unfinished, still emerging, but we can see the beginnings of this in some of the flashpoints of the autism controversies.

The legal case (*Auton v. British Columbia*) that pitted mothers of autistic children against the provincial government of British Columbia wended its way through provincial courts (trial and appeals courts) and up to the Supreme Court of Canada. The Supreme Court stunned many in the mainstream autism advocacy community, namely the proponents of the Lovaas technique, when it overturned two lower court judgments. The Supreme Court argued that the failure of the provincial government to cover the costs of this therapy did not constitute a violation of equality rights as defined in the Canadian Charter of Rights and Freedoms, as had been claimed by the parents of four autistic children who launched the legal action. News of the legal defeat was met with anger and disappointment. Sabrina Freeman, the founder of the British Columbia (BC) chapter of Families for Early Autism Treatment (FEAT) and the mother of an autistic teenage daughter, commented on the decision: "Why do we have a Supreme Court of Canada, if they cannot uphold the Constitution and they cannot protect the most vulnerable members of society from the vagaries of government?" (CBC 2004). Freeman wrote a book on the case in 2003, well before the appeal was heard by the Supreme Court. In *Science for Sale in the Autism Wars*, she decries the BC government and its "academic mercenaries" in the BC Office of Health Technology Assessment for trying to convince the court that autism treatment is "purportedly experimental, unsubstantiated therapy, unworthy of health insurance coverage" (Freeman 2003, 2). Although both BC courts sided with the parents on the merits of the treatment, Freeman declared that the report commissioned by the BC government "will haunt parents of children with autism fighting for their children's rights around the world. Justice will elude these children as governments work to save money and academics pad their curriculum vitae" (Freeman 2003, 212). By the time it reached the Supreme Court, the *Auton* case had attracted a total of 19 interveners, including ten governments, eight organizations, and one individual (Michelle Dawson). Dawson was the only intervener actually named in the Supreme Court decision. A vocal critic of ABA and of the unethical treatment of autistic people in general, Dawson believes there is no scientific basis on which to claim that this therapy actually helps autistic children. In its decision, the Supreme Court Chief Justice mentions on three occasions the controversial or unproven nature of the treatment for which state support was being sought (Manfredi and Maioni 2005, 19):

> Objections range from its reliance in its early years on crude and arguably painful stimuli, to its goal of changing the child's mind and personality. Indeed one of the interveners in this appeal, herself an autistic person, argues against the therapy. (*Auton* 2004, para. 5)

In her own factum, Michelle Dawson compares the situation of autistic people to Aboriginal people in Canada; both groups, she claims, are "denigrated and infantilized by those deemed qualified to decide their future":

> It would be reprehensible to perform a statistical analysis to prove that aboriginal people are a burden on society because they are aboriginal, then to propose that society would profit greatly if only aboriginal people became less aboriginal or not aboriginal at all. (Dawson 2004, 16)

Issues surrounding representation and communication take on a particular resonance when dealing with autism, since one of the claims of mainstream autism advocates concerns the supposed inability of autistics to communicate appropriately. Dawson herself pointed to the fact that none of the organizations that claim to speak for autistic people actually involves them in any significant way in decision-making or priority setting. She adds:

> It is striking that not one of the intervener groups indicated in their Applications to intervene that actual autistic individuals were represented on their boards or on their staff. Therefore, services sought for autistics reflect the needs and agendas of parents and other non-autistics. The services are those which attempt to teach autistics to be "normal" such that they can participate in society by passing as non-autistic. (Dawson 2004, 17)

In a joint factum filed in the Supreme Court case, two organizations presented a gendered perspective on autism. Although autism is more commonly diagnosed in boys, one of the interveners argued that the court was overlooking, at its peril, the gendered dimensions of autism. The two organizations, DisAbled Women's Network (DAWN) and the Legal Education and Action Fund (LEAF), each of which has intervened in a number of landmark court cases in the past, argued that the court should pay particular attention to the differential impact of autism on girls, especially if they require institutionalization once they become adults. The factum claims that women with autism who are institutionalized may be physically and sexually abused there, although they do not provide any evidence to substantiate their claim with regard to the prevalence of such abuse. The interveners nonetheless urged the court to think of gendered disability in a different light: "Gendered disability discrimination is not the additive experience of sex plus disability discrimination; it is a distinct experience, more than the sum of its parts" (LEAF/DAWN 2004, 5). In addition, the interveners stress that it is important to recognize the gendered nature of caregiving and how the retreat of the state from funding treatment places undue responsibility onto the backs of parents, namely mothers. In a book chapter reflecting on the court decision's failure to uphold the equality rights guaranteed in the Canadian Charter, Fiona Sampson, a lawyer for the interveners, argued that part of the problem with the court's decision is apparent in Justice McLachlin's opening statement that she "sympathized" with the petitioners, autistic children and their parents: "The emotion of sympathy provides a convenient cover for what's really happening relationally between the non-disabled and the disabled; that is, between the dominant norm and the oppressed group. To declare sympathy for the disabled allows the person making the declaration to portray her/his self as a benevolent humanitarian" (Sampson 2006, 261).

In the next section, I draw on the notion of "biological citizenship" to reflect on the important challenges raised by autistic citizens clamouring to speak for themselves, and to represent "autism" to other autistic people and to society at large in ways that are authentic and grounded in the lived experience. It is not insignificant that the internet has been an important mobilizing force for autistic citizens throughout the world, as it provides a safe space for individuals who may have difficulty with social interaction or who are non-verbal, to communicate with others.

Biological Citizenship and Autistic Subjectivities

Adriana Petryna describes biological citizenship as "a massive demand for but selective access to a form of social welfare based on medical, scientific and legal criteria that both acknowledge biological injury and compensate for it" (2002, 6). As she explains in her examination of the aftermath of the Chernobyl disaster, "the damaged biology of a population has become the grounds for social membership and the basis for staking citizenship claims" (2002, 5). Nikolas Rose and Carlos Novas use the term "to encompass all those citizenship projects that have linked their conceptions of citizens to beliefs about the biological existence of human beings, as individuals, as families and lineages, as communities, as population and races, and as a species" (2005, 440).

Biological citizenship has been discussed in the context of efforts to responsibilize citizens in the age of ever-present risk, urging them to take measures to manage their lives in ways that are productive, and, ultimately, health-enhancing (Rose and Novas 2005, 450). Biological citizens are expected to do more than take care of themselves, however. The discourse of the "new genetics," for instance, urges citizens to learn more about their genetic selves and to make prudent choices in light of this knowledge. Rose and others have gone to great lengths, however, to distance themselves from simplistic critiques of genetic determinism. As Rose notes: "There is little evidence that modern genetic biomedicine reduces the genetically risky person to a passive body-machine that is merely to be an object of a dominating medical expertise" (2006, 129). In a nuanced reading of the genetics of autism, Silverman argues that autism "has become genetic, but it has become so in the wake of a long history of theorizing about autism as a form of organic emotional deficit in those diagnosed, or as caused by a deficit of emotion in their parents" (Silverman n.d., 9). There is no doubt, however, that the current debates about genetic research in the field of autism have provoked fierce opposition from autistic activists who fear this is a short step toward a new form of eugenics. Some activists fear that, just as in the case of Down syndrome, if technology could detect the presence of an autistic gene or genes *in utero*, many parents would opt to terminate the pregnancy.

In earlier work on biological citizenship in the context of Hepatitis C activism, I described the process of citizen/patient contestation in three ways (see Orsini 2008). For the purposes of this chapter, I apply this threefold process to understand contestation in the field of autism. First, individuals, as individuals or as members of organizations, may challenge society and its institutions to take seriously autism in the first place. Part of this is accomplished by some advocates with repeated reference to the so called "autism epidemic," which has penetrated media and popular discourses to the point of being virtually incontestable. Indeed, it is the success with which these advocates have been able to frame autism, especially childhood autism, in epidemic terms that has spawned a countermovement of activists who rail against the culture of fear and ignorance they believe this type of discourse exacerbates. It does little, they counter, to address the real concerns of autistic people, including autistic adults. Parents of autistic children and some autistic individuals themselves have done this by becoming experts in the science and politics of autism. One popular website, neurodiversity.com, run by Kathleen Seidel, provides an exhaustive and highly informative review of an array of legal, medical, and policy issues related to autism.

Second, some autistic people contest the stigma attached to the autistic label, or to an autism diagnosis. This is evident in the discourses of activists who celebrate their autistic pride, and who reject the idea that they have "autism," as if it were a horrible affliction they needed to rid themselves of. Autism, in this construction, is not something one *has*, it is something one *is*. Finally, contestation takes place collectively when individuals locate the cause of their disability, or their inability to deal with it effectively, in outside forces. Therefore, it can be useful—and necessary—to mobilize an "injustice frame" that locates blame. In the field of autism, this has been most pronounced in the bitter debates about the role of vaccines in autism prevalence, specifically a potential link between autism and the MMR vaccine and to vaccines made with thimerosal, a preservative that contains mercury (Blume 2006; Fombonne et al. 2006).

The issue of vaccine safety has been at the centre of a recent court challenge in the US by parents seeking compensation for the harms they claim their children suffered after being vaccinated. The representative plaintiff in the case, 12-year-old Michelle Cedillo, was recently wheeled into the courtroom at the start of the trial. Her parents claimed she was healthy when she received the MMR vaccine at the age of 15 months. Soon after, the few words in her still limited vocabulary all but disappeared: "She developed a high fever one week after the shot and went rapidly downhill. Today, she does not speak and is totally dependent on caregivers. She suffers from seizures, arthritis and inflammatory bowel disease and is nearly blind" (Vedantam 2007). In April 2008, a federal compensation court for people injured by vaccines agreed to settle with the family of a nine-year-old who claimed their daughter developed autism following a round of shots against infectious diseases (Harris 2008). In the UK, fears over a study linking the MMR vaccine to autism in a group of 12 children led to widespread panic and a dramatic drop in the number of parents opting to vaccinate their children. Even the former British

Prime Minister Tony Blair entered the fray when he refused to reveal whether his son Leo had been vaccinated against MMR.

Biological citizenship, whether in its individualizing or collectivizing form, operates in a "political economy of hope," in which "[b]iology is no longer blind destiny or even a foreseen but implacable fate. It is knowable, mutable, improvable, eminently manipulable. Of course, the other side of hope is undoubtedly anxiety, fear and dread at what one's biological future ... might hold" (Rose and Novas 2005, 442). In his own work, Novas has argued that "it is the relational qualities of hope that make it possible to consider studying it in a political economy context." As he explains, "The hopes for cures or treatments that are expressed and acted upon by participants in patients' associations have distinctly biopolitical dimensions in the sense that, through working alongside scientists, health professionals and political authorities, they attempt to shape in the present the future health and well being of specific populations" (Novas 2006, 302).

What do we make of the forms of activism that have emerged in the wake of the "autism epidemic"? Indeed, the term itself is largely the product of tireless advocacy in North America. Websites abound with organizations lamenting the epidemic, and speculating about the factors that might help to explain the spike in the rate of children diagnosed. As noted earlier, several factors have fuelled support for the "autism epidemic" theory, including the fact that doctors and psychiatrists are more aware today of the signs of autism, children are being diagnosed earlier, and the concept of autism has broadened somewhat to include a range of neurological disorders (Grinker 2007). What is particularly interesting—and indeed controversial—about autism is who is doing the majority of the advocacy. In the case of autistic children, it is their parents, in particular their mothers, who have been the most vocal. They have immersed themselves in the literature, in the science, challenging doctors and the healthcare system itself. Parents "have been essential in advancing research" and questioning the received wisdom on autism (Silverman and Brosco 2007, 393). An activist associated with the popular neurodiversity.com website recently forced a scientific journal, *Autoimmunity Review*, to retract an article by two geneticists claiming that thimerosal was largely responsible for an increase in diagnoses of behaviour disorders (Deer 2007). In the case of Canada, autism advocates took their concerns to the highest court in the land, in the name of their autistic children, even though courts had earlier rejected a class action claim on behalf of thousands of autistic children.

Thinking about autism advocacy/activism through the lens of biological citizenship forces us to confront important questions about agency, since, in the case of parents agitating for state support of behavioural interventions for their children, the parents are speaking for their children. These children do not necessarily have the opportunity to articulate their own positions, but they are important political symbols in their own right.

The figure of the child has been central to the creation of the so-called "social investment state" of the last decade that is the hallmark of Third Way politics. Such a state is built on the premise that we must view social programmes aimed at, for instance, combating social exclusion or addressing poverty, as investments in the future. This halfway house between unbridled capitalism and state sponsored socialism is purported to be a marriage of the best of both worlds. Not surprisingly, the new found focus on the child as the centrepiece of a host of policy initiatives has been greeted with widespread support; to be sure, there is very little, if any, organized opposition to pro-child policies. In an age of neoliberalism and the never-ending struggle to justify support for robust social programmes, the child has emerged as an important symbolic tool to hammer home the message that failing to "invest" in children can have disastrous effects on the economy and on society. As Chen explains: "The symbol of suffering children has worked as a way of keeping unpopular issues like poverty on the public agenda in the midst of the New Right backlash against the welfare state" (Chen 2003, 190). In recent years, there has been an increasing focus on children and families as the privileged target of welfare state intervention (Chen 2003; Dobrowolsky and Jenson 2004). A central pillar of the new "child-focused" welfare state architecture is a focus on alleviating child poverty, sometimes but not always with an explicit reference to the family in which the poor child is embedded. In Canada and in other countries, much effort has been placed in early childhood intervention programmes for "at risk" families, a descriptor or catch all that is at once inclusive but also vague. It is not always clear what or who is at risk—the family, the child, or the capitalist economy that depends upon productive worker citizens?

Autistic adults, in contrast to the non-autistic parents of autistic children, partly derive their legitimacy from the fact that they are speaking for themselves, that they are indeed reclaiming a "spoiled identity" (Goffman 1963). They are exercising their citizenship rights as members of democratic societies, using the internet or other fora to counter what they see as an avalanche of advocacy in the name of, but not for, autistic children. How, therefore, do we distinguish this form of political activity from the activism of parents agitating for state support of behavioural therapy and greater recognition of the negative effects of autism on families and society in general? Is parental activism a form of biological citizenship, or biological citizenship by proxy, since the parents in question are intervening on behalf of their children? What about those parents who do not support the pro-treatment agenda, and are instead more interested in supporting their autistic children without necessarily "curing" them? And what impact are these forms of collective action in the name of autism and autistic people having on the way in which we understand autism itself?

In *The Social Construction of What?*, philosopher Ian Hacking addresses the latter question in the context of a discussion of what he calls "interactive kinds." Although he is admittedly vague with regard to a precise definition, he does note that the notion of an interactive kind helps us to think about how classifications "make up" citizens, to borrow a term from Rose and Novas. That is,

> We are especially concerned with classifications that, when known by people or by those around them, and put to work in institutions, change the ways in which

> individuals experience themselves—and may even lead people to evolve their feelings and behaviour in part because they are so classified. Such kinds (of people and their behavior) are interactive kinds. This ugly phrase has the merit of recalling actors, agency and action. The inter may suggest the way in which the classification and the individual classified may interact, the way in which the actors may become self-aware as being of a kind, if only because of being treated or institutionalized as of that kind, and so experiences themselves in that way. (Hacking 2000, 104)

The key difference between interactive kinds and indifferent kinds such as quarks is that "calling a quark a quark makes no difference to the quark" (Hacking 2000, 105). Such is not the case with autism. Autistic labels, characterizations, or classifications have a "looping effect" on autistic people, on non-autistics, and on the ways in which we understand the autistic descriptor.

Biological citizenship as it relates to autism thus appears to be studded with contradictions. It is at once empowering and affirming to find others who share your neurological distinctiveness, and to build the requisite networks of mutual support, be they online or offline. As Nadesan points out, however, to suggest that autistic people are biologically different—genetically and neurologically—"is simultaneously divisive and affirmative in its representation of autistic difference" (Nadesan 2005, 208). While attempts by autistic people to celebrate their neurodiversity in a world of neurotypicals (the term used by autistics to describe others unlike them) help to counter the stigma attached to an autism diagnosis, they can also essentialize autistic people as "ontologically different beings" (Nadesan 2005, 209). The contradiction lies in the efforts by advocates/activists to embrace, indeed reclaim, the autistic label, while at the same time "advocating for understanding of and special care for the more troubling autistic deficits or symptoms" (Nadesan 2005, 209). Moreover, there is a need for greater recognition of how the autistic "experience" is mediated by other factors, such as class, race, and gender. With regard to the latter, Davidson's illuminating analysis (2008) of the autobiographies of autistic women sheds some necessary light on the gendered nature of autism diagnoses, or the lack thereof. It was common for women or girls expressing concern about their health to be dismissed as "neurotic" or "hysterical," which often led to misdiagnoses (Davidson 2008, 247).

Conclusion

This chapter has only begun to sketch the contours of autistic subjectivity. As part of a larger project on health social movements, I am only at the starting point here in thinking about the significance of autism to the field of health and disability, and about the struggles over how to conceptualize the autistic subject in these discourses. Certainly, the autistic subject is multifaceted and constantly evolving. While the dominant constructions of autism have always included children, recently autistic adults are beginning to articulate their own distinctive identities, reminding society at large that autistic children might be the focus of popular media attention, but the unique needs and demands of autistic adults, many of whom speak on their own behalf, require the attention of society at large. After all, autistic children will soon become autistic adults.

Autistic advocates are correct to point out the pitfalls inherent in a view of treatment as "medically necessary" and constitutionally protected, as it further pathologizes a disability and positions parents who opt out of treatment/therapy as virtual pariahs: "[T]he deprivation of 'medically necessary' treatment will be seen as the mistreatment or neglect of that child" (Dawson 2004, 18). Autism advocates, on the other hand, are rightly concerned about what they see as the limits of the welfare state as it pertains to policies that have the potential to improve the quality of life of disabled citizens living with autism. In an age in which governments are looking for ways to opt out of the provision of universal programmes and services, the suggestion that ABA should not be funded because it is unproven scientifically may seem particularly disingenuous given the range of programmes and services that are financially supported by governments even though they may be lacking the sufficient evidence base.

Acknowledgements

This chapter is part of a larger project, titled "Health Policy from Below: Social Movements and Contested Illness in Canada and the US." Activism in the field of autism is one of three case studies. The author would like to acknowledge the support of the Social Science and Humanities Research Council of Canada, #410–2007–0256, and Miriam Smith, the co-investigator on this project. The author would also like to thank the editors for helpful suggestions and Jonathan Simon for comments on an earlier version of the chapter, which was presented at the Law and Society Association meeting in Berlin, July 2007.

References

Autism Every Day (2006), Documentary. Directed by L. Thierry. Produced by Autism Speaks, USA.

Auton (Guardian ad litem of) v. British Columbia (Attorney General, (2004) 3 SCR 657, 2004 SCC 78).

Baron-Cohen, S. (1997), *Mindblindness: An Essay on Autism and Theory of Mind* (Cambridge, MA: MIT Press).

Bettelheim, B. (1967), *The Empty Fortress: Infantile Autism and the Birth of the Self* (New York: Free Press).

Blume, S. (2006), "Anti-Vaccination Movements and Their Interpretations," *Social Science and Medicine* 62: 628–42.

CBC (2004), "Top Court: B.C. Doesn't Have to Fund Autism Treatment," *CBC News* [website], (updated 22 Nov. 2004), <http://www.cbc.ca/canada/story/2004/11/19/autism_supremecourt041119.html>.

Chen, X. (2003), "The Birth of the Child-Victim Citizen," in J. Brodie and L. Trimble (eds), *Reinventing Canada: Politics of the 21st Century* (Toronto: Pearson Education Canada), 189–202.

Davidson, J. (2008), "More Labels Than a Jam Jar: The Gendered Dynamics of Diagnosis for Girls and Women with Autism," in P. Moss and K. Teghtsoonian (eds), *Contesting Illness: Processes and Practices* (Toronto: University of Toronto Press), 239–58.

Dawson, M. (2004), "An Autistic at the Supreme Court," Factum of the Intervener, Michelle Dawson [website], <http://www.sentex.net/~nexus23/naa_fac.html>.

Dawson, M. (2005), "An Autistic Victory: The True Meaning of the Auton Decision" [website], (updated 30 March 2005), <http://www.sentex.net/~nexus23/naa_vic.html>.

Dawson, M. (2007), "Autism Research Rogues Gallery" [website], (updated 28 March 2007), <http://autismcrisis.blogspot.com/search?q=autism+research+rogues>.

Deer, B. (2007), "What Makes an Expert?" *British Medical Journal* 334:31 (March), 666–7.

Dobrowolsky, A. and Jenson, J. (2004), "Shifting Representations of Citizenship: Canadian Politics of 'Women' and 'Children'," *Social Politics* 11:2 (summer), 154–80.

Don't Speak for Me (n.d.), online petition [website], <http://www.autism-hub.co.uk/autism-speaks-dont-speak-for-me/index.php>.

Fombonne, E. et al. (2006), "Pervasive Developmental Disorders in Montreal, Quebec, Canada: Prevalence and Links with Immunizations," *Pediatrics* 118:1 (July), e139–e150.

Freeman, S. (2003), *Science for Sale in the Autism Wars: Medically Necessary Autism Treatment, the Court Battle for Health Insurance and Why Health Technology Academics are Enemy Number One* (Langley, BC: SFK Books).

Goffman, E. (1963), *Stigma: Notes on the Management of Spoiled Identity* (Eaglewood Cliffs, NJ: Prentice Hall).

Greschner, D. and Lewis, S. (2003), "*Auton* and Evidence-Based Decision-Making: Medicare in the Courts," *Canadian Bar Review* 82, 501–35.

Grinker, R.R. (2007), *Unstrange Minds: Remapping the World of Autism* (New York: Basic Books).

Gross, J. and Strom, S. (2007), "Autism Debate Strains a Family and its Charity," *New York Times*, 18 June.

Hacking, I. (2000), *The Social Construction of What?* (Cambridge, MA and London: Harvard University Press).

Harris, G. (2008), "Deal in an Autism Case Fuels Debate on Vaccine," *New York Times*, 9 March.

Hobson West, P. (2003), "Understanding Vaccination Resistance: Moving Beyond Risk," *Health, Risk, and Society* 5:3 (November), 273–83.

Jackman, M. (n.d.), "Under the Knife? Charter Equality and the Right to Publicly Funded Health Care," unpublished manuscript.

Manfredi, C. and Maioni, A. (2005), "Litigating Innovation: Health Care Policy and the Canadian Charter of Rights and Freedoms." Paper presented at the annual meeting of the Canadian Political Science Association, London, Ontario, 1–4 June.

Nadesan, M.H. (2005), *Constructing Autism: Unravelling the "Truth" and Understanding the Social* (London and New York: Routledge).

New York Times (2007), "Editorial: Autism in the Vaccine Court," 24 June.

Novas, C. (2006), "The Political Economy of Hope: Patients' Organizations, Science and Biovalue," *BioSocieties* 1, 289–305.

Orsini, M. (2008), "Hepatitis C and the Dawn of Biological Citizenship: Unravelling the Policy Implications," in P. Moss and K. Teghtsoonian (eds), *Contesting Illness: Processes and Practices* (Toronto: University of Toronto Press).

Petryna, A. (2002), *Life Exposed: Biological Citizens After Chernobyl* (Princeton, NJ: Princeton University Press).

Picard, A. (2006), "The Postie and the Prof Dispute Perceptions of Autism," *The Globe and Mail*, 20 February.

Rabinow, P. (1996), *Essays on the Anthropology of Reason* (Princeton, NJ: Princeton University Press).

Rose, N. (2006), *The Politics of Life Itself: Biomedicine, Power, and Subjectivity in the Twenty-First Century* (Princeton, NJ: Princeton University Press).

Rose, N. and Novas, C. (2005), "Biological Citizenship," in A. Ong and S.J. Collier (eds), *Global Assemblages: Technology, Politics and Ethics as Anthropological Problems* (London: Blackwell), 439–63.

Sampson, F. (2006), "The Law Test for Discrimination and Gendered Disability Inequality," in F. Faraday, M. Denike, and M.K. Stephenson (eds), M*aking Equality Rights Equal: Securing Substantive Equality Under the Charter* (Toronto: Irwin Law), 245–74.

Schreibman, L. (2005), *The Science and Fiction of Autism* (Cambridge, MA and London: Harvard University Press).

Silverman, C. (n.d.), "Brains, Pedigrees, and Promises: Lessons from the Politics of Autism Genetics," unpublished manuscript.

Silverman, C. and Brosco, J.B. (2007), "Understanding Autism: Parents and Pediatricians in Historical Perspective," *Archives of Pediatrics and Adolescent Medicine* 161 (April), 392–8.

Sinclair, J. (1993), "Don't Mourn for Us," *Our Voice*, the Newsletter of Autism Network International 1:3 [website], <http://web.syr.edu/~jisincla/dontmourn.htm>.

Sinclair, J. (2005), "Autism Network International: The Development of a Community and its Culture" [website], <http://web.syr.edu/~jisincla/History_of_ANI.html>.

Standing Senate Committee on Social Affairs, Science, and Technology (2003), Proceedings, 26 February 2003 (Ottawa: Canadian Government Publishing).
Standing Senate Committee on Social Affairs, Science, and Technology (2007), *Pay Now or Pay Later: Autism Families in Crisis*, Final Report, March 2007 (Ottawa: Canadian Government Publishing).
Vedantam, S. (2007), "Fight Over Vaccine-Autism Link Hits Court," *Washington Post*, 10 June, A06.
Women's Legal Education and Action Fund and Disabled Women's Network (2004), Factum of the Intervener, Auton v. British Columbia.

PART III
Gendered Interventions

Chapter 8
The View from Inside: Gendered Embodiment and the Medical Representation of Sex

Shelley Wall

> For hundreds of years, the anatomist and artist did ventriloquism with cadavers, making them speak, sing, dance, and tell jokes. Eventually the tables turned: the images of anatomy became part of us, started speaking through us. We became the ventriloquist's dummy, an effigy of the anatomical self. Anatomical identity inhabits us, even as it coexists with, and infuses, other representations of the body. (Sappol 2006)

Introduction

Visual images figure centrally in the discourse of biomedicine. In Western healthcare, anatomical images of the human body make legible our invisible, visceral regions as well as our visible selves. If I am a patient, I may be shown representations of my individual anatomy—produced by imaging technologies such as mammogram, ultrasound, or MRI—in the context of a clinical encounter focused on my body's conformity with, or deviation from, normative health or shape. Alternatively, I may be shown or encounter a generalized anatomical representation in the form of an illustration, with the implication that my body constitutes an instance of, or a deviation from, that representative anatomy. And because "the being, or rather the becoming, of the self is always intricately interwoven with the fabric of the body" (Shildrick 2005, 2), these images we see of (our) bodies influence how we live in our bodies—that is, these external representations in part construct our embodied subjectivity (see, for instance: Birke 2000; Butler 2004; Dreger 2004; Gatens 1996; Howson 2001). That construction of corporeal subjectivity may, in turn, influence our health status and healthcare decisions. As Cassandra Aspinall, a medical social worker with her own history of physical difference, writes: "I know that your image of your insides affects intimately how you make decisions, including decisions about surgery" (2004, 170). Health information, including visual information, can be empowering. But there is also the possibility that certain pictures of the anatomical body, when used and reproduced uncritically, can perpetuate alienating conceptions of a normative, mechanistic body. In many instances, there may be a disjunction between the subjective experiences of patients and the objectifying visual rhetoric of conventional anatomical imagery.

This chapter considers the genealogy of the anatomical images used in patient counselling and consumer health education and the assumptions about embodied life that they encode. Specifically, it looks at two related and particularly charged aspects of anatomical illustration: representations of female anatomy and the presumption of normative sexual dimorphism. My perspective on this topic is at least three-fold: that of an embodied female subject, an academic in a medical discipline, and a professional creator of anatomical images. As an embodied subject I experience my body from "inside"; my direct visual experience of my external body is partial (I have never *seen* my own chin directly, for instance), does not adhere to accepted representational conventions (when I look down at my body, my toes are at the top of the visual field), and so has been supplemented over a lifetime with various representations—in mirrors, photographs, and categorical images of "the body." As for my internal structures, the only visual images I have come from mediated representations. As an academic, I consume analyses of visual representations of the body—from feminist, anatomical, bioethical, historical, artistic, clinical, and activist viewpoints, to name only a sample of the interests that converge on this topic. And as a professional medical illustrator, I participate in and contribute to the discursive production of the biomedical body with every drawing I make. It is this concatenation of perspectives that leads me to consider how we might effect a critical intervention in the language of biomedical illustration, rethink the body from the inside out, and become more aware of the importance of "doing justice" (Butler 2004) to the diverse embodied experience of patients.

The Anatomical Self

Let me begin with three examples of simple anatomical images intended for consumer or patient information.

Figure 8.1 is adapted from the kind of image commonly used to map areas of sensation on the body in the course of a clinical encounter. Figure 8.2 is the kind of image conventionally used to convey information about vulvar anatomy or health. And Figure 8.3 is adapted from illustrations of the female and male urogenital systems.[1]

We are supposed to know how to read these images—and I suspect that most of us do. Where does that literacy come from? In industrialized Western culture, we are surrounded by the visual discourse of biomedicine, whether it be to teach us about "health" in school, to explain diagnoses or procedures in a healthcare

1 These figures are drawn by the author, based on typical examples found in consumer health information or patient education and on images created in the course of her work as a medical illustrator.

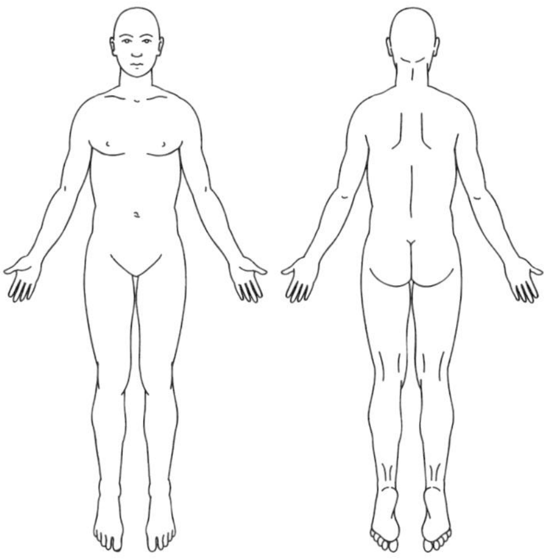

Figure 8.1 Areas of sensation on the body

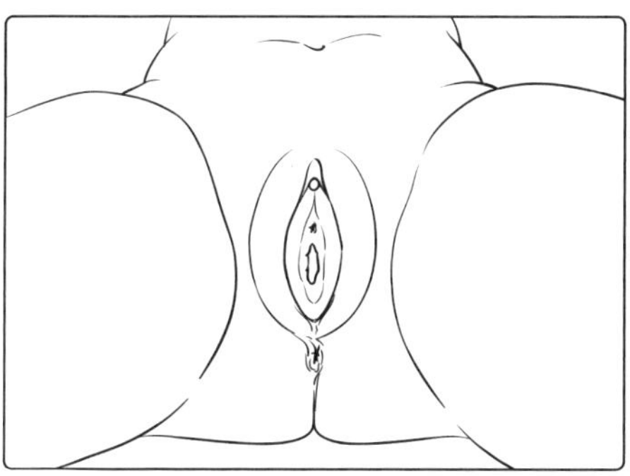

Figure 8.2 Vulvar anatomy

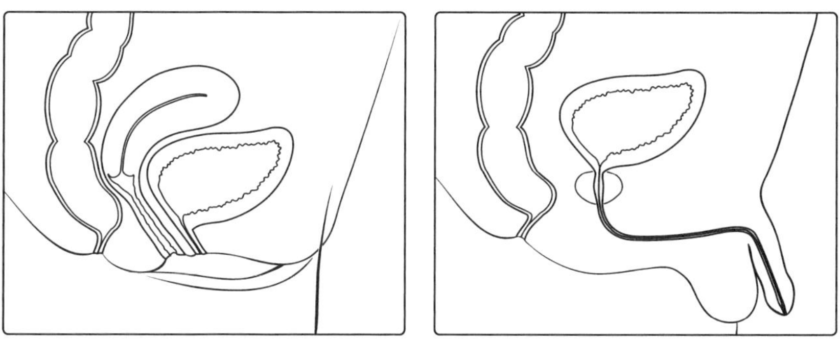

Figure 8.3 Female and male urogenital systems

provider's office, to explain medical topics in the popular press, or to sell us medication for the relief of sore joints. This bath of imagery teaches us that we are to read these diagrammatic, fragmentary, bisected images as representations of our own bodies, and thereby to gain some understanding of ourselves (Birke 2000). Art historian James Elkins suggests that depicted bodies "may be understood as opportunities for a peculiar kind of response that can be difficult to name—although it might be called 'visceral seeing' or 'thoughtful embodiedness'" (1999, vii). When we see a body we respond physically, feeling that body mapped along our own, whether that body shows vitality or passivity, agency or vulnerability, wholeness or fragmentation. Anatomical imagery has the authority of biomedical knowledge behind it, and so has all the more persuasive power to activate and inform our body image. The result, in Michael Sappol's words, is that we become "an effigy of the anatomical self" (2006).

Body of Knowledge

Since the time of Andreas Vesalius (1514–64), the discipline of anatomy in the West has been about making the material architecture of the human body visible and comprehensible. During the same period, illustrations to document and disseminate knowledge of the body have been central to anatomical science (Roberts 1996). Vesalius argued for the importance of cadaveric dissection—work of the hand and eye—to corroborate or refute the canonical anatomy teachings of Galen (131–201 CE), and he was the first to insist on the primacy of visual documentation; his seven-volume *De Humani Corporis Fabrica* (1543) is a watershed in both anatomical inquiry and illustration. As Vesalius notes in his Preface, the volumes of the *Fabrica* "include pictures of all the parts inserted in the text in such a way that they place the dissected body, as it were, before the eyes of those studying the works of Nature" (Vesalius 2003). Illustrations or schemata of the body can depict shape, size, volume, structure, spatial relationship, and measurement, among other features. That the cadaver becomes a source of manipulable data subject to visual articulation is made clear by Vesalius through analogy: "How much pictures aid the understanding of these things and place a subject before the eyes more precisely than the most explicit language, no one knows who has not had this experience in geometry and other branches of mathematics" (2003).

Contemporary imaging technology allows the detailed, interior observation of living bodies, but anatomical science for most of its history has been bound up with the exploration of dead bodies. The complex and geographically specific histories of cadaver acquisition and dissection form in themselves an extended chapter in the history of bioethics (see, for example: Jones 1998; Richardson 1987; Roberts 1996; Sawday 2006). Ultimately, anatomical knowledge derived from cadaveric dissection is extrapolated (and interpolated) back onto the living body (Roberts 1996), but it is not an untroubled transfer. Anatomist D.G. Jones articulates anatomy's position as a liminal discipline, in the borderlands between life and death, between what is socioculturally acceptable and what is not, and notes that "procedures on the cadaver have the potential to objectify, and hence depersonalize, the cadaver" (1998, 101). Because of their intimate relationship to dissection, the pictorial conventions of Western medical illustration have evolved in the context of this object-body—no longer the embodiment of a living being, but rather an inert physical quantity, literally reducible to component parts. The dead body functions, in effect, as a 1:1 scale model of the living body. Through the arts of dissection, prosection, and cross-section—whereby elements of anatomy are isolated, removed or foregrounded, arranged so as to articulate specific hierarchies and relationships—the cadaver itself is transformed into a series of compositions. Thus even before a drawing, woodcut, engraving, photograph, or other two-dimensional image is made, the cadaver is already an image of itself, composed and arranged in accordance with evolving or established representational conventions.

Michael Sappol traces a trend toward increasing austerity in the aesthetics and meanings of anatomical conventions from Vesalius to the present. Whereas early anatomical illustrations sometimes incorporated elements of the *danse macabre* and "animated" their cadavers, by the eighteenth century "anatomical realism" dictated the depiction of the cadaver exactly as it appeared on the dissection table, complete with ragged, cut flesh, the apparatus of the dissector's trade, and signs of decay. This "realism" gave way over the course of the nineteenth century to "anatomical universalism," the depiction, as in *Gray's Anatomy*, of isolated, idealized organs and regions of the body (Sappol 2006). Although anatomical and pictorial conventions have shifted over time, certain broad categories persist. For example, both dissection and illustration transform the structure of the body through dismemberment into sections, through removal of progressive layers of tissue, or through isolation of individual organs or systems (such as skeletal, vascular, nervous). Certain postures are conventional: the "anatomical position" (the body supine, symmetrical, arms at sides, palms out, viewed frontally) has become standard. It maximizes the visibility of the internal organs, allows for ready comparison among similar images, and replicates the position of the body on the dissection table. The cataloguing function of anatomical study requires images that assemble organs or features in pairs or series to enforce comparison or contrast: the pairing of "normal" with "abnormal" or "pathological" anatomy is a common version of this visual convention. And another convention is the cross-sectional view, which became widespread only when preservation and refrigeration technologies had advanced to a certain point. A cross-sectional view—a slice through a single plane—figures the body as a landscape and, more specifically, the cadaver as a map of the living body. As the Preface to Nicolaus Rüdinger's 1873 *Topographisch-chirurgische Anatomie des Menschen* puts it, cross-sectional anatomy "giv[es] a deeper insight into the topographical relations of the organs, and … enabl[es] one to carry over from the cadaver to the living body the total picture thus obtained" (quoted in Eycleshymer and Schoemaker 1911, xi). Cross-sectional atlases, which depict the body as a kind of geological section, anticipate the planar anatomies of magnetic resonance imaging. They also, in their flattened cartography, epitomize the body as what Foucault describes as a "medical field" "pervaded wholly by the gaze": "a space whose lines, volumes, surfaces, and routes are laid down, in accordance with a now familiar geometry, by the anatomical atlas" (2003, 3, 38). Illustrations such as Figure 8.3 rely upon a viewer's understanding of this convention: her ability to conceptualize the body as sliced in half, like a pastry, to shed light on the interior.

Such conventions encode the "anatomo-clinical gaze" (Foucault 2003): the gaze of the subject in possession of power/knowledge, surveying and classifying the territory of the body. Jonathan Sawday draws attention to the shared tropes of exploration/colonization that characterized early modern European attitudes toward both the body and the world: "To 'open' a body, or a continent, was not only to know it, but also to own it in some way" (2006). Such penetrating exploration has long been the province of explicitly masculine subjects. Vesalius's work represents an approach to scientific investigation that is self-consciously "male"—virile, empirical, and practical (Birke 2000). But at the same time this tradition of gendered empiricism presents itself as neutral: pure seeing. For example, Vesalius's ambition to "place the dissected body, as it were, before the eyes of those studying the works of Nature" (2003) is echoed over two centuries later by anatomist/man-midwife William Hunter in the Preface to *The Anatomy of the Human Gravid Uterus Exhibited in Figures* (1774) when he claims that "the art of engraving" in his atlas supplies "an universal language" and "to every person conversant with the subject, gives an immediate comprehension of what it represents" (quoted in Massey 2005, 80). Each work emphasizes the *immediacy*, or transparency, of its representations. And yet each of these statements also qualifies its claim in specifying its audience: "those studying the works of Nature" (scientists) and "every person conversant with the subject" (anatomists, medical men, and "man-midwives"). The anatomical knowledge available in these representations is gendered and exclusive. Rather than being "universal," it is only available to those "conversant with the subject"—that is, those who already understand the structure of its visual language.

Although anatomist Jakob Henle (1809–85) declared that "[t]he questions which the clinician demands that anatomy shall answer, have first of all the purpose, as it were, of making the body transparent" (quoted in Eycleshymer and Schoemaker 1911, xiv), anatomical imagery is *not* transparent (Grosz 1994). "From the first anatomical prints and engravings to the earliest microscope, stereoscope, daguerreotype, x-ray, and photograph and on to contemporary medical visualization methods, technologies of envisioning the body simultaneously have mediated, defined, and naturalized what constitutes knowledge of the body" (Adelson 2006, 367). And yet there remains an assumption that anatomical imagery is somehow neutral (Barilan 2007). The contemporary Visible Human Project (VHP), Naomi Adelson's subject, would seem to epitomize the unbiased collection of "raw" anatomical data. In the VHP, the US National Library of Medicine has undertaken "the creation of complete, anatomically detailed, three-dimensional representations of the normal male and female human bodies" through the collation of magnetic resonance imaging data, computed tomography data, and digital scans of paper-thin sections through two frozen cadavers (US National Library of Medicine 2008). And yet, as Lisa Cartwright, Catherine Waldby, and Naomi Adelson have demonstrated, the VHP is embedded in and perpetuates assumptions about gender, the body, technology, and visuality (Adelson 2006; Cartwright 1998; Waldby 2000). The conventions of anatomical illustration carry their origins with them: "Positivist empiricism does not, in fact, yield neutral and universally valid conceptions of knowledge. Instead, knowledge is indelibly shaped by its creators and attests to the specificities of their epistemic locations" (Goldenberg 2006, 2624).

Patient Embodiment and Biomedical Visual Conventions

Naomi Adelson comments on the process articulated by Foucault whereby "anatomical drawings serve to 'subtract' the person/patient both from disease as well as from his or her body" (Adelson 2006, 366). Until the latter part of the twentieth century, the primary audiences for anatomical illustrations were, with few exceptions, anatomists, doctors, surgeons, students, sometimes midwives, or others within a learned elite. The visual canon of anatomy from its earliest days carried the authoritative weight of "anatomy's symbolic capital" (Massey 2005) born of the fear-tinged respect accorded to anatomical science. In relation to the corpse-body featured in these illustrations, the implicit viewer stands as knowing subject to object of knowledge, active mover to passive matter. In this scenario, when the knowledge gained from anatomical study is applied in medical practice, the patient's body may be seen as a more or less successful instantiation of that normative "imaginary body" (Gatens 1996) discovered through dissections and documented in images, and the patient as individual particularity disappears, or rather, must be "placed in parentheses" so that disease may be seen clearly (Foucault 2003). The patient's body remains an object-body and the unequal power relations embedded in the image carry over into the clinical encounter.

What happens when, in the context of contemporary consumer or patient education, the audience for these images becomes the lay person or patient her/himself—a first-person rather than a third-person observer—and the illustration is supposed to function not just as a map, but as a mirror? The result is a third-person view of one's own body. Repeated exposure to these kinds of images (and we are exposed to them continually) can lead to "self-objectification"—that is, the process whereby a person "internalize[s] an observer's perspective on self" (Fredrickson and Roberts 1997, 179). Fredrickson and Roberts use this term to refer primarily to women's and girls' acculturation to perceive themselves as sexualized objects; but the term applies as well—and not without overlap—to the perception of oneself as a medicalized object. The clinical gaze is insinuated into the body schema of patients themselves. Like the sexualizing gaze, it can lead to feelings of vulnerability, violation, and self-alienation. Alexandra Howson, building on previous feminist scholarship, argues that "women's sense and understanding of our 'bodily insides' is governed by the imagery and discourses of the biological sciences" and that, moreover, "such imagery and discourses contribute to and structure a fragmented, objectified, and alienated embodiment" (2001, 97). In interviews with Scottish women who had undergone routine cervical smears, for example, Howson found that most respondents viewed their own cervix, imaged on a TV monitor, as an object external to them and suggests that this kind of screening reinforces the idea of the female body as a body "at risk" (2001). Similarly, a Danish study found that being shown the results of their bone scans for osteoporosis actually altered women's body image and sense of embodiment—by, for example, creating a sense of distance between body and self, and increasing the women's sense of fragility (Reventlow et al. 2006). It is a curious double movement whereby graphic representations of the body both construct and trouble a person's sense of embodiment. They provide cognitive information that, like ill-fitting clothing, sits uncomfortably with how a person inhabits her body and alters how she moves and feels in it.

Picturing "Normal"

The human body, as Moira Gatens remarks, is "unrepresentable" because each body is unique and "the selection of a particular image of the human body will be a selection from a continuum of differences" (1996, vii). Nevertheless, anatomical atlases and the generations of images derived from them do, relentlessly, represent the human body. They attempt, moreover, to represent the "normal" body. However, the definition of "normal" in medical or anatomical contexts varies widely (Gilbert 2005; Murphy 1997). "Normal" within anatomical study may mean, among other things: morphology that falls within a normal range of variation; the morphology that is most typically or commonly encountered; an "ideal," the most perfect or optimum form of a given feature; or anatomy that is not pathological or diseased—normalcy as health (Murphy 1997; Gilbert 2005). Like definitions of what is ideal or what is pathological, the definition of normalcy is value-laden, contentious, political, and underpinned by assumptions about gender, race, age, and ability. Anatomical norms are also social and cultural norms (Dreger 2004).

One long-standing anatomical and social norm is the presumption of the male body as the standard and the female body as a variation on it (Cartwright 1998). This presumption is reflected in anatomical illustrations, both historical and contemporary. Historically, the masculinist bias in anatomical observation and illustration intertwines with the gendered nature of both science and crime: male scientists produced "pictures of themselves," in Lynda Birke's words (2000, 51); and an important source of cadavers—the gallows—also produced more male than female "specimens." But these historical circumstances only embody the embedded gender imbalance that, among other things, perceived women as lesser or imperfect versions of men—the "one-sex" model, as Thomas Laqueur (1990) articulates it. Laqueur reproduces numerous Renaissance anatomical illustrations that portray Galen's notion of a woman's sexual organs as the same as a man's, turned inside out: the vagina corresponds to the penis; the uterus to the scrotum; and the ovaries to the testes.[2] The signal difference in a woman's body—and the only reason to represent it especially—was its capacity for pregnancy: "Whereas the male body carried the burden of explaining the greater part of normative human anatomy, the pregnant female body served to illustrate the reproductive system and human generation" (Massey 2005, 75). The "one-sex" conceptualization of human sexuality may not have persisted beyond the seventeenth century, but this imbalance in representation endures into the present. A team of American researchers analyzing widely-used anatomy texts, atlases, and diagnostic manuals in 1994 found that male bodies were depicted far more often than female bodies in illustrations of non-reproductive anatomy, and that female bodies featured primarily in chapters on reproduction. They argue that this disproportion "may create the perception [among medical students] that the male body is 'normal' and the female body 'abnormal'" (Mendelsohn et al. 1994, 1267). Use of the Visible Human Project dataset reflects the same gender bias: as of 2000, the male dataset primarily was used to represent standard human anatomy, whereas the female dataset was used mainly for gynaecological information (Waldby 2000). The category of age as well as sex figures here: the anonymous woman whose body was donated for the project was post-menopausal. Catherine Waldby notes that "the age of the Visible Woman's body renders its status as normal problematic, departing as it does from an implicit equation of the normal female body with the youthful and the reproductive" (2000, 18). In fact, a separate digital dataset implicitly supplies the deficiency in the VHP: the Stanford Visible Female provides data from scans of the pelvis of a woman of reproductive age (Chase et al. n.d.).

"The exclusion of women's bodies from anatomical textbooks, except the specifically obstetrical, reveals the phallocentricity of anatomical discourse, even in the 20th century. The male body is understood to be the 'universal' anatomical model" (Petherbridge and Jordanova 1997, 63). This phallocentricity is reflected in the supposedly androgynous figure reproduced in Figure 8.1. It lacks an actual phallus, but its proportions reflect typical male morphology in every other way. This figure is deliberately neutered, but one does not have to look far among consumer health images to find explicitly male bodies depicting, for instance, the location of the pancreas in diabetes brochures, the airways in decongestant advertisements, or the skeleton in back-pain information. I know that, as a woman, I have learned to make the automatic translation and understand such images as proxies for myself, in the same way I translate gender-biased language to include myself. It becomes

2 Contemporary anatomy also identifies homologues between typical female and typical male genital anatomy—e.g., ovaries/testes, clitoris/glans penis, labia majora/scrotum—but these homologies are based on a common origin from tissues in the undifferentiated genital primordium.

an automatic translation but not a completely smooth one; there is always that snag, that instant of friction as I jump the cognitive gap. This same dissonance will affect anyone, indeed, whose body does not approximate that able, adult, usually white, male standard.

When specifically female anatomy is represented in anatomical atlases and in the educational images derived from them, the depiction often takes the form of Figure 8.2, which replicates the perineal view typically seen by clinical specialists, for instance, as the patient lies, legs spread and elevated, on the examination table. Historically, it harkens back to graphic obstetrical images of sectioned and dissected pregnant female pelvises in the illustrated atlases of William Smellie and William Hunter. The current image is problematic symbolically, in the power relations it inscribes for the viewer and the woman viewed: the (dismembered) woman is supine and supremely vulnerable, and the borders between this image and pornography are contingent and indistinct. It is also problematic practically for the purpose of communicating with women about their own bodies, in that it is an unfamiliar view of one's own body. A woman needs a mirror and freedom from certain cultural constraints to see herself from that perspective. Like Figure 8.1, this image functions in patient education as a visual icon we usually recognize, not from our own embodied awareness, but because we've seen it in other visual representations of the body. For me the image provokes simultaneously a curious sense of detachment from my own anatomy and a feeling of inhabiting, or being inhabited by, the image—of being "an effigy of the anatomical body" (Sappol 2006). Elkins's term "visceral seeing" describes the discomfort I feel in looking at conventional medical illustrations of the vulva because of the context they imply. At some level I feel vulnerable myself; I feel the stirrups cupping my heels, and anticipate the speculum. The image I see shapes my embodied experience. In fact, the experience of *having* a vulva isn't primarily visual at all, although visual images are one of the languages we use to talk about it. In the words of Petra Kuppers, "Western medical science tells different stories about our insides than the narratives common sense can make knowable" (2004, 125).

Another issue arises in connection with this image, and bears, once again, on questions of normativity. The vulva depicted may be typical, but while it purports to represent "woman" it does not reflect the bodies of all women. Even beyond the implicit power relations, this image encodes normative cultural assumptions. For women whose cultural practices, such as genital cutting, can profoundly alter their anatomy (see, for instance: Einstein 2008), normative gynaecological images also produce dissonance between the image and the embodied self supposedly represented in that image. (In images of the penis, as well, cultural assumptions are embedded in the choice to depict it as circumcised or uncircumcised.) And beyond cultural assumptions, most anatomical illustrations encode normative assumptions about biological sexual dimorphism. Figure 8.3, for instance, may be pragmatically useful, but should not be taken to represent the only possibilities for human anatomy. Not only is male anatomy not the standard measure for all bodies; the "ideal" female and male bodies that represent the two sexes in anatomical manuals are in fact typical poles in a spectrum of possibilities for sexual anatomy, as the intersex movement and research into the complexities of foetal sexual differentiation have made clear. Nevertheless, in anatomical representations, sexual bodies outside the binary norm remain practically invisible. Recent decades have seen a feminist reclaiming of the body—for instance, in the vogue for cervical self-examination and the attendant politicization of the cervix (Howson 2001). But what about the woman with androgen insensitivity syndrome (AIS) who does not have a cervix? For that matter, what about the man with hypospadias, whose urethral opening may fall anywhere between the base and the corona of the penis, when he is confronted with normative illustrations of male anatomy? Intersex conditions, or "disorders of sex development" as they are now known clinically,[3] are not uncommon: one baby in every 4,500 born may have some kind of genital "anomaly" (Hughes et al. 2006); some estimates put the figure as high as 1.7 per cent of live births (Fausto-Sterling 2000). Where can people whose bodies differ from the binary anatomical norm find representations that reflect *their* embodied experience? At present, only in the annals of pathology. Variations from the norm do not necessarily pose any physiological health risk, and yet this is the only category open to them within the "normal/abnormal" binary system reinforced in biomedical visual discourse.

Conclusion

What it means to be human, and what counts as a "normal" body, are important questions in contemporary ethical debate (Butler 2004; Shildrick 2005) that relate directly to the messages conveyed in anatomical illustration. Anatomical representations teach us to recognize, compare, and categorize the body: the bodies of others, and also our own. Judith Butler observes, with regard to the operation of social norms, that "recognition becomes a site of power by which the human is differentially produced," and that the "norms that govern idealized human anatomy ... work to produce a differential sense of who is human and who is not, which lives are livable, and which are not" (Butler 2004, 2, 4). These norms pervade social interactions: they are also embodied in biomedical visual discourse about the body. Intersex activist and theorist Morgan Holmes asserts that "[t]hrough their dominant position in Western culture, the particular biomedical metaphors of bodies and their 'functions' threaten to become, if they have not already, the only *legitimate* symbolic and interpretive system mediating how we understand ourselves and our place in the social order" (2008, 25). Anatomical images may

3 "Disorders of sex development" (DSD) became in 2006 the official clinical designation for conditions marked by variations on the usual conjunction of chromosomal, gonadal, and anatomical sex (Hughes et al. 2006). Since that time there has been debate about use of the word "disorder," since many intersex conditions do not pose specific threats to health.

appear neutral by reason of their "empirical" content and clinical context, but in fact they assert their values through a visual rhetoric that is all the more powerful for having been naturalized over the course of centuries. Thus, those who create, disseminate, and use biomedical images bear an ethical responsibility. First of all, we must become critically aware of the assumptions about gender, normativity, and the fragmentable object-body embedded in much contemporary anatomical imagery. And, after that, we must find ways to consciously renovate the visual vocabulary we use to communicate about bodies, to represent the living, varied, integrated flux that we are as embodied human beings.

References

Adelson, N. (2006), "Visible/Human/Project: Visibility and Invisibility at the Next Anatomical Frontier," in A.B. Shtier and B. Lightman (eds), *Figuring It Out: Science, Gender, and Visual Culture* (Hanover, NH: Dartmouth College Press).

Aspinall, Cassandra (2004), "The Scaffolding of the Self," *Perspectives in Biology and Medicine* 47:2, 169–72.

Barilan, Y.M. (2007), "Contemporary Art and the Ethics of Anatomy," *Perspectives in Biology and Medicine* 50:1, 104–23.

Birke, L. (2000), *Feminism and the Biological Body* (New Brunswick, NJ: Rutgers University Press).

Butler, J. (2004), *Undoing Gender* (New York: Routledge).

Cartwright, L. (1998), "A Cultural Anatomy of the Visible Human Project," in P.A. Treichler et al. (eds), *The Visible Woman: Imaging Technologies, Gender, and Science* (New York: New York University Press).

Chase, R.A. et al. (n.d.), "Stanford Visible Female," Stanford University School of Medicine, [website] <http://summit.stanford.edu/ourwork/PROJECTS/LUCY/lucywebsite/home.html>.

Dreger, A.D. (2004), *One of Us: Conjoined Twins and the Future of Normal* (Cambridge, MA: Harvard University Press).

Einstein, G. (2008), "From Body to Brain: Considering the Neurobiological Effects of Female Genital Cutting," *Perspectives in Biology and Medicine* 51:1, 84–97.

Elkins, J. (1999), *Pictures of the Body: Pain and Metamorphosis* (Stanford, CA: Stanford University Press).

Eycleshymer, A.C. and Schoemaker, D.M. (1911), *A Cross-Section Anatomy* (New York: D. Appleton-Century).

Fausto-Sterling, A. (2000), *Sexing the Body: Gender Politics and the Construction of Sexuality* (New York: Basic Books).

Foucault, M. (2003), *The Birth of the Clinic: An Archaeology of Medical Perception*. A.M. Sheridan (trans.) (London: Routledge).

Fredrickson, B.L. and Roberts, T.-A. (1997), "Objectification Theory: Toward Understanding Women's Lived Experiences and Mental Health Risks," *Psychology of Women Quarterly* 21:2, 173–206.

Gatens, M. (1996), *Imaginary Bodies: Ethics, Power and Corporeality* (London: Routledge).

Gilbert, S.F. (2005), *Bioethics and the New Embryology: Springboards for Debate* (Sunderland, MA: Sinauer Associates).

Goldenberg, M.J. (2006), "On Evidence and Evidence-Based Medicine: Lessons from the Philosophy of Science," *Social Science and Medicine* 62:11, 2621–32.

Grosz, E. (1994), *Volatile Bodies: Toward a Corporeal Feminism* (Bloomington, IN: Indiana University Press).

Holmes, M. (2008), *Intersex: A Perilous Difference* (Selinsgrove, PA: Susquehanna University Press).

Howson, A. (2001), "'Watching You—Watching Me': Visualising Techniques and the Cervix," *Women's Studies International Forum* 24:1, 97–110.

Hughes, I.A. et al. (2006), "Consensus Statement on Management of Intersex Disorders," *Archives of Disease in Childhood* 91:7, 554–63.

Jones, D.G. (1998), "Anatomy and Ethics: An Exploration of Some Ethical Dimensions of Contemporary Anatomy," *Clinical Anatomy* 11, 100–105.

Kuppers, P. (2004), "Visions of Anatomy: Exhibitions and Dense Bodies," *Differences: A Journal of Feminist Cultural Studies* 15:3, 123–56.

Laqueur, T. (1990), *Making Sex: Body and Gender from the Greeks to Freud* (Cambridge, MA: Harvard University Press).

Massey, L. (2005), "Pregnancy and Pathology: Picturing Childbirth in Eighteenth-Century Obstetric Atlases," *The Art Bulletin* 87:1, 70–91.

Mendelsohn, K.D. et al. (1994), "Sex and Gender Bias in Anatomy and Physical Diagnosis Text Illustrations," *JAMA* 272:16, 1267–70.

Murphy, E.A. (1997), *The Logic of Medicine* (Baltimore, MD: Johns Hopkins University Press).

Petherbridge, D. and Jordanova, L. (1997), *The Quick and the Dead: Artists and Anatomy* (Berkeley, CA: University of California Press).

Reventlow, S.D. et al. (2006), "Making the Invisible Body Visible: Bone Scans, Osteoporosis and Women's Bodily Experiences," *Social Science and Medicine* 62:11, 2720–31.

Richardson, R. (1987), *Death, Dissection and the Destitute* (London and New York: Routledge and Kegan Paul).

Roberts, K.B. (1996), "The Contexts of Anatomical Illustration," in *The Ingenious Machine of Nature: Four Centuries of Art and Anatomy* (Ottawa: National Gallery of Canada).

Sappol, M. (2006), *Dream Anatomy* (Bethesda, MD: US Department of Health and Human Services, National Institutes of Health, National Library of Medicine).

Sawday, J. (2006), "The Paradoxes of Interiority: Anatomy and Anatomical Rituals in Early Modern Culture," in A. Patrizio and D. Kemp (eds), *Anatomy Acts: How We Come to Know Ourselves* (Edinburgh: Birlinn).

Shildrick, M. (2005), "Beyond the Body of Bioethics: Challenging the Conventions," in M. Shildrick and R. Mykitiuk (eds), *Ethics of the Body: Postconventional Challenges* (Cambridge, MA: MIT Press).

Treichler, P.A. et al. (1998), "Paradoxes of Visibility," in P.A. Treichler et al. (eds), *The Visible Woman: Imaging Technologies, Gender, and Science* (New York: New York University Press).

US National Library of Medicine (2008), *The Visible Human Project: Overview*, [website], (Bethesda, MD: National Institutes of Health) <http://www.nlm.nih.gov/research/visible/visible_human.html>.

Vesalius, A. (2003), "On the Fabric of the Human Body," in *An Annotated Translation of the 1543 and 1555 Editions of Andreas Vesalius' De Humani Corporis Fabrica* [website], D. Garrison and M. Hast (trans.) (Evanston, IL: Northwestern University), <http://vesalius.northwestern.edu/flash.html>.

Waldby, C. (2000), *The Visible Human Project: Informatic Bodies and Posthuman Medicine* (London: Routledge).

Chapter 9
The Politics of Medico-Legal Recognition: The Terms of Gendered Subjectivity in the UK Gender Recognition Act

Sarah Burgess

Introduction

The concept of transsexuality, from its beginning, has been linked to medical and psychological discourses that attempt to identify and diagnose "abnormal" or "aberrant" practices of sex and gender. In the late nineteenth and early twentieth centuries, sexologists, attempting to understand the legal implications of "sexual deviance," began investigating the causes and effects of behaviours such as cross-dressing, transvestism, and homosexuality (Hausman 1995, 112). It was not until the 1950s that the desire to become the "other" sex emerged as a distinct and differentiated phenomenon; previously, it was considered little more than a version of homosexuality, whether a phenomenon of behaviour (as in the work of Richard von Krafft-Ebing) or of physiology (as in the work of Havelock Ellis). During this time, the term "transsexual," first introduced in David O. Cauldwell's 1949 article "Psycopathia Transexualis," came to signify a medical syndrome in which an individual profoundly identifies with the opposite sex—an identification that cannot be classified as a fetish or as the intermittent desire to cross-dress (Hausman 1995, 118–19). Harry Benjamin, considered to be the father of modern transsexualism, further advanced an understanding of transsexuality when he "advocated surgical 'treatment' for transsexualism—that is the treatment 'below the belt'—for what he believed manifestly to be 'above' it" (Hausman 1995, 125). Claiming that transsexuality was a "gender problem," Benjamin argued against the psychotherapeutic models of treatment popular at the time, wishing instead to surgically alter the body to "fit" the psychological sex of the individual. His findings were significant because they, first, suggested that the primary symptom of transsexuality was the demand for a sex change and, second, laid the groundwork for a significant change in the way the *Diagnostic and Statistic Manual for Mental Disorders* (*DSM*) classified transsexuality—changing it from its original classification as "sexual deviation" to "gender dysphoria" in the 1970s and, finally, to "gender identity disorder" (GID) in the 1980 *DSM III*.

The emergence of the terms of transsexuality in these medical and psychiatric discourses, according to several scholars, has created the possibility for trans individuals to seek and receive treatment while validating their experiences and (gender) identities. Bernice Hausman argues more strongly that it is in and through these discourses that transsexual people become agents:

> It is important to underscore the agency of transsexual subjects insofar as they forced the medical profession to respond to their demands. Transsexuals needed the services of professional physicians to achieve their goals, and their ability to work with physicians to create a discourse describing their condition and advocating surgical and hormonal interventions was central to realizing those goals. Transsexual agency is not unproblematic, but to acknowledge its significance to the emerging diagnostic categories in psychiatric sexology is to recognize that transsexuals were (and are) not the passive recipients of medical intervention. (1995, 110)

Emphasizing the dialectical relationship between transsexual individuals and doctors, Hausman celebrates the agency that emerges when transsexual people help define the terms through which they become (trans)gendered subjects.[1] Dean Spade adds that the diagnosis of transsexuality as an "illness" also creates the conditions for trans individuals to receive social recognition. He explains, "A model premised on a disability—or disease—based understanding of deviant behaviour is believed by many to be the best strategy for achieving tolerance by norm-adherent people for those not adhering to norms" (2006, 328–9). The medicalization of transsexuality thus appears to offer individuals social standing and, as such, access to resources.

Contemporary social, political, and academic discourses, however, have started to question the effects of thinking about trans identity in solely medical or psychiatric terms. The transition in terminology from "transsexuality" to "transgenderism" itself signals this social change. Influenced by Virginia Prince's work in the late 1970s, many have adopted the more inclusive term "transgenderism" to signify a range of identities and practices that

> challenge various aspects of the psychomedical construction of "gender identity" and of transsexuality. Here, transgenderism may be understood as referring to a political positioning that draws from post-modern notions of fluidity (for both bodies and genders). Transsexuality may be understood, in more modernist terms, as a (psychiatrically defined) state of being that assumes the preexistence of two sexes between which one may transition. (Roen 2002, 501–2)

1 Hausman argues more specifically that it is through the demand for a sex change that individuals become transsexuals. She writes, "it is through this demand that the subject presents him/herself to the doctor as a transsexual subject; the demand for sex change is an enunciation that designates a desired action and identifies the speaker as the appropriate subject of that action" (1995, 110).

The resistance to the terminology of "transsexuality" follows from the resistance to a psycho-medical binary paradigm of sex. Spade, while recognizing the potential benefits of characterizing non-normative gender identities as "illnesses," argues that the cost of this characterization might be too great because this binary vision imposes norms on trans individuals. He explains, "the medical approach to gender variance, and the creation of transsexuality, has resulted in a governance of trans bodies that restricts our ability to make gender transitions which do not yield membership in a normative gender role" (2006, 329). Facing the medical complex, trans individuals must then "fit" within a pre-determined concept of what it means to be (or to have or live in) a particular gender—ostensibly relinquishing the agency to re-define the terms of medical discourse that regulate bodies. The result, as Spade demonstrates, is that trans individuals seeking medical information and treatment omit "information which would disrupt the version of normative femininity or masculinity that they were presenting to the doctors, including homosexuality and enjoyment of sex practices in the unaltered body" (2006, 326).[2]

While this normative medical discourse affects the ability of trans individuals to demand medical care on their own terms, it also affects their standing before law. That is to say, another difficulty with the medicalization of trans identity is that law invokes and depends on the binary medical definitions of sex and gender in order to define rights and access to resources for trans people. The history of the way law has responded to trans people's demands demonstrates that this invocation has been pernicious. Around the world, medical evidence becomes the basis on which trans people either are denied rights altogether or have their rights restricted. In his book *Transgender Jurisprudence: Dysphoric Bodies of Law*, Andrew Sharpe claims that laws regulating sex and gender employ a "(bio)logic" that:

> serves to reproduce the view that there exists an immutable, binary and oppositional division of sex which precedes, and therefore provides an apparent foundation for, gender. It also serves to reveal how "coherent" gender identity in law is linked to the state of genitalia thereby demonstrating that this approach to bodies is founded on phallocentric and aesthetic concerns. (2002, 56)

This "(bio)logic," according to Sharpe, is problematic because it locates the foundation or the truth of one's (gendered) subjectivity in scientific evidence that purports to authenticate who one is by examining the appearance of his or her genitals—an appearance that can only be classified in a "traditional" binary of male and female. In other words, law's use of medical discourse to find out who

2 In "Trans Health Crisis: For Us It's Life or Death," Leslie Feinberg issues a stronger charge, claiming that "our standing before medical audiences to tell personal stories as patients has not been effective in ushering in change" (2001, 899). Here, Feinberg points to the fact that the dialectic that Hausman championed has failed; in the face of medical professionals, trans people have effectively lost their voices.

one "authentically" is betrays the way law depends on and constructs identity as a ground for an individual's actions, agency, and subjectivity.

The critique of the ways in which law employs medical evidence is hard to deny. To be recognized by medical professionals, one must appear recognizable—one must meet certain established criteria. Although I am persuaded by this critique and understand the stakes of it for those individuals who seek care within a medical system that operates as if the binary vision of sex were simply true, I worry that the various critiques of law's relation to medicine rest on a presumption that, within legal realms, medical evidence enjoys an absolute, unquestioned authority. It is this presumption that leads some, perhaps too quickly, to call for the elimination of medical evidence or gender categories from law. What is lost in these arguments is the real way trans individuals—in fact, all individuals—depend on medical discourses to construct a sense of what it means to be a gendered subject. This chapter seeks, then, to understand how law might critique, upset, or challenge the authority of medical evidence while recognizing how this form of evidence provides the conditions in and through which individuals stand before the law in the first place.

To this end, this chapter closely reads the parliamentary debates surrounding the United Kingdom's 2004 Gender Recognition Act. An Act meant to offer trans people a legal status that conforms to their present gender identity, it establishes a process through which individuals may be granted a "gender recognition certificate"—a public document that marks the legal recognition of an individual in his or her "new" or "acquired" gender identity. An administrative rather than judicial process where individuals submit evidence to a panel of medical and legal experts, it requires that applicants demonstrate that they have lived in their "acquired gender" for at least two years, are currently living in that gender, and plan to continue living in that gender permanently. Applicants must provide documentation from at least two medical and/or psychiatric professionals who confirm that the applicant experienced (or experiences) Gender Identity Disorder (GID). If individuals can meet these requirements while also demonstrating that they are at least eighteen years of age and unmarried, then, from the moment of legal recognition forward, they will enjoy rights of marriage and parenthood, pension and social security benefits, and succession rights that formerly had been denied them because of the difference between their lived gender identity and their sex assigned at birth.

Different from previous legislation addressing trans rights, the Gender Recognition Act does not require individuals to undergo any form of body modification, including but not limited to hormone therapy, sex re-assignment surgery, mastectomy, or hair removal. This provision of the Act opens a discussion in Parliament about what constitutes sufficient evidence to prove that one is "living in" a gender. These debates, held in late 2003 and early 2004, offer a site to examine how legislators understand and value medical evidence while defining the terms of law that regulate bodies, identities, and lives. Throughout this chapter, I will argue that the criteria employed to determine whether an individual should receive a gender recognition certificate opens a space for trans individuals to challenge the authority of medical evidence to define their lived experiences. More specifically, the law's requirement that individuals show that they have been living in their acquired gender for at least two years, are "living in a gender now," and "intend to continue to live in the acquired gender until death" (Gender Recognition Act, Section 2(1)(c)) resists universal, stable, coherent, binary visions of gender articulated by both legal and medical discourses. As such, the Gender Recognition Act recognizes that, like trans people, law and medicine are contingent and transitioning bodies, unable to articulate with absolute authority what it means for a life to be lived in a gender.

Setting the Scene: The Implications of *Corbett* for Trans Law in the United Kingdom

Conceived as a way to offer trans individuals an equal legal status, the Gender Recognition Act ostensibly signals a departure from the standard set in the 1971 case *Corbett v. Corbett*. In this English probate case, the court argued that sex—for legal purposes—would be defined by chromosomal, gonadal, and genital congruency tests. That is, a determination of sex was to be based on an individual's genetic make-up and the appearance of his or her genitals. The sex determined and recorded at birth could not (legally) be changed—even in the event of a surgical intervention that altered the appearance of an individual's genitals. According to this case, the sex assigned at birth is an "historical fact." The practical consequences of this case were devastating for trans people. *Corbett*'s standard affected marriage rights,[3] conditions of imprisonment,[4] pension allocation, succession rights, parental rights, rules governing participation in sporting events, and insurance coverage. Reaching into almost every aspect of daily life, the *Corbett* standard placed trans people's access to rights (and, more generally, their safety and quality of life) in jeopardy.

For scholars and activists, *Corbett* established a dangerous precedent precisely because it over-medicalized the lived experiences and subjectivities of trans people. Employing this logic until 2003, British law could not recognize the demands of trans people because their demands seemed to issue from a subject position that was, in the eyes of the law, impossible. As one trans activist explained,

---

3 The decision in *Corbett* was used in subsequent cases to support a ban on marriages between a male-to-female transsexual and a male, as well as between a female-to-male transsexual and a female. Because these marriages failed to produce "ordinary and complete sexual intercourse," the courts found that marriages involving trans people were not legitimate marriages according to the 1973 Matrimonial Causes Act.

4 Following *Corbett*, individuals who were sentenced for crimes were detained in prisons according to their sex as determined at birth (even if they had undergone sex re-assignment surgery).

> There is a whole generation who had no voice, no language and thus no way of articulating their profound sense of disability .... By defining us as medical objects, as "transsexuals," it denies us our human identity, denies us our individuality and removes from us the reasonable right of any minority community—the right to speak for ourselves. (P. 1996)

Although many trans individuals had challenged the *Corbett* standard in British courts, it was not until the European Court of Human Rights (ECHR) intervened that the Government changed the way they define and regulate sex and gender for legal purposes. The ECHR handed down its decision in *Christine Goodwin v. The United Kingdom* on 11 July 2002. It found that British laws defining sex according to a set of biological criteria applied at birth prevented trans people from enjoying the full spectrum of rights guaranteed by the European Convention of Human Rights. Barring individuals from changing their sex for legal purposes on official documents, such as birth certificates and insurance forms, these laws, according to the court, created discordance between the lived experience of trans individuals—who they present themselves to be—and their legal status—who the law says they are. The ECHR recognized the potential and real harm of this disjunction "between social reality and law" (*Christine Goodwin v. The United Kingdom* 2002, para. 77); left in an "anomalous position," trans people were subject to discrimination and misrecognition without the protection of law. To rectify this injury—the "lack of legal recognition of the gender re-assignment of post-operative transsexuals" (*Christine Goodwin v. United Kingdom* 2002, para. 120)—the ECHR demanded that the United Kingdom change its laws. Responding to their mandate, the British Parliament first issued a draft bill of the Gender Recognition Act on 11 July 2003; it received royal assent on 1 July 2004.

Within this historical context, the introduction of the Gender Recognition Act held out the possibility for trans individuals to speak for themselves and to speak in a way that resists the (bio)logic that the law had employed for 33 years. Following the demands of Press for Change, the United Kingdom's leading organization for the promotion of trans rights, Parliament drafted the Bill in such a way that seemed to eliminate or at least minimize the importance of surgical or hormonal treatment as a condition for gender recognition. Critics have a wide range of opinion about whether and to what extent Parliament succeeded in this task. For some, this provision effectively shifts the legal thinking about sex and gender from a biological, medical, and psychological paradigm to a more open, fluid sense of what it means to "live in" a gender. In this view, the Act has the potential to "interrupt the orthodoxies of gender that law has peddled to a greater extent than any other development in recent times" (Sandland 2005, 44–5). Proponents view this part of the Act not only as a victory for trans rights but a victory over discourses that understand sex and gender to be natural or given binaries. There are those, however, who are suspicious about whether there *is* a shift in legal logic. Sharon Cowan, for one, is particularly concerned with the way in which a binary emerges in the Act's requirement that individuals demonstrate that they are not married or that they have obtained or are in the process of obtaining a divorce. For her, "the UK case law leaves intact not only the sex/gender distinction *per se*, but also the notion that marriage is based on sex (the natural fixed biological body), as opposed to gender (socially constructed masculinity/femininity)" (Cowan 2005, 75). Sharpe extends these claims by pointing out that "a biological understanding of sex persists as an important subtext within the legislation" (2007, 60). He finds this subtext in "a biological understanding of sex for the purposes of comprehending the pre-operative body, the insulation of marriage from the effects of some reform decisions pertaining to other legal subject matters, and judicial anxiety over non-disclosure of gender history prior to a marriage ceremony" (Sharpe 2007, 60). According to Sharpe, then, even in the face of the non-surgery criterion, the law re-inscribes a biological understanding of gender—in many cases an understanding that presumes this biology tells who one "really" is—in the conditions and terms through which trans people receive rights. For both authors, the point is that the Act reproduces and upholds a binary (and biological) vision of sex and gender—ushering in the same logic found in *Corbett* through the back door. They cite the fact that the Act requires individuals to dissolve any existing marriages and the unstated presumptions that "genital surgery functions as a threshold requirement for legal recognition" (Sharpe 2007, 8) to show that, even without a surgery requirement, there remains a gender and/or sex binary that works to guarantee that an individual's identity appears as coherent and stable over time.

Although the stakes of this debate are significant—they speak to whether this practice of legal recognition significantly alters the standing of trans individuals in law—the purpose of this chapter is not to argue whether or to what extent the standard for assessing gender set out by the Gender Recognition Act re-inscribes the anatomical and chromosomal standard delineated by *Corbett*. The parliamentary debates demonstrate that this question might rest on the false presumption that law either wholly defers to or completely rejects medical discourses. In what follows, I argue instead that the parliamentary debates both invoke and critique medical discourses, suggesting that this practice of legal recognition operates to challenge the very norms on which it depends.

The Terms of Debate

To make their case for the Gender Recognition Act, several members of the Labour Party invoked a familiar "right gender/wrong body" narrative to describe the lived experiences of trans people. In this narrative, a trans person's "acquired gender" is cast as his or her "real" gender—a descriptive that suggests there is a truth or a stability to the gender that is acquired. Lynne Jones, one of the most vocal supporters of the Act, argued that transsexual people are "living in the wrong body, and their brain identity [is] different from their chromosomal identity" (HC deb. 23 February 2004, col. 64). To unify an individual's gender identity, then, is to alter the appearance of the "wrong body" so that it reflects the "right gender" known or felt by the individual. Transgenderism is thus figured as a "fix," a way to make the body fit the truth of the person. "Correcting" the body in this way, in the words of parliamentary member Ann Widdecombe, allows "a woman who has lived her life as a woman … [to] change gender to become fully a man" (HC deb. 23 February 2004, col. 52). Within this economy of gender identity, the transition between man and woman is one made without a remainder or excess. A zero-sum game, an individual occupies "fully" the "opposite" gender—trading or exchanging one gender for the other.

Although this narrative is offered in service of passing the Act to grant trans individuals rights they had been denied for years, it does so in a way that seems to re-institute a binary conception of gender. As Cowan argues, the right gender/wrong body narrative "depends on the dichotomous framework of sex and gender in order to make sense of the non-sense of transsexuality" (2005, 72). If this is the case, then recognition seems to be offered to individuals only insofar as they "fit" or conform to certain (dominant) norms of gender. Cowan underscores the way in which such a practice of recognition might strip individuals of their agency rather than bolster it. She argues that transsexual people—and here she is discussing post-operative transsexuals—"are, literally, 'made to fit' within existing sex and gender structures" (2005, 72). Recognition thus serves the dominant norms that define sex and gender. Practically, this means that the gender recognition panels operate to shore up dominant gender structures—structures that depend on the aesthetics of the body—how one (or at least one's genitals) appear.

At the outset of the second reading of the Bill, however, David Lammy, Under-Secretary of State for Parliamentary Affairs, insists that the aesthetics of the body could be neither the referent nor the standard for assessing whether an individual should be offered a gender certificate. According to Lammy, the gender recognition panel must decide instead "whether the person has taken decisive steps to live fully and permanently in their acquired gender" (HC deb. 23 February 2004, col. 53). Lammy explains:

> That must be the test for legal recognition in the acquired gender, not whether the person's physiology fully conforms to the acquired gender and not whether they "look the part." Such tests are inappropriate and inconsistent with our broader ambition to respond to the needs and concerns of a small minority group. (HC deb. 23 February 2004, col. 53)

The criterion for recognition, here, is that one must appear in a gender without having to "look the part." A counter-intuitive claim, this provision, when read closely, suggests that the language of this law makes it possible to re-signify rather than reproduce dominant gender norms that are based on a biological binary. In other words, what Lammy's comment demonstrates is that the state offers recognition to those who appear fully in a particular gendered identity. In this case, however, the parameters or forms of this appearance are not already constituted or given. In the context of the Gender Recognition Act, this means that the practice of recognition determines not only who counts *as* a man or woman—that is, who can take up a defined legal status or lay claim to rights *as* a man or woman—but, also, what it means to *be* a man or woman.

This double task of recognition in which gender norms are created and applied demonstrates that there is an ontological question at stake in this Act that exceeds the problem of finding a set of criteria for determining gender roles. To put it another way, the significant shift that occurs in the Gender Recognition Act might not be the shift from a medicalized view of sex to a cultural construction of gender as some theorists have pointed out. Instead, the shift seems to take place when we stop thinking about gender as a category of knowledge—what we might know about an individual's identity—represented in the "historical fact" of sex at one's birth and begin thinking about gender as a set of practices that condition who we can say we are.

The parliamentary debates enact this shift by demonstrating how this "historical fact" employs a medical discourse of chromosomes and sex that does not provide an authoritative or complete set of criteria for determining who counts as a man or woman in the eyes of the law. This discussion emerges in response to the expressed anxiety of parliamentary members over the loss of what they understand to be a clear indicator of gender identity: a scientific and foundational measure of what constitutes a man or woman. Baroness O'Cathain for one expresses her worry that

> a great deal of difficulty arises. If people say that they have always felt that they wanted to be man [*sic*] and that they will live as such for two years, they can then go to the gender recognition panel and say, "I am a man, please give me recognition. That is the way I feel." (HL deb. 29 January 2004, col. 363)

For O'Cathain as well as parliamentary members who both support and oppose the Bill, the question of whether there are standards or evidence for this judgment of recognition determines whether positive law will be reduced to what Lammy calls a "rubber stamp" (HC deb. 9 March 2004, col. 13). That is, without established criteria for what counts as "living in" a gender not only is there confusion about who can receive a certain legal status, there is great concern that this law no longer has the force to regulate the terms of recognition—the terms that, in this case, name individuals as a man or woman.

For some parliamentary members, the response to this anxiety is to pin down gender in a clear way, to locate an Archimedean point where we might not only see clearly the truth of one's gender but judge it as well. Tim Boswell, a Conservative Party member, hopes to accomplish this task by proposing a "double lock on the system of gender recognition" (HC deb. 9 March 2004, col. 57). An almost literal attempt to confine and limit the legal status of gender, Boswell's proposal targets the make-up of the gender recognition panel. He argues that panels should be formed not only by trained members of the medical and psychiatric community, but also by lay members, family members or lawyers—someone who will bring "an ordered mind to the matter and will also in a sense stand in on behalf of the general public and ensure that doctors … are given some check and balance" (HC deb. 9 March 2004, cols 57–8). The introduction of those with no expertise in the field of transgenderism into the scene of recognition, for Boswell, theoretically works to confine what can and cannot be done within these scenes. Boswell's point is that the panels cannot be trusted; they must be checked by the presence of a third figure who possesses an "ordered mind." Although we might point to the obvious problems of constructing family and lawyers as those with an abstract "ordered mind," Boswell's proposal is interesting, in part, because it demonstrates that, while the law requires individuals seeking recognition to obtain medical documentation in order to come before the panel, the opinion of medical experts within the panel is not given absolute authority. For Boswell, the doctors and psychiatrists do not check or limit recognition practices; instead, they are part of the threat to a stable, coherent gender order.

Medical evidence thus appears, throughout the debate, not as an authoritative source of information, but as a form of knowledge that is contingent and changing—much like society, law, and trans people themselves. Robert Key, a Conservative Party member, pointed out the extent to which the medicalized binary view of sex that the law invokes is, in fact, incomplete and inconsistent with current medical knowledge:

> I had always taken my sex and the sex of others for granted. It all seemed so obvious, but it is not. Perhaps the most enlightening debate in the other place, where the Bill started, took place on 3 February when an amendment to schedule 4 sought to prohibit marriage between two persons each possessing XX chromosomes or each possessing XY chromosomes, or each possessing genitalia appropriate to the same sex. After all, it was argued that that is the undoubted determinant of biological sex, but it is not. What about Turner's syndrome, which affects women with only one X chromosome? Is one X chromosome enough to count as a woman? What of Klinefelter's syndrome, which affects men who have two Xs and a Y? Should they be classified as men or women? (HC deb. 23 February 2004, col. 83)

Key points out that the science of chromosomes—what many take to be the determining factor or ground of gender identity—cannot in every case determine who counts as a woman and who counts as a man. As an inexact form of knowledge, medicine too appears to be in a state of flux. Parliamentary Member Kali Mountford remarks, "Our society is in transition, as, indeed, is our medical profession and this House. And the same is true of some of the people whom we are talking about" (HC deb. 23 February 2004, col. 85). If we draw out the implications of this statement, the analogy between trans people, law, society, and medicine suggests that all are seeking some sort of re-cognition, a way to be understood and make sense as they change over time. As such, none enjoys an absolute authority to define once and for all what constitutes gender.

If we are to understand how law might upset the authority of medical evidence, then this identificatory moment within the debate is critical. It demonstrates that, in the face of a trans individual's demand for recognition, both medical and legal discourses lose their status as "two powerful and privileged discourses" (Sharpe 2002, 8). This is not to say that both are rendered impotent. Rather, both medicine and law, in the context of the Gender Recognition Act, are called into question, asked to explain what they mean and why their explanation is true, good, or right. As the debates show, this question is posed at the level of definition. For many parliamentary members, the terms employed in the language of the Bill and the debates—especially concerning "sex" and "gender"—fail to invoke a clear referent. Unwilling to accept a now commonplace distinction between gender as a cultural construct and sex as a biological characteristic, Parliament turned to the problem of the transitional nature of language itself. Lord Turnberg argues that "It all seems so straightforward and black and white, but unfortunately this is not quite the whole picture. One's sex is only a part of one's gender. It is an important and essential part but not the only part" (HL deb. 29 January 2004, col. 360). The ambiguity of this relation between sex and gender is, according to Lord Filkin, an ambiguity in the terms themselves. He claims, "Our sense of the words 'sex' and 'gender' has changed over time and no doubt will do so in the future. While the meaning of the word 'sex' is not the same as that of 'gender,' the word 'sex' is increasingly in use in ways that go beyond a narrow biological definition" (HL deb. 29 January 2004, col. 366). Understanding language as something that is "mobile" (HL deb. 29 January 2004, col. 365) and "fluid" (HL deb. 29 January 2004, col. 366), Lord Filkin reasoned that there was no sense in debating the specific language as it would undoubtedly change over time (HL deb. 29 January 2004, col. 365). Here, the language of law appears unable to clearly identify the subject of recognition—that is, the person to whom recognition is granted—because this subject does not remain constant over time.

In this context, the gender identity of a trans person exceeds the language of both law and medicine. In other words, the terms employed do not and perhaps cannot render intelligible the identity of the one who demands recognition. The language of the law fails, then, not only to bring about a universal standard for defining gender as in *Corbett*, but also to make sense of an individual's gendered subjectivity in terms that others already understand or with which they already identify. Lord Tebbit, responding to Lord Filkin's "'linguistic relativism,'" illustrates this point quite clearly. He argues that without this standard Parliament is forced to "legislate using words whose meanings we do not understand and which mean different things to different people" (HL deb. 29 January 2004, col. 367). Unable to offer words that clearly define what gender is, Lord Tebbit renders the law silent on this problem. Although he declares that he "find[s] the matter profoundly unsatisfactory," he moves to withdraw the amendment and "move on with the debate on other amendments" (HL deb. 29 February 2004, col. 367). This movement to end the debate on the definition of gender is telling. Acknowledging that Parliament might not be able to define gender once and for all, he defers the question, leaving it to be answered by something or someone outside the law.

Silencing the law on this issue, the linguistic confusion is untenable, according to Tebbit, because ignorance of the meaning of terms could "prejudice life" (HL deb. 29 January 2004, col. 367). A curious phrase, it suggests that the language of law affects (and possibly effects) how we understand and judge life itself. If the terms of life—in this debate, the terms of gender—are contingent, what life is and how law regulates it are called into question.

It is in this way that the Gender Recognition Act's criterion of "living in" a gender unsettles the medical and legal definitions of gendered subjectivity. It is the act of living in a gender—or being alive in it—for which law and medicine fail to account. The debates thus turn us to a question of who gives voice to this life. Who speaks for the subject of recognition? Read literally, the question asks who might bear witness to the transition and lived gender identity (both past, present, and future) of trans people. A question of incredible import in the parliamentary debates, it asks who might provide reliable evidence for the "truth" of a subject's identity as the law's record of this identity, "the historical fact" of one's birth, and medical evidence seem to offer little insight. Thus, while medical evidence is a condition or criteria for a gender recognition certificate, it does not authorize (the truth of) life. By this I mean it is neither the authority that guarantees the truth of the subject nor the discourse that authors the meaning of this life. The question of who gives voice to this life is one that concerns the ways trans people communicate their gendered history to the gender recognition panels in order to receive recognition.

This communicative act in which trans individuals give voice to their life—a speech act addressed to panel members who operate in the name of law—is a paradoxical moment in which gendered subjectivity is both constituted and recognized. By this, I do not mean to suggest that trans individuals define their gender identity apart from medical or legal norms. Instead, it is in the address—we might say more specifically in the demand for recognition—that individuals articulate themselves *to others* in a way that marks this statement as contingent and transitional. That is to say, in this address trans individuals appear as subjects who speak in transition. As Parliamentary Member Kali Mountford explains, "none of us can be absolutely sure of who we are at any point" and, as such, any claim articulated on the basis of or in service of a stable, coherent identity cannot bring about a "sensible and logical conclusion about who we are" (HC deb. 23 February 2004, col. 85). The question of who speaks, therefore, is not answered by thinking about the ways an individual takes up an already established gender position. Rather, the structure of the Gender Recognition Act demonstrates that any attempt to define what it means to live in a gender is created when trans individuals and the members of a gender recognition panel negotiate the meaning of this life at a particular time.

In this framework, two significant points become apparent. First, medicine and law appear as a set of competing discourses through which individuals articulate and negotiate a lived sense of self. Yet, neither captures the way in which gender appears as a set of practices and experiences that change over time. Coming to terms with the contingency of human identity, law, and medicine too are rendered contingent bodies that are, at times, unintelligible and in need of recognition. As Sharpe points out, laws addressing trans identity in the past have viewed "the transgender body as the locus of dissonance, ambiguity and contradiction," however, law itself "more accurately fits that description" (Sharpe 2002, 4). Parliament recognizes the limitation of the Gender Recognition Act and, as such, cedes the law's ability to construct and regulate a universalizable set of gender norms.

Second, and as a result of the first, this act of legal recognition opens spaces in which individuals may challenge the very medical evidence that allows them to demand recognition from the law. Individuals are invited to present evidence from a variety of sources, including utility bills addressed to the individual in his or her new name, letters from family or friends, or personal narratives, to demonstrate that they are living in a gender. These various forms of evidence articulated alongside the medical evidence demonstrate the ways different discourses run under, around, and through the language of law. That is, the debates over what it means to live in a gender suggest that law is not the singular site at which gendered identities are defined and judged. Scholars and legal commentators often misunderstand the way law opens up a space in which individuals might challenge (medical) definitions of gender because they only examine the rule articulated in the law. Cowan, for instance, speaks in terms of "legal regulation": "the legal regulation of sexual identity [does not] acknowledge that there is a spectrum of possibilities of sex/gender, the existence of which confounds the binary sex and gender system" (2005, 72). It is, for her, the principle generated by law that should be read, analysed, and critiqued. Such a reading, however, leaves the language of law intact. That is, it does not address *how* the law defines these terms in the context of other discourses. The effect of this kind of reading is that scholars accept that (positive) law frames the scene of recognition. As the structure in which recognition takes place, the conditions under which law articulates the terms of gender recognition, as well as the way in which these terms affect medical, social, and interpersonal practices are left unexamined.

To read the law for the way it challenges the authority of medical evidence is therefore to understand how the demand for legal recognition emerges in a cycle of demand and response that continuously alters not only what law can say about gendered identity but also how medical professionals treat trans individuals. In other words, the debates show that the Gender Recognition Act is but one discourse that shapes and limits the language in which bodies of law and bodies of subjects come to mean something. Understanding this point, we see that the meaning of gendered identity does not belong solely to legal or medical discourses. It is instead developed over time through various discourses that overlap, agree, compete, and clash with one another. This law, unlike the ones before it, provides a space for this debate to take place and, in doing so, opens the possibility to define the terms of life itself while recognizing that these terms are relational, contingent, and unstable. It is in this scene of recognition that trans individuals might demand rights and resources in terms they make their own.

References

Christine Goodwin v. The United Kingdom, (2002), Application No 28957/95 ECHR, *Press for Change* [website], <http://www.pfc.org.uk/node/350>, accessed 5 August 2006.

Corbett v. Corbett (1970) 2 All ER 33.

Cowan, S. (2005), "'Gender is No Substitute for Sex': A Comparative Human Rights Analysis of the Legal Regulation of Sexual Identity," *Feminist Legal Studies* 13, 67–96.

Feinberg, L. (2001), "Trans Health Crisis: For Us It's Life or Death," *American Journal of Public Health* 91, 897–900.

"Gender Recognition Act," United Kingdom. Parliament. House of Commons. *Parliamentary Debates, Official Report (Hansard)* 6th Series, 418 (23 February 2004).

"Gender Recognition Act," United Kingdom. Parliament. House of Commons. *Parliamentary Debates, Official Report (Hansard)* 6th Series, 418 (9 March 2004).

"Gender Recognition Act," United Kingdom. Parliament. House of Commons. *Parliamentary Debates, Official Report (Hansard)* 6th Series, 418 (11 March 2004).

"Gender Recognition Act," United Kingdom. Parliament. House of Commons. *Parliamentary Debates, Official Report (Hansard)* 6th Series, 418 (16 March 2004).

"Gender Recognition Act," United Kingdom. Parliament. House of Lords. *Parliamentary Debates, Official Report (Hansard)* 6th Series, 415 (18 December 2003).

"Gender Recognition Act," United Kingdom. Parliament. House of Lords. *Parliamentary Debates, Official Report (Hansard)* 6th Series, 416 (13 January 2004).

"Gender Recognition Act," United Kingdom. Parliament. House of Lords. *Parliamentary Debates, Official Report (Hansard)* 6th Series, 416 (14 January 2004).

"Gender Recognition Act," United Kingdom. Parliament. House of Lords. *Parliamentary Debates, Official Report (Hansard)* 6th Series, 417 (29 January 2004).

"Gender Recognition Act," United Kingdom. Parliament. House of Lords. *Parliamentary Debates, Official Report (Hansard)* 6th Series, 417 (3 February 2004).

"Gender Recognition Act," United Kingdom. Parliament. House of Lords. *Parliamentary Debates, Official Report (Hansard)* 6th Series, 417 (10 February 2004).

Hausman, B.L. (1995), *Changing Sex: Transsexualism, Technology, and the Idea of Gender* (Durham, NC: Duke University Press).

P. (1996), “Living Truth: P Tells Her Story,” *Press for Change* [website], <http://www.pfc.org.uk/node/367>, accessed 26 September 2006.
Roen, K. (2002), “‘Either/Or’ and ‘Both/Neither’: Discursive Tension in Transgender Politics,” *Signs* 27:2, 501–22.
Sandland, R. (2005), “Feminism and the Gender Recognition Act 2004,” *Feminist Legal Studies* 13, 43–66.
Sharpe, A. (2002), *Transgender Jurisprudence: Dysphoric Bodies of Law* (London: Cavendish).
Sharpe, A. (2007), “Endless Sex: The Gender Recognition Act 2004 and the Persistence of a Legal Category,” *Feminist Legal Studies* 15, 57–84.
Spade, D. (2006), “Mutilating Gender,” in S. Stryker and S. Whittle (eds), *The Transgender Studies Reader* (New York: Routledge).
United Kingdom. Parliament, House of Lords, 2003–04 Sess. *Gender Recognition Act*. As introduced 28 November 2003.

Chapter 10
Journeys of Choice? Abortion, Travel, and Women's Autonomy

Christabelle Sethna and Marion Doull

Introduction

On 28 January 1988, the Supreme Court of Canada in *R. v. Morgentaler* struck down the country's abortion law as contrary to the *Charter of Rights and Freedoms*. The court ruled that the law violated a woman's security of person not only by forcing her to carry a foetus to term under threat of criminal sanction, but also by causing lengthy delays in obtaining an abortion, thereby increasing her risk of physical and psychological harm. The Crown had argued that women who had difficulty procuring a legal abortion in their home communities could travel to access pregnancy termination elsewhere. Yet in rendering the decision of the majority, Chief Justice Brian Dickson countered that the law, which invested only hospital-based Therapeutic Abortion Committees (TACs) with the power to grant a legal abortion based on their assessment of the threat the continuation of the pregnancy posed to the life or health of the pregnant woman, burdened women unduly. He recognized that as a result of the law, many women were forced to travel, often at enormous emotional and financial expense, to seek abortion services in other jurisdictions.[1]

In the 20 years since the Morgentaler decision, there has been no federal law regulating abortion in Canada. Now abortion is purportedly fully funded under the *Canada Health Act* as a "medically necessary" service. Abortion services are available domestically in public sector hospitals as well as in private and public sector for-profit and non-profit clinics. Dr Henry Morgentaler, the figure at the centre of *R. v. Morgentaler*, has even received the Order of Canada for his services to women and leadership in civil liberties (CBC 2008). Understandably, the case is celebrated as enshrining the right of Canadian women to choose to have an abortion. Nevertheless, abortion services exist today as a "patchwork quilt with

1 With Justice Lamer, Dickson stated: "The argument that women facing difficulties in obtaining abortions at home can simply travel elsewhere would not be especially troubling if those difficulties were not in large measure created by the procedural requirements of s. 251. The evidence established convincingly that it is the law itself which in many ways prevents access to local therapeutic abortion facilities." See *R. v. Morgentaler*, [1988] 1.S.C.R.30, p.7.

many holes" (Eggertson 2001). Consequently, many Canadian women continue to travel for abortion services. While there is no doubt that some women want to journey away from their home communities for an abortion in order to protect their anonymity, the geographical distance to abortion services remains one of the major barriers to abortion access. Indeed, there is international evidence to indicate that the further a woman has to go to for an abortion the less likely she is to obtain one and the more likely she is to be young and underprivileged (Henshaw 1991; Wiebe 2008).

Although a stream of reports has identified a steady diminution of public sector hospital abortion services across the country (Shaw 2006), there have been few investigations of the role abortion clinics currently play in providing women with the choice to terminate their pregnancies. Defined commonly as having "the power, right or liberty to choose an option" (The Free Dictionary 2008), "choice" remains the battle cry of pro-choice activists seeking to safeguard abortion access. Nevertheless, some critics, such as American historian Rickie Solinger, suggest that choice is a poor substitute for rights (Solinger 2001). Others contend that by using the language of choice, women are lulled into believing that their rights to abortion are secure. Thus, women remain silent when those choices are infringed upon and become implicated in their own oppression (Baker 2008).

As the first step in the development of a cross-Canada research project focused on tracking women's travel to abortion clinics, the authors conducted a pilot study. The study tested a questionnaire intended to gather information from women who journeyed for abortion services to the Toronto Morgentaler Clinic (TMC) in 2006 (Sethna and Doull 2007). In this chapter, the data from the pilot study are used to examine whether standard bioethical conditions of individual autonomy may be applied to the respondents. According to the bioethics discourse, an individual seeking health services makes decisions believed to be autonomous if he or she:

1. is deemed to be sufficiently competent (rational) to make the decision at issue;
2. makes a (reasonable) choice from a set of available options;
3. has adequate information and understanding about the available choices;
4. is free from explicit coercion toward (or away from) one of these options. (Sherwin 1998, 26–9)

However, as these standard conditions are limited by the very structural systems within which they are exercised, the concept of choice may be criticized as unstable and highly dependent upon the circumstances of the choice maker (Baker 2008). Abortion is a controversial issue that challenges any universal application of bioethics (Hedayat 2007). Consequently, each of the aforementioned conditions will be evaluated within the context of women's access to abortion services at the TMC in order to determine whether there exists a distinction between women's presumed autonomous right to choose and their actual ability to exercise that choice autonomously.

The Pilot Study

The TMC is a well-known abortion clinic that first opened in 1983. It is based in mid-town Toronto, Canada's largest and most multicultural city, located in the province of Ontario. The clinic is a non-profit, licensed facility, fully funded by the province. It is one of seven non-profit and for-profit abortion clinics operating alongside a number of public sector hospitals that also provide abortion services in and around the Greater Toronto Area (GTA). Women with an Ontario Health Insurance Plan (OHIP) card do not pay for abortion services performed at the clinic. Women from outside Ontario may or may not pay and may or may not be reimbursed according to the regulations of the health insurance plan effective in their home province. The TMC usually requires one appointment that includes a counselling session, an ultrasound, a medical examination, and the abortion itself. It provides detailed post-abortion instructions and recommends that women have their own doctors perform a medical check-up two to three weeks after the abortion. If need be, the TMC will supply the name of a physician near the women's place of residence who could perform this check-up.[2]

Acting upon the advice of TMC staff and an Advisory Committee consisting of medical personnel, pro-choice groups, and women's health advocates, the authors developed a questionnaire for women seeking abortion services at the TMC. The questionnaire sought demographic, logistical, and experiential data on respondents' travel. At the end of the questionnaire, an open-ended section encouraged the respondents to write more detailed notes evaluating their journeys to the TMC.[3] The questionnaire was distributed twice, each time over two consecutive months in 2006. After the first distribution period ended, the questionnaire was revised to gather more precise information. In total 1,256 original and revised questionnaires were distributed. A total of 81 per cent of these questionnaires were completed and returned, representing a very high response rate. This response rate indicates a major interest in the study and, perhaps, a desire by the women to tell their abortion stories in a culture that shrouds the experience of abortion in silence and stigma (Cochran 2008).

Demographically, 54 per cent (the majority of the respondents) were between the ages of 21 and 30, 56 per cent were partnered, and 51 per cent were employed full-time. Despite the latter statistic, 68 per cent of the respondents earned less than \$30,000 annually, while almost 30 per cent earned less than \$10,000.[4] Immigrants to Canada constituted 28 per cent of the entire sample. When asked to self-identify ethnic background, 56 per cent said they were White/Caucasian, with another 8 per cent claiming European ancestry. Thirteen per cent self-identified as having Black,

2 Such details are available on the TMC's website. See <http://www.morgentaler.ca/abortion.asp>, accessed 7 May 2007.

3 The questionnaire and research methodology were approved by the University of Ottawa Ethics Board (file #01–60–07).

4 All dollar figures in this chapter are Canadian dollars.

African or Caribbean heritage and 7 per cent as South Asian. Women citing Asian, South American, biracial, First Nations/Métis or Middle-Eastern backgrounds ranged over 3 to 5 per cent. Most of the respondents were Canadian born (70 per cent), spoke English at home (90 per cent), and had a high school (40 per cent) or university/college (38 per cent) education.

Eighty-two per cent of the respondents contacted the TMC as their first choice. The clinic's good reputation was cited as the main reason at 40 per cent. It was followed by a doctor's referral at 29 per cent, knowing someone who had already been to the clinic at 24 per cent, and proximity of clinic to place of residence at 19 per cent. Additional reasons offered less often included previous visit(s) to the TMC; no extra fees charged; inadequate services at other clinics or hospitals; imposition of gestational limits at other clinics or hospitals; lack of confidentiality at other clinics or hospitals; and satisfaction with the TMC's safeguards against anti-abortion activists as compared to other clinics.

The minority of women (19 per cent) who first contacted other clinics or hospitals for abortion services found that timely appointments were unavailable at these facilities (34 per cent), the abortion fees were prohibitive (18 per cent), safeguards against anti-abortion activists were inadequate (15 per cent), staff were rude (13 per cent), and that the other facility contacted was located too far from their place of residence (10 per cent). Hand-written comments overwhelmingly expressed frustration with the inability to obtain an appointment at the facility they first contacted within a gestationally-sensitive timeframe: "Couldn't get an appointment for 3 weeks and that would have been too late"; "It was too long to have the abortion. It was not done on the first visit and the first visit was over 3 hours"; "Small city, the procedure takes weeks between family doctor, ultrasound, pre-op, op. 4 weeks. I am too sick/too busy to deal with morning sickness for another month"; "The appointment wasn't immediate in [city of residence]"; "Too far along when doctor comes. Only comes to my town [to perform abortions] once a month"; "They needed an initial exam on one day and then the procedure would be on another day, so 2 days would be lost from work and travel cost doubled"; "There were three separate days, it was very confusing, unlike Morgentaler clinic which was very helpful."

Approximately 74 per cent of the respondents travelled one or more hours to the TMC from their place of residence. The other 26 per cent needed less than half an hour to reach the clinic, reflecting the fact that women who live in or near the GTA have ready access to abortion services. However, women earning less than $30,000 annually were more likely to have travelled the longest distances, anywhere from 200 km to over 1,000 km. Over 60 per cent of the respondents made their way to the clinic in a car driven by a companion. The next most popular mode of transportation was a city or regional bus, taken by 16 per cent of the respondents. Although TMC instructions insist that women do not drive themselves to or from their abortion appointments, nearly 12 per cent of the respondents indicated they drove themselves. The remaining respondents took a taxi, a train, a streetcar, an airplane, or simply walked.

Travel costs were impossible to pin down accurately because just under half of the respondents did not give out any such information. As well, some reported costs for their one-way journey to the clinic while others detailed expenses for a return trip. Approximately 90 per cent reported spending less than $50 on transportation to and from the clinic. Nearly 20 per cent said they spent nothing. Almost 10 per cent reported spending more than $50 to over $100. When overnight accommodation was necessary, the majority of women (94 per cent) recorded paying nothing; however, the majority of those who did pay, paid more than $100. When travel costs were tabulated, they varied greatly: "$150 for gas"; "$20.92 Greyhound [bus] one way"; "$300 to buy a return flight ticket to Toronto"; "$2.50 for the bus and $2.50 for the train"; "$84.36 x 2, have to get back home"; "3 nights hotel downtown Toronto $2,000"; "$4,445.05 for 3 nights." One respondent indicated that she "couldn't find a motel, got in too late, had to sleep in the car." Another commented that she rented "a hotel room for two days so I could check in right after the procedure. I got a room last night so I wouldn't have to wait until 4pm to check in. I will stay overnight as to wait out the anaesthetic so I can drive home after the suggested 12 hours." Some respondents had additional costs because they travelled with a companion: "Me and my boyfriend paid $208 to get here on the bus." Additional costs extended to child-care, phone calls, meals, loss of wages (often for travel companions as well), and parking.

Twelve per cent of the sample agreed that their journey was "difficult" or "very difficult"; respondents under 30 years of age were more likely to say so. Travel to the TMC was found to be difficult because of the length of the journey, the total costs incurred, the mode of transportation or the physiological discomfort involved: "It was hard because of the cost and also, it's a six hour bus ride"; "It is almost four hours travel time total"; "It takes a long time especially in rush hour go back. Feeling nausea it's worse to travel by car, more discomfort, pricey as well." Occasionally the difficulties were related to emotional conflicts associated with the journey: "Expensive, emotional, do not like traffic, very nervous, leaving other children at home"; "I was lonely. I had a headache. I feel hungry and hate travelling alone"; "I have one more credit at [school] to complete … but I am 26 and I feel like the timing is not right although I am getting older."

Eighty-eight per cent of the respondents believed that their journey was "easy" or "very easy" because, for example, they "just followed the directions [provided by the clinic]," because "someone drove them," because the clinic was "close to home," or because "a friend had been there before." Nevertheless, many of these responses could easily have been categorized as "difficult" or "very difficult." One respondent stated, "We travelled all night, so there wasn't much traffic, went by fast." Another said that the journey was "easy because I wasn't really thinking about the [abortion] procedure, but rather worried about the distance, traffic, and getting here on time. No time to worry." Still others reported that the journey was "expensive, I don't have the money," or that it was "easy, other than the distance 100+ km." Such responses could be attributed to the possibility that these respondents assessed the journey mainly in terms of logistical ease: "Before

I left [city of residence] I mapped all my routes out and estimated the amount of time it would take. I memorized the maps and found my way to the clinic easily." Others included an emotional point of view which complicated their assessment of the journey: "I mean easy as in it took 20 min. with a cab, but in my head I was thinking about what I was gonna go through so that wasn't easy." In some cases, the women claimed that the journey was "easy" because they were content with the decision to abort: "I am making the right decision."

Abortion, Travel, and Autonomy

As stated earlier, the bioethics discourse holds that in order for an individual to be deemed an autonomous subject, capable of exercising choice, four standard conditions must be met. Each of these conditions of autonomy is now evaluated in the context of the respondents' travel to the TMC. This evaluation considers the historical and current limits on Canadian women's putative right to choose.

Condition (1): Being a Competent (Rational) Decision-Maker

The respondents made decisions about whether or not to carry a pregnancy to term within structural systems that work *against* an unfettered choice to have an abortion (Sherwin 1992). Women have not been treated traditionally as competent decision-makers, especially in regard to laws pertaining to the regulation of reproduction. "For too long," notes legal scholar Joanna N. Erdman, "the mere physical fact of pregnancy—the unique capacity to reproduce—justified the discriminatory treatment of women" (2007, 1155). Abortions used to be performed as a back-up method of birth control by the woman herself or by physicians or by non-medical personnel. However, in the late nineteenth century, the Canadian government joined Britain and the United States to outlaw the sale, dissemination, and advertisement of birth control. Penalties for providing or procuring an abortion included incarceration. The law permitted abortions to save the life of the mother, leading some non-Catholic hospitals to strike TACs composed of physicians who would rule whether or not to grant a woman an abortion. Fearful of legal consequences, many doctors refused to perform any abortions (Jenson 1992; McLaren 1986).

The practice was driven underground. While most women survived their abortions, many others died from sepsis. Beginning in the 1960s, women who could afford the expense went to countries with more liberal abortion laws; Canadian women travelled to the United States, England, and to Japan (see for instance: Sethna forthcoming). The federal government under Prime Minister Pierre Trudeau passed Criminal Code reforms in 1969. These reforms decriminalized contraception, homosexual acts between consenting adult men, and legalized abortion. Ironically, the new abortion law made access a convoluted and lengthy procedure. Canadian women had to have a doctor's referral to a TAC, a TAC could only be established at accredited hospitals, no hospital was obligated to strike a TAC, and those hospitals that did were located in the larger cities. Furthermore, TACs were at liberty to interpret the "health" criterion the law set forth as they wished, resulting in arbitrary decision-making. Although the new abortion law was intended to alleviate the problem of illegal abortion, it failed. It also did not succeed in curtailing Canadian women's travel to abortion services in other jurisdictions. Indeed, in the 1970s abortion referral agencies burgeoned into a cross-border business, luring Canadian women who could afford to travel to pay for quick, safe, and legal abortions in the United States (Badgley et al. 1977).

As Kathleen McDonnell (1982) has stated, the legalization of abortion did not win women the "right" to abortion. Feminists, pro-choice activists, students, lawyers, physicians, clergy, and laypersons who did believe that abortion was a reproductive right women should be able to exercise without criminal sanction, increasingly opposed the new abortion law. Their figurehead was Morgentaler, a physician who openly performed abortions in his Montreal clinic before the Criminal Code reforms of 1969 took effect. Despite imprisonment and numerous legal battles, Morgentaler opened the TMC in 1983 and another clinic in Winnipeg that same year. Clinic abortions contravened the requirement that only a TAC in an accredited hospital could grant an abortion. Repeated attacks on the validity of the law eventually reached the Supreme Court, culminating in the victorious Morgentaler decision of 1988.

Given these shifts in the abortion law, the decision of the respondents to have an abortion cannot be viewed as an exercise in autonomy because abortion has been and still is perceived as intrinsically related to societal concerns about women, men, sexuality, the foetus, and the state (Hewson 2007). Attempts to unpack such relationships in constructive ways are, even today, stymied by the ongoing dearth of official attention paid to women's reproductive healthcare needs in federal and provincial health policy and health systems research. For example, the *Romanow Report*, upheld as the most comprehensive review of healthcare in Canada to date, acknowledges its own failure to "discuss the critical role reproductive health services, such as fertility control, abortion access, the prevention and treatment of sexually transmitted infections and maternity care play in primary health care for women" (Romanow 2002). Neither does the *Report* approach gender as a social determinant of health. It does consider geography to be a social determinant of health, suggesting that Canadians who live in rural or remote locales are disadvantaged because of the travel distance to a healthcare provider. However, by not taking gender into account, the *Romanow Report* misses an important opportunity to investigate just how women's reproductive healthcare needs may be compromised by the very same geographical factors that negatively affect populations living in rural or remote areas (National Coordinating Group on Health Care Reform and Women 2003).

Condition (2): Making a (Reasonable) Choice from a Set of Available Options

Once the respondents made a decision to have an abortion, they were faced with accessing abortion services. The act of making a choice implies that an individual has options from which to choose. Yet in regard to abortion services, the options available to a number of the respondents were limited. The minority of respondents who contacted other hospitals or clinics before they contacted the TMC, discovered that access to abortion services was a challenge primarily because of the other facility's inability to set up an appointment within a gestationally-sensitive timeframe and, secondarily, because of the prohibitive fees the other facility charged for an abortion.

From the beginning, the TMC served as an important "site and symbol of resistance" to the 1969 abortion law (Rebick 2008). Today it is said to provide a medically necessary service. The Canada Health Act governs all health services delivered by a physician or within a hospital setting in Canada. Decisions regarding what is and is not funded as a medically necessary service are made by the provincial and federal governments in collaboration with the governing body for physicians in Canada. Clinics have traditionally been excluded from this funding arrangement due to the "hospital" restriction in the Act. In some Canadian provinces abortion clinics are an exception to this rule. Private health services usually disadvantage women because they are less able to pay for them. Still, abortion clinics like the TMC, especially if they are provincially funded, have given women an important healthcare alternative (Rodgers 2006).

Such an alternative is all the more important given the documented diminution of access to abortion services in public sector hospitals. The 1969 legislation mandated that only hospital-based TACs could grant a legal abortion. Yet the *Badgley Report* (1977), the first comprehensive study on abortion access since the passage of the abortion law, found that only 20.1 per cent of all public sector hospitals performed abortions. Since then, pro-choice organizations as well as various government bodies have released their own findings. The Canadian Abortion Rights Action League, also known by its acronym, CARAL (2003), established that the 20.1 per cent figure first recorded in the *Badgley Report* had fallen to 17.8 per cent. On behalf of Canadians for Choice (CFC), Jessica Shaw (2006) asserted that only 15.9 per cent of Canadian hospitals offer abortion services, representing an even further drop in access in just three years. Moreover, women in rural areas and the Maritimes are underserved; no hospitals on Prince Edward Island perform abortions, whereas in the large cities of Toronto, Vancouver, and Montreal women have access to several major hospitals when seeking abortion services (Badgley et al. 1977; CARAL 1998; 2003; Shaw 2006).

The decrease in the availability of abortion services in public sector hospitals has contributed to a rise in the establishment of abortion clinics across the country. To date, there are approximately 25 clinics scattered from coast to coast. Despite their existence, abortion access remains uneven for the following reasons. Some provinces' reciprocal billing agreements may exclude abortion, whether it is performed in the public or private sector, as a medically necessary service under the Canada Health Act. Other provincial governments refuse to fund abortions performed outside hospitals. Like hospitals, most abortion clinics can be found in larger urban centres as opposed to rural areas or the Maritime provinces. There exists little or no training in abortion techniques in medical schools. Ageing and retirement have shrunk the pool of available abortion providers (CARAL 1998; 2003; Shaw 2006).

Under such circumstances, some of the respondents may have had no choice but to travel to the TMC because the clinic was able to provide abortion services in a timely manner and charged no prohibitive fees. Notably, those respondents who reported the lowest incomes also reported travelling the farthest to the clinic. Yet even when a lengthy journey, physiological and emotional discomfort, logistical worries, and financial expenses for accommodation, child-care, parking, and lost wages for themselves and for a travel companion were involved, some of the respondents were still willing to identify their travel to the TMC as very easy or easy. For many respondents, travel to a reputable clinic that offers women a timely abortion appointment at no additional fee outweighed the considerable inconveniences they experienced.

Condition (3): Has Adequate Information and Understanding of the Available Choices

The responsibility for gathering information about physicians, clinics, hospitals, appointments, fees, travel, and accommodation, and making the necessary arrangements belonged to the respondent. This responsibility would be all the more difficult to exercise should the respondent be a new immigrant or have language difficulties or be unable to communicate directly with a physician, clinic, or hospital. In spite of the recognition that access to safe, legal, timely, and cost-efficient abortion services is a key aspect of reproductive and sexual health and gender equity that can reduce maternal mortality substantially (WHO 2004), abortion services do not always meet the needs of women. Information about abortion services in a wide range of languages is lacking. Moreover, deliberate failure to provide women seeking accurate information about abortion services is commonplace.

One 1992 study outlining the limits on access to abortion services in public sector hospitals in the Canadian Northwest Territories detailed practices that showed rampant disregard for women seeking abortions, especially when these women were Aboriginal. Women were not provided with adequate information about the abortion procedure, their options for anaesthesia or about post-abortion care (Government of the Northwest Territories 1992). Shaw provided further evidence of the lack of information women across the country continue to receive regarding abortion services. In addition to travel distance, two of the key barriers to abortion access in public sector hospitals as outlined in her CFC report are "unknowledgeable hospital staff members" and "judgmental gatekeepers" (2006). She found that staff answering phones at 41 per cent of the hospitals contacted did not know if abortions were offered at their hospital and did not know to whom to transfer the call in order to obtain this information. Shaw discovered that in some cases not only was the staff member (the first point of contact for a woman seeking assistance) unaware of the abortion services available but he or she was unwilling to assist the caller in getting this information. In fact, Shaw, posing as a young woman deliberating whether or not to have an abortion, was hung-up on, laughed at, told that no one would want to speak to her about abortion and was deliberately misled about the health effects of having an abortion.

Moreover, staff pointedly directed her to anti-abortion agencies (Shaw 2006). These agencies, known as Crisis Pregnancy Centres (CPCs) in Canada, often operate in the vicinity of clinics and hospitals providing abortion services. Well-funded by fundamentalist Christian organizations with links to the right-wing anti-abortion movement in the United States, CPCs actively conduct a disinformation campaign. They counsel women by giving out graphic information about the supposed negative health effects of abortion: breast cancer, infertility, substance abuse, eating disorders, suicide, and depression. Significantly, these organizations, which have an anti-abortion, anti-gay, anti-feminist, anti-contraception, and anti-sex education agenda have co-opted the language of choice and rights to proclaim that women have a right to control their own bodies. Carrying to term a God-given precious life in the form of a foetus is, therefore, framed as the best choice they can make (Johansen 2004).

Condition (4): Having Freedom from Explicit Coercion

Some of the respondents claimed they chose the TMC because of the its safeguards against anti-abortion activists. Others decided against going to another facility because they determined that the safeguards were inadequate. The respondents were no doubt aware that both abortion providers and abortion facilities have been targeted for violence. Morgentaler was physically assaulted and has received many death threats. The TMC itself was the target of two fire bombings, the first in 1983 and the second in 1992. For the safety and security of staff and patients, the TMC has an unobtrusive appearance, a video surveillance system, a locked front door, and security guards. Entrance to the TMC is possible only when the intake officer verifies the photo identification and the appointment of every visitor from behind a bullet-proof glass window.

Violence on the part of anti-abortion activists is an explicit coercive practice that can intimidate women into carrying a pregnancy to term. However, coercive practices can also be implicit. Partners, friends, and family can dissuade a woman from having an abortion. Anti-abortion billboards, websites, pamphlets, and leaflets designed to sway public opinion can spread disinformation about foetal development, the negative health effects of abortion, as well as practices and laws related to abortion. Doctors can refuse to provide information on, or referrals for, an abortion. Pharmacists can resist dispensing the morning-after pill. Anti-abortion activists can harass women entering hospitals or clinics offering abortion services. Provincial governments can make getting an abortion an obstacle course. For example, the province of New Brunswick pays for abortions only if they are approved by two obstetricians or gynaecologists and are performed in a hospital. Accessing abortion services under such conditions is very difficult even for the most resourced woman (Cooke 2008; Rodgers and Downie 2006).

In Canada, attempts to de-list abortion as a medically necessary service, to elect anti-abortion members of government, or to recriminalize abortion are popular tactics of anti-abortion activists (Pro-choice Action Network 2004; Rankin 2004; Sallot 2004). Short of rescinding *Roe v. Wade*, the landmark 1973 American Supreme Court decision that protects abortion as a constitutional right, keeping abortion legal but under ever narrowing conditions is a favourite legislative strategy of anti-abortion activists in the United States. Various states have enacted laws that limit women's right to choose. Some states require mandatory pre-abortion counselling that may include disinformation that the foetus may feel pain during the procedure. Others demand parental consent for minors wanting abortions, insist on prosecution of adults accompanying minors out of state to obtain abortion services, and threaten with incarceration doctors who perform late term, or what has come to be known as "partial birth abortions" (Abrams 2004; Planned Parenthood 2004; Reuters 2003; Sonfield 2004; Taylor 2004; The White House 2002).

More than 30 American states have also passed laws that categorize the murder of a pregnant woman as a double homicide, thereby giving the life of the woman and that of the foetus equal legal weight. Canadian private member's legislation, Bill C-484, also known as the Unborn Victims of Crime Act, makes it a criminal offence to harm the foetus of a pregnant woman subjected to violence. Opponents argue that if Bill C-484 is passed, it could be used to accord legal status to the foetus. By technically granting "personhood" to the foetus, pro-choice activists believe that the legislation will be used to prosecute pregnant women seeking abortions in addition to those doctors performing them. As the American experience shows, such laws do not protect women against violence. Rather, they can result in punitive "policing of pregnant women" especially for illegal drug consumption believed to cause the death of the foetus (National Advocates for Pregnant Women 2008). When faced with the possibility of a federal election, Prime Minister Stephen Harper's government dropped Bill C-484 because of the criticism it has generated, notably from the Canadian Medical Association. In an apparent compromise, the government promised to introduce new legislation that will punish violence against pregnant women but without introducing the spectre of foetal rights (Fenlon 2008).

Autonomy, Travel, and Inequality

Susan Sherwin rightly acknowledges that each of the four standard conditions characteristic of the bioethics discourse discussed above "is more problematic than is generally recognized" (1998) when it comes to disadvantaged populations in society. If women are considered to be a disadvantaged population, then access to abortion services, particularly for marginalized women, inevitably complicates the question of women's autonomy even further. As critics have articulated, "choosing" is never completely autonomous in situations of inequality (Baker 2008).

Widespread concern about women's travel to access abortion services is largely absent from fierce national debates about wait times for domestic health services. Indeed, travel to access health services, popularly labelled "medical tourism," is not exclusive to abortion. The mainstream media have been filled with accounts of Canadians who have to or choose to travel abroad to India, Thailand, Malaysia, and Mexico, often paying personally for private sector health services like hip replacements, dental surgery, experimental cancer remedies, organ transplants, and general diagnostics, rather than face lengthy wait times for treatment in the public sector at home (CBC 2004). Medical tourism brokers emphasize that as a healthcare consumer, Canadians have the autonomy to make a choice.[5] Herein, choice is situated within a neoliberal market perspective. Like other forms of exploitative tourism, medical tourism can illustrate a unidirectional privilege because only those with economic resources can take advantage of health services offered at competitive prices, timelines, and conditions (Nowicka 2007).

Whereas some Canadians travel for elective procedures, others journey for more urgent care. The choices made by the latter may resonate with the experiences of pregnant women who have to or choose to travel for an abortion. Nevertheless, travel to access abortion services is a unique type of medical tourism. Abortion is exclusive to women, involves an extremely sensitive timeframe, resists interpretation as a solely medical procedure, and, unlike the vast majority of health services, is regularly the subject of ethical controversy. Moreover, Canadian women's travel to access abortion services has a direct relationship to gender, race, and class inequalities. By contrast, overseas health services located chiefly in developing countries, allow Canadians who travel to these locations to exercise choices underpinned by class and/or race privileges within a complex system of globalized disparity (Eggertson 2006; Hutchison 2005).

Conclusion

Given the ongoing difficulties accessing abortion services, legal abortion rights can appear somewhat of a hollow achievement (Palley 2006). "Choice," while perhaps a shakier substitute for rights, is still preferable to no choice at all. However, women, healthcare professionals, governments, and policymakers need to recognize that the barriers placed in the way of women's ability to exercise that choice autonomously

5 For examples of web advertisements for medical tourism brokers in Canada, see for instance: <www.timelymedical.ca> and <www.medsolution.com>, accessed 14 July 2008.

is, in fact, restrictive of women's rights. As Solinger clearly articulates: "I am convinced that choice is a remarkably unstable, undependable foundation for guaranteeing women's control over their own bodies, their reproductive lives, their motherhood, and ultimately their status as full citizens" (2001, 7).

Women who travel for abortion services give the lie to standard conditions of individual autonomy according to bioethics discourse. The combination of women's inequality in society and uneven access to abortion services makes the realization of women's autonomy difficult and the exercise of choice impossible in some cases. Interestingly, in their assessments of their journeys to the TMC, the respondents to the questionnaire in the pilot study did not express misgivings about their decision to travel. Even when travel resulted in myriad inconveniences, it was neither problematized nor politicized. It may be that the respondents counted themselves fortunate because they managed to access abortion services after all; indeed, there was no way in the pilot study to account for the responses of those women who were unable to journey to the TMC for an abortion because of the barriers they undoubtedly encountered.

Furthermore, the marginalized status of the respondents represented in the questionnaire—the younger respondents, the respondents from lower-income brackets, the immigrant respondents, and non-English-speaking respondents—may help explain just why there exists such a lack of official attention paid to women's reproductive healthcare needs in federal and provincial health policy and health systems research. Conversely, the noticeably high 81 per cent overall response rate to the questionnaire may indicate that women seeking abortions do wish to have their experience of abortion made known to the public but in circumstances that ensure them a fair measure of respect, security, and privacy.

Some progress has been made provincially to support Canadian women's choice to have an abortion as evidenced by recent legal decisions. The Supreme Court of the province of Manitoba has ruled that women who had abortions at the province's private clinics because they could not obtain a timely appointment for an abortion in the public health sector should be reimbursed for their expenses. A similar ruling was rendered by the Québec Supreme Court. It ordered the Québec government to reimburse 45,000 women who were charged extra fees between 1999 and 2005 for provincially-funded abortion services at a total of 13 million dollars. Both courts ruled that women's rights under Canada's Charter of Rights and Freedoms were violated because they were forced to pay for a medically necessary service under the Canada Health Act (Bourque 2006; CBC 2004).

These victories, as in the Morgentaler case, cannot be the end of the story. A false sense of autonomy hides the fact that Canadian women's right to choose remains seriously limited. Canada's vast geography and east-west, north-south, and urban-rural divides mean that travel to access health services for many individuals will remain a necessity for the foreseeable future. However, provincial and federal governments must work together to ensure that access to abortion services is legally protected, available in a timely fashion, and financially feasible for every woman who seeks them in this country.

Acknowledgements

The authors would like to thank the director and staff at the Toronto Morgentaler Clinic for their cooperation as well as the Advisory Committee members for their assistance. Marion Doull is funded by a doctoral scholarship from the Institute of Gender and Health at the Canadian Institutes for Health Research. Funding for this research was provided by the Faculty of Health Sciences, the University of Ottawa and the Social Sciences and Humanities Research Council of Canada.

References

Abrams, J. (2004), "Conservatives Win Big with Fetus Bill," *Associated Press* [website], (published online 26 March 2004), <http://story.news.yahoo.com/news?tmpl=story&u=/ap/20040326/ap_on_go_co/fetus_rights>, accessed 31 March 2004.

Badgley, R.F. et al. (1977), *Committee on the Operation of the Abortion Law* (Ottawa: Minister of Supply and Services Canada).

Baker, J. (2008), "The Ideology of Choice. Overstating Progress and Hiding Injustice in the Lives of Young Women: Findings from a Study in North Queensland, Australia," *Women's Studies International Forum* 31, 53–64.

Bourque, O. (2006), "Quebec Told to Reimburse Women for Abortions," *Globe and Mail*, 19 August 2006.

CARAL (1998), *Access Granted: Too Often Denied* (Ottawa: Canadian Abortion Rights Action League).

CARAL (2003), *Freedom of Choice: Protecting Abortion Rights in Canada* (Ottawa: Canadian Abortion Rights Action League).

CBC (2004), "Medical Tourism: Need Surgery, Will Travel," *CBC News Online* [website], (published online 18 June 2004) <http://www.cbc.ca/news/background/healthcare/medicaltourism.html>, accessed 13 July 2008.

CBC (2007), "Manitoba Must Pay for Private Abortion Judge Rules," *CBC News Online* [website], (published online 24 December 2004) <http://www.cbc.ca/canada/story/2004/12/24/abortion-041224.html>, accessed 7 May 2007.

CBC (2008), "Ontario Premier Supports Honours for Morgentaler," *CBC News* [website], (published online 8 July 2008) <http://www.cbc.ca/canada/story/2008/07/08/morgentaler-order.html?ref=rss>, accessed 13 July 2008.

Cochran, C. (2008), "Why Not Just Talk About It?" *Globe and Mail*, 19 July 2008.

Cooke, P. (2008), "Why Is a Pro-Choice Canada so Important?" *Voices for Choice* 2:1 (Special Edition).

Eggertson, L. (2001), "Abortion Services in Canada: A Patchwork Quilt with Many Holes," *Canadian Medical Association Journal* 164:6, 847–9.

Eggertson, L. (2006), "Wait-Weary Canadians Seek Treatment Abroad," *Canadian Medical Association Journal* 179:9, 1247.

Erdman, J.N. (2007), "In the Back Alleys of Health Care: Abortion, Equality and Community in Canada," *Emory Law Journal* 56, 1155.

Fenlon, B. (2008), "Tories Abandon 'Unborn Victims' Bill," *Globe and Mail* [website], (published online 25 August 2008), <http://www.theglobeandmail.com/servlet/story/RTGAM.20080825.wnicholson0825/BNStory/National/home>, accessed 26 August 2008.

The Free Dictionary (2008), *Definition of Choice* [website], <www.thefreedictionary.com>, accessed 27 May 2008.

Government of the Northwest Territories (1992), *Report of the Abortion Services Review Committee* (Northwest Territories: Government of the Northwest Territories).

Hedayat, K.M. (2007), "The Possibility of a Universal Declaration of Biomedical Ethics," *Journal of Medical Ethics* 33, 17–20.

Henshaw, S.K. (1991), "The Accessibility of Abortion Services in the United States," *Family Planning Perspectives* 23:6, 246–52.

Hewson, B. (2007), "Reproductive Autonomy and the Ethics of Abortion," *Journal of Medical Ethics* 27, suppl. II, ii10–ii14.

Hutchison, J. (2005), "Sun, Surf and Surgery," *Reader's Diges*t (November), 124–31.

Jenson, J. (1992), "Getting to *Morgentaler*: From One Representation to Another," in J. Brodie et al. (eds), *The Politics of Abortion* (Toronto: Oxford University Press).

Johansen, S. (2004), "Who Are the Crisis Pregnancy Centres?" *Pro-Choice Press* [website], (spring/summer 2004) <http://www.prochoiceactionnetwork-canada.org/articles/who-are-cpcs.shtml>, accessed 13 July 2008.

Lewis, C. (2008), "Fetal Rights Stir Debate on Abortion," *National Post*, 1 March 2008.

McDonnell, K. (1982), "Claim No Easy Victories: The Fight for Reproductive Rights," in Maureen Fitzgerald et al. (eds), *Still Ain't Satisfied* (Toronto: Women's Press).

McLaren, A. and McLaren, A.T. (1986), *The Bedroom and the State: The Changing Practices and Politics of Contraception and Abortion in Canada, 1880–1980* (Toronto: McClelland and Stewart).

National Advocates for Pregnant Women (2008), *Lessons from the U.S. Experience with Unborn Victims of Violence Laws* [website], (published online April 2008) <http://www.arcc-cdac.ca/action/LessonsfromUS.pdf>, accessed 30 June 2008.

National Coordinating Group on Health Care Reform and Women (2003), *Reading Romanow: The Implications of the Final Report of The Commission on the Future of Health Care in Canada for Women* (Toronto: National Coordinating Group on Health Care Reform and Women).

Nowicka, P. (2007), *The No-Nonsense Guide to Tourism* (Toronto: New Internationalist Publications).

Palley, H.A. (2006), "Canadian Abortion Policy: National Policy and the Impact of Federalism and Political Implementation on Access to Services," *Publius: The Journal of Federalism* 36:4, 565–86.

Planned Parenthood Federation of America (2004), "Press Release: Federal Abortion Ban Struck Down in Court, Judge in Planned Parenthood Lawsuit Declares Dangerous Law Unconstitutional," 1 June 2004.

Pro-Choice Action Network (2004), "Press Release: Conservative Party Can't Hide Their Anti-Abortion Agenda," [website], <www.prochoiceactionnetwork-canada.org>.

Rankin, D. (2004), "Editorial: Canada Needs Informed Consent Law on Abortion: Fundamental Principle of Patient Care Women Need Complete Information When Making Reproductive Choices," *The Montreal Gazette*, 16 May 2004, A13.

Rebick, J. (2008), "Celebrating the 20th Anniversary of the Morgentaler Decision," Oral Presentation, in *Event to Commemorate 20th Anniversary of Morgentaler Decision*, 28 January 2008, Canadians for Choice, Ottawa.

Reuters (2003), "House Passes Ban on Abortion Procedure," <www.medscape.com/viewarticle/456786>, accessed 18 June 2003.

Rodgers, S. (2006), "Abortion Denied: Bearing the Limits of the Law," in C. Flood (ed.), *Just Medicare: What's In, What's Out, How We Decide* (Toronto: University of Toronto Press).

Rodgers, S. and Downie, J. (2006), "Abortion: Ensuring Access," *Canadian Medical Association Journal* 175:1, 9.

Romanow, R. (2002), *Building on Values: The Future of Health Care in Canada* (Ottawa: Government of Canada).

Sallot, J. (2004), "Abortion Creeps Back on to the Political Agenda," *Globe and Mail*, 2 June 2004, A4.

Sethna, C. (forthcoming), "All Aboard? Canadian Women's Abortion Tourism, 1960–1980," in Cheryl Krasnick Warsh (ed.), *Women's Health History in North America, 1800–2000* (Waterloo, ON: Wilfred Laurier University Press).

Sethna, C. and Doull, M. (2007), "Far from Home? A Pilot Study Tracking Women's Journeys to a Canadian Abortion Clinic," *Journal of Obstetrics and Gynaecology Canada* (August), 640–47.

Shaw, J. (2006), *Reality Check: A Close Look at Accessing Abortion Services in Canadian Hospitals* (Ottawa: Canadians for Choice).

Sherwin, S. (1992), "Abortion," in S. Sherwin (ed.), *No Longer Patient: Feminist Ethics and Health Care* (Philadelphia, PA: Temple University Press).

Sherwin, S. (1998), "A Relational Approach to Autonomy in Health Care," in S. Sherwin (coordinator), *The Politics of Women's Health: Exploring Agency and Autonomy* (Philadelphia, PA: Temple University Press).

Solinger, R. (2001), *Beggars and Choosers: How the Politics of Choice Shapes Adoption, Abortion and Welfare in the United States* (New York: Hill and Wang).

Sonfield, A. (2004), "New Refusal Clause Shatter Balance Between Provider 'Conscience,' Patient Needs," *The Guttmacher Report on Public Policy* 7:3, <http://www.guttmacher.org/pubs/tgr/07/3/gr070301.html>.

Taylor, D. (2004), "Does a Foetus Have More Rights Than Its Mother?" *The Guardian*, 23 April 2004.

The White House (2002), "National Sanctity of Human Life Day 2002: Press Release," *White House: Office of the Press Secretary* [website], (published 18 January 2002) <www.whitehouse.gov/news/releases/2002/01/20020112-10.html>, accessed 27 January 2003.

Wiebe, L. (2008), "The Abortion Puzzle: It's Been Legal for 20 Years, But Getting One Remains a Challenge," *Winnipeg Free Press*, 27 January 2008.

World Health Organization (2004), "Sexual Health—A New Focus for WHO," *Progress in Reproductive Health Research* 67, 1–8.

PART IV
Cultural Interventions

Chapter 11
The Code of Ethics in Medicine: Intertextuality and Meaning in Plato's *Sophist* and Hippocrates' *Oath*

Twyla Gibson

Introduction

Technological advances in medicine and biology raise profound ethical questions about the nature and potential of human beings. Bioengineering, pharmacology, cloning, genetic engineering, enhancement technologies, and other body and brain modifications hold the possibility of changing the species (Parens 1998). While many point to the benefits of technology, anti-technology activists and critical social theorists of science and technology are deeply concerned that interfering with nature will cause irreparable harm (Young 2000, 407–10). Finding a way to work through the moral issues and ethical dilemmas presented by new technologies is an urgent priority for parties on all sides of this debate. The problem is particularly pressing because the bioethical principles of autonomy, beneficence, non-maleficence, and justice (see Beauchamp and Childress 2009) have proven to be an overly simplistic framework for dealing with complex ethical issues emerging from the intersection of technology and medicine (Keenan 1999, 104–20). Scholars are therefore returning to the Hippocratic tradition in an effort to shed new light on the philosophical underpinnings of ethics in healthcare (Miles 2004; Takala 2001, 72–7).

Given that so many ethical dilemmas in biomedical technology today are unprecedented, it is fair to ask, why continue to investigate the ethical code of an ancient society so different from our own? What justification is there for continuing to research a tradition that many view as an anachronism that should be set aside? (Carrick 2001, xix).

I begin by formulating a response to this question concerning the relevance of the *Oath* to the history of medicine and to current and emerging problems in medical ethics. I also point to the complexity and virtuosity of the *Oath*, and argue that this work is worthy of study in its own right. I then describe some of the issues that have until recently stood in the way of new analyses of the *Oath* and explain how these barriers impact current meaning-making and interpretation. I note that the earliest surviving references to Hippocrates occur in Plato's dialogues (*Phaedrus* 270c; *Protagoras* 311b), and describe recent advances in the study of intertextuality—the comparative investigation of connections among texts from different collections and traditions—that are revolutionizing our understanding of the origins and influence of significant works of ancient literature. I develop a set of criteria for identifying connections between Hippocrates and Plato by drawing upon media and information theory to adapt the principles devised by researchers working on intertextuality in other ancient Greek collections. Next, I turn to Plato's *Sophist*, a dialogue that explains the procedure for distinguishing multiple sequences of classifications that make up the different branches of the definition of art or technique (*technē*). I delineate the topics in the definition of the Merchant of Learning, and then use this Platonic sequence as a template for comparing the organization of topics and ideas in the *Oath*. I show that the sequential order of topics in the *Oath* corresponds point by point to the serial order of the topics in the various classifications of the definition explained in Plato's *Sophist*. The presence in the *Oath* of the same sequence described in Plato makes it possible to line up the classifications in the two works and to cross-reference and compare information in corresponding categories. Cross-referencing of topics and ideas allows us to bring information presented in Plato to bear on the interpretation of the *Oath*. This new information provides the resources for dealing with issues of interpretation that have gone unresolved due to lack of evidence concerning the meaning and context of words and ideas. The discovery of connections between Plato and Hippocrates adds to our understanding of the meanings communicated in the *Oath* by linking the Greek medical tradition to the wider context of ancient thought and expression. This broadened context sheds new light on the foundations of Western medical ethics and provides the evidence and insights needed to reconstruct and reassess the history of our ethical tradition. It is my argument that the expanded horizons of meaning gained though the study of intertextual connections among Hippocratic and Platonic texts and traditions provides a rich resource for reevaluating the history of Western medical ethics, and for defending and critiquing the possibilities entailed by biomedical technologies today.

Hippocrates' *Oath*, Bioethics, and Analytic Philosophy

Turning to the question of why we should continue to investigate the Hippocratic *Oath* and tradition, I would point out that confidence in physician's ethics among the general public today stems from a widespread impression that doctors have sworn the Hippocratic *Oath*. Even among "the educated public," many still "profess an almost reverential admiration for the ethical teachings of Hippocrates" (Carrick 2001, xx). However, the views held by many members of these publics are frequently at odds with major tenets of the *Oath* that proscribe abortion, euthanasia, and even surgery (ibid.). This gap between public perception and fact indicates that additional research and public education concerning the Hippocratic ethic and tradition is warranted.

In addition, Hippocrates' *Oath* was the template for all subsequent revisions to codes of medical ethics (Jonsen 1998; Orr et al. 1997). To understand and re-envision contemporary professional ethics, we must look to the long history of amendments and updates to the ethical code—all of which owe a debt to the Hippocratic *Oath* and tradition. Again, these facts highlight the centrality of the *Oath* to our tradition of ethics in medicine and indicate that continued research is justified.

In contrast with the millennia-long history of the Hippocratic code of ethics, both the field of bioethics, and the four principles it espouses in popular versions of principlism, are recently manufactured constructions. Bioethics is a new discipline that was formed to study the moral dimensions of issues in healthcare. Though bioethicists bring a variety of ethical methodologies to bear on problems, the field relies primarily on the intellectual tools associated with analytic philosophy. In his review of John H. Evans's *Playing God: Human Genetic Engineering and the Rationalization of Public Bioethical Debate*, Robert Baker (2002) compares this work with two other books that trace the origin, growth, and success of the discipline. He describes how differing accounts all emphasize the same phenomena as being central to the development of North American bioethics: the research scandals that took place in the 1970s; the investigations and commissions created to address them; and the designation of philosophers to the commissions. David Rothman's *Strangers at the Bedside* (1991), claims that as physicians became more powerful and concentrated on technology, they also became estranged from their patients and hence "strangers at the bedside." His account is consistent with the argument of Albert Jonsen (1998), who describes the expansion of biomedical technology controlled by scientific and medical elites that were unresponsive to requests for accountability from patients and public funding sources. Those public bodies reacted by supporting a new field—bioethics—which had the aim of holding scientific and medical establishments accountable to the values and priorities of patients and the public. As a consequence, philosophers—previously strangers to the bedside—moved into the social space formerly occupied by physicians. The end result was that the discourses of medicine and theology were displaced by a new bioethical discourse dominated by the argument forms and discourse styles derived from analytic philosophy (Baker 2002, 65–9).

Not surprisingly, the movement of bioethicists into a position of authority over physicians touched off a crisis in the medical profession. The current "revival of interest in medical ethics … in medical history, the Hippocratic corpus" and various other kinds of literature is an indication that "physicians are reexamining the foundations of medicine and what it is that gives meaning to medicine" (Young 2000, 407–10). This crisis has coincided with mounting concerns about the professionalism of physicians (Connelly 2003, 178–83; Doukas 2003, 147–54; Kuczewski 2003, 144–5). The central issue is how to reevaluate and update the Hippocratic ethic in light of current issues and new technological developments.

Analytic philosophy is not suited to this task of reassessing the principles of Hippocratic ethics and the history of revisions to its code. For analytic philosophy is self-designated as an anti-historical, epistemologically-based approach to research. Thus, the analytic approach to bioethics is by definition not equipped to deal with questions of interpretation that emerge from the historical roots of medicine. Nor is it an appropriate tool for investigating the way medical codes of ethics have developed over time. Indeed, analytic method gives priority to argumentative form over context, even though context often has a crucial bearing on the persuasiveness of an argument. For these reasons, a new generation of philosophers—including many who trained at analytically oriented schools—have questioned this ahistorical way of doing philosophy. These thinkers are now actively challenging the analytic approach that has dominated the discipline (Romano 2003).

In contrast to the imposition of recently formulated terms and principles by Anglo-American analytic philosophers, a number of Continental philosophers have turned to the ancient Greek tradition in order to rediscover the original character of philosophy and to re-conceive the Western tradition as a whole (Zuckert 1996, 2). Continental theorists maintain that revitalizing our traditions of meaning surrounding moral choices in order to think differently about our ethics and values entails going back to the beginning, learning from the ancient source texts that ground our traditions, and adopting and adapting these insights to imagine new terms and possibilities.

The Hippocratic *Oath* in Historical and Cultural Context

Until recently, however, there has been a significant barrier to new interpretation of the *Oath*. Little direct evidence has survived concerning its origins and authority, its connection to the seventy-odd other works in the *Corpus Hippocraticum*, its relation to other ancient collections, or its influence on the history of ancient medicine (Carrick 2001, 78–9). Since the first references to Hippocrates appear in Plato's dialogues, we do know that by 400 BCE, Hippocrates the Asclepiad was regarded as the paradigm of the physician (Jones [1923] in Hippocrates 1995, xii). Otherwise, the record of the early history of the *Oath* "is nearly blank." It is "this lack of context for the *Oath* [that] greatly complicates any effort to understand its meaning" (Miles 2004).

However, significant breakthroughs over the last decade—both in our technologies for analyzing texts and other media, as well as in the comparative and interdisciplinary research on intertextuality—have opened new avenues for interpreting and understanding ancient writings. Media and information theory have advanced the study of the organization and representation of information in texts, art, and artefacts. New techniques of intertextuality have provided ways of gaining access to the meanings ancient texts held for the cultures and societies that produced them, and for re-conceiving their history and influence. The term "intertextuality" (first coined by Julia Kristeva in 1966) has come to be used in a variety of ways to describe the relationship of a text to other writings dated to the same or earlier time periods. Intertextuality "has given new life to the old search for sources" by "radically" shifting the emphasis from reconstructing sources out of a single book to connecting entire books with other extant writings (Brody et al. 2006, 4–5). Major progress has been made on the intertextual relations between Homer's epics and Old and New Testament narratives, for example. The works of Mary Douglas (2007) and Dennis R. MacDonald (2003) are representative of this research. Douglas brings together a number of studies showing that ancient texts from different traditions are all organized into ordered sequences of topics using techniques such as "parallelism." She explains how sequencing of information functioned as a "framing device" or "code" for communicating meaning. She points out that neither the sequencing of information nor the communication purpose served by these patterns has been recognized in the modern period, and argues that antique texts from around the world must be reassessed and reinterpreted. Similarly, serial patterning of topics is a major component in MacDonald's studies of repetition and influence among Homer, New Testament narratives, and Plato's dialogues. Arguing for important connections among traditions previously considered distinct, he too asserts that ancient texts must be reinterpreted. Along with MacDonald, a handful of studies have identified in Plato's dialogues the ordered arrangement of topics associated with parallelism (Brumbaugh 1989, 17–22; Notomi 1999, 39–42; Pritzl 1999, 60–83; Thesleff 1999, 143). Studies have also identified parallel sequences in the Hippocratic collection (Garcia 1995; van Groningen 1960). However, these studies have not recognized the communication purpose of serial patterning. Nor has there been any systematic effort to connect sequencing in Plato's philosophy with the sequences in the Hippocratic texts, even though the texts manifest the same organizing patterns, Plato is the earliest and closest source to reference Hippocrates, and the dialogues align themselves with that venerable medical tradition. In what follows, I begin to make these connections.

Order and Repetition: The Organization and Representation of Information in Ancient Texts

Scholars working on intertextuality have argued that repeating sequences have been overlooked because modern readers approach ancient writings with a radically different "cultural competence from those for whom they were written" (MacDonald 2003, 2). The first step to reassessment and new interpretation, they maintain, involves explicitly identifying the rules that shape the organization of information in ancient treatises. In this section, I develop the criteria most relevant to spotting comparable sequences in Plato and Hippocrates. I rely on media and information theory to refine the principles and techniques developed through comparative work on other ancient Greek texts and traditions. I concentrate on two fundamental principles governing the organization and representation of information in ancient texts and other media: order and repetition.

Order

The ordering of information in ancient literature manifests in a number of different sequential patterns. The first criterion for identifying sequences is the presence in a text of certain formula *types* which involve a fixed progression of words and details that proceeds from beginning to end treating each stage in a nearly identical order, for example, A-B-C-D (Parry 1971, 357). *Themes* are defined as "groups of *ideas* regularly used … in the formulaic style" (Lord 1964, 68). Whereas *types* entail identical words and phrases, the *theme* is not limited to exact word-for-word repetition. Thematic progressions involve instances of one or more reiterations of a chain of events, acts, or objects. Every journey, for instance, reiterates a consistent order in the formal and ideational sequence of (A) loading; (B) embarking; (C) disembarking; and (D) unloading of ships, i.e., A-B-C-D. Though the wording changes in different passages, thematic progressions duplicate a consistent series of topics (*topoi*, literally "places") and forms, ideas, appearances (*ideas*). *Parallelism* is a more complex thematic form that involves the duplicate ordering of sequences in an A-B-C-A*-B*-C* pattern (the asterisk represents a repeated idea) where there is a step-by-step progression of topics after which the series is repeated in identical order. The repetition establishes a relation of meaning between parallel places in the series, i.e., A and A*.

Repetition

The organization of information in texts is consistent with a fundamental principle governing representation in Greek art and iconography of the Archaic period (600–480 BCE): *repetition*. Homer's *Iliad* and *Odyssey*, for example, manifest highly conventionalized formulaic sequences typical of visual representation in black- and red-figure Athenian vases (Steiner 2007, 5; Whitman 1958, 249–84). Thus, media theory may be employed to compare the principles governing the organization and representation of information in ancient writings with the conventions governing representation in another medium of the same time period. Based on the premise that information theory can be applied to "any system in which a 'message' can be sent from one place to another" (Steiner 2007, 11), scholars have applied information theory to a comparative analysis of ideational repetition in texts and visual repetition of images and motifs on vases. Both "verbal and visual messages are expressed through codes—languages" and messages conform "to the rules of the code" (ibid.). Since disorder, high entropy, and therefore noncommunication is the natural state, information theory identifies repetition or redundancy as the fundamental mechanism separating messages from noise, and order from disorder, in a communication system. Repetition is "more than a formal aesthetic principle; it is an enabler of communication" (ibid.) that is central to the code employed by ancient Greek painters, poets, and writers. Repetition constructs meaning, reduces ambiguity, eliminates alternative interpretations, and decreases transmission errors in the communication of messages.

Further, repetition over a number of different texts and across different media through time typically leads to the creation of certain conventionalized ways for expressing information, a kind of language of representation that is shared and understood by people living in a society as part of the core of their cultural competence. A number of devices serve this representational code. *Antonymy* refers to instances where topics and motifs are presented as polarities, as with day and night; *synonymy* is created by "reiteration," a cohesive device that involves not exact repetition, but the substitution of a related item that has equivalence of meaning; *ellipsis* is something left unsaid or not depicted that the listener or reader must fill in themselves. Whereas in synonymy something equivalent is placed in a position, in other cases the place is left empty. Viewers or readers must possess a high level of cultural competence in the "signs" of the conventionalized language, so they know the standard formula well enough to notice when something has been omitted.

Thus images on particular vessels and ideas in specific texts belong to a wider cultural context. Any one representation resonates with a host of related connotations that proliferate in the culture during a time period, so that ideas, images, and texts are interconnected in a repertory that has a cumulative cultural meaning that exceeds any particular example. In comparative research, it is the density of the parallels between the model text and the one under examination that determines the strength of the connection. I will be using the ordering and repetition of information as the major criteria for examining intertextual connections between Plato and Hippocrates.

On my reading, repetition of traditional formulas such as types, themes, and parallelisms were conventions that served as an expressive language for a wide range of compositions and media in Greek culture during the late Archaic period. If information in prose texts participates in the same artistic principles and conventions as poetry and vase painting of the era, then it should be possible to detect the presence of similar sequences, as latent organizing patterns, in passages from different works that deal with the same topics, ideas, and themes. In other words, if different texts composed by way of this conventionalized language discuss similar notions, we should anticipate finding similar sequential formulas related to those particular subjects as an underlying organizational matrix in the discourse. The Hippocratic *Oath* conforms to the standard, three-part pattern for all oaths sworn in Greek culture during this time frame: there is a promise for future action; there is an invocation to "powers greater than oneself" as witnesses; and there is a curse which the swearer calls upon him- or herself in the event that the promise is broken (Sommerstein 2007, 2). Given that the *Oath* conforms to the patterned format followed by all oaths in this era, we should anticipate that it is organized in accordance with other conventions associated with prose compositions as well. In the next section, I demonstrate, through the comparison of sequences in Plato and in the *Oath*, that this expectation is satisfied.

Plato's Definitions

Plato's *Sophist* offers explicit instructions for distinguishing the topics and ideas in a number of different definitions that make up the overall definition of the arts as well as guidelines for using the definitions to create discourse. The value of these instructions in the *Sophist* is that they provide an accurate account of the order and arrangement of topics and ideas so the definitions presented in this dialogue can serve as a basis for comparison with the sequence of ideas in the Hippocratic *Oath*.

It is my argument that Hippocrates' *Oath* is a discourse of extraordinary virtuosity and complexity created by twining together at least seven of the definitions described in Plato's *Sophist*, including the sequences of divisions of Acquisition and Production pertaining to the Hunter (219b–223a); the Merchant of Learning (223c–224c); the Retail Dealer (224d–e); Purification (226b–231c); and Imitation (265a–268c). It is not possible to explain in this study how all these different definitions manifest in the *Oath*. Here, I am only able to hint at the *Oath*'s complexity by tracing one of these definitions.

The series for the Merchant of Learning is most relevant to the professional ethics of physicians, nurses, and other healthcare practitioners because it deals with exchanges of money for professional services; with teaching knowledge of arts and technologies to appropriate students; with nourishments and remedies for the body as well as treatments for ailments of the soul; and with wrong-doing that stems from errors or a lack of knowledge as distinct from wrong-doing that results from an intention to do harm. The Merchant definition therefore holds the most potential as a basis for meaning-making and interpretation of contemporary ethical issues and concerns at the intersection of technology and medicine.

Accordingly, I begin by delineating the topics in Plato's definition of the Merchant of Learning. Next, I use this series as a template for viewing the organization of information in the *Oath*, showing how it manifests a sequence of topics that corresponds point by point to the serial order of ideas in Plato's definition of the Merchant. This exercise demonstrates the density of the parallels between the two discourses. Recognition of a repeating sequential order is preliminary to identifying the wider range of meanings and associations communicated by the conventions that give shape to these two ancient texts. Comparison of the order of topics in Plato with the corresponding divisions in the *Oath* makes it possible to line up the sequences and to index and cross-reference information.

I present this material in English translation. Since this study examines a thematic sequence rather than a type, this pattern does not rely on verbatim repetition, but rather, on repetition of a series of ideas. However, when there are some keywords common to both the instructions for the definition in Plato's *Sophist* and the text of Hippocrates' *Oath*, I have indicated these keywords in transliterated ancient Greek.

Initial instructions for the definition of the Merchant of Learning are given at *Sophist* 223c–224c. The sequence is then repeated two more times, at 224d, and after that, at 224e, so it is presented three times in total. In Table 11.1, I map the statements in this passage into a parallelism, using ***boldface italics*** to designate the classes in the series and *regular italics* to indicate the ideas in the text that correspond to these topics. The instructions for making the divisions that separate the topics and ideas are fairly straightforward. For example, the directions for dividing *exchange* are "And of the *art* of *exchange* there are two divisions, the one of *giving* and the other of *selling*" (*Soph.* 224c). I have indicated this information in shortened form as "*exchange* ÷ *giving* + *selling*." In addition, the dialogue states outright that in spelling out the definitions, parts have been omitted and that few sequences are "comprehensive in all details" (*Soph.* 235c). With this warning, learners are instructed to attend closely to the procedure, to note consistencies and departures from this routine, and to use the information that is given and the patterns that are demonstrated to figure-out the missing pieces for themselves. Where ellipses occur in the discourse, I have noted these absences by way of square brackets [ ]. Finally, when the dialogue mentions new topics and ideas when it reiterates the series, and these topics and ideas were not mentioned in the previously given instructions for the divisions, I have indentified this new information by underlining.

Let us turn now to the definition of the Merchant of Learning in Plato's *Sophist* (see Table 11.1).

The definition of the Merchant is presented by way of a triple parallelism; the initial series and the two repetitions all have the same shape based on reiteration of a sequence of 18 classifications. The second and third renditions of the series frequently paraphrase rather than present a verbatim repetition of words, so this series satisfies the criterion for a thematic sequence. In addition, the two reiterations manifest many ellipses even as they provide confirmation of a number of classes in the initial series. According to information theory, ellipses in any one of the three series may be filled-in through comparison with the other two series to build up a composite picture of the definition. For example, the first repetition at 224d reiterates key classes from the initial sequence and adds new information that was not mentioned previously (i.e., part of the class that *serves the soul* is "*concerned with words*"). Similarly, both the initial series and the first repetition move from *art* directly to *acquisition*. However, new information is added when the series is reiterated for a third time. Apparently, retailers and merchants may be in the business of *making* as well as buying, selling, bartering, and giving as ways of acquiring goods. The appearance of a topic for which there was no overt reference in the first and second presentations of the sequence allows us to identify an ellipsis in the series and to fill-in this empty slot with *production* of wares (*Soph.* 219b–e), a topic that was described earlier in the dialogue as entailing an *art* that "brings into existence something that did not exist before"—through *making*—and this class includes "the care and tendence of mortal creatures" (*Soph.* 219a–b). Thus *production* comes after *art* and before *acquisition* in the order of the divisions. Putting together the information from all three repetitions of the series for the Merchant of Learning builds an amalgam of this thematic parallelism, clarifying ambiguities and reducing errors in the transmission of information (see Table 11.2).

Table 11.1 The definition of the art of the Merchant of Learning in Plato's *Sophist* 223c–224c

A	***art***: Let us take another branch of his genealogy, for he is a professor of a great and many-sided *art* (*technēs*).
B	[ ] …
C	***acquisition***: There were two sorts of *acquisitive art*—the one the division of *hunting* the other of *exchange*.
D	***hunting***: [ ]
E	***exchange***: And of the *art of exchange* there are two divisions,
F	***giving***: the one of *giving* gifts …
G	***selling***: the other of *selling*. Next, the art of exchange by *selling* is divided into two parts.
H	***one's own productions***: one part which is distinguished as the *sale of a man's own productions*;
I	***the work of others***: and another, which is the *exchange of the works of others*. The part of *exchange* …
J	***retail***: *which takes place in the city*, being about half of the whole, is *retailing*. And the one which …
K	***merchant***: *exchanges goods of one city for those of another by selling and buying is the merchant.*
L	***serves the body***: *The merchant* is of two kinds, part serves the body (*sōma*) for its support and needs …
M	***serves the soul***: and part serves the soul, which includes the liberal arts, music, and painting.
N	***play***: Things that affect the soul are divided into a part that is imported and sold for entertainment and …
O	***serious***: a part for its serious needs. This merchandising in *knowledge* (*mathēmatopōlikēis)* is …
P	***other kinds of knowledge***: divided into the sale of *knowledge* (*mathēmata*) of the other arts …
Q	***knowledge of virtue***: and that which has to do with *virtue*. And so this trader in *virtue* …
R	***sophist***: again turns out to be our friend the sophist …
First Repetition	
A*	***art***: Let us summarize the matter by saying that sophistry has appeared a second time as …
B*	[ ] …
C*	***acquisition***: that part of *acquisitive* art …
D*	***exchange***: through that art of *exchange*,
E*	***hunting***: [ ]
F*	***giving***: [ ]
G*	***selling***: of trafficking …
H*	***one's own productions***: [ ]
I*	***the work of others***: [ ]
J*	***retail***: *trade* …
K*	***merchant***: of *merchandising* …
L*	***serves the body***: [ ]
M*	***serves the soul***: of soul-merchandising …
N*	***play***: [ ]
O*	***serious***: which deals in words and knowledge (*mathēmata*) …
P*	***other kinds of knowledge***: [ ]
Q*	***knowledge of virtue***: and the knowledge (*mathēmata*) of virtue …
R*	***sophist***: [ ]
Second Repetition	
A**	***art***: But there is a third case: a man may settle in a city and …
B**	***production***: make his living by selling wares of *knowledge* (*mathēmata*), buying some and *making others himself.*
C**	***acquisition***: Then also that part of *acquisitive art* …
D**	***exchange***: which proceeds by *exchange* …
E**	***hunting***: [ ]
F**	***giving***: [ ]
G**	***selling***: and by *sale* …
H**	***one's own productions***: *of one's own productions*;
I**	***the work of others***: [ ]
J**	***retail***: or as mere *retail* trade, as the case may be, so long as it is the class …
K**	***merchant***: of *merchandising* …
L**	***serves the body***: [ ]
M**	***serves the soul***: [ ]
N**	***play***: [ ]
O**	***serious***: specifically, merchandising in *knowledge* (*mathēmatopōlikon*) …
P**	***knowledge of virtue***: [ ]
Q**	***other kinds of knowledge***: [ ]
R**	***sophist***: you would again term sophistry?

Table 11.2 Composite of the definition of the Merchant of Learning based on three repetitions

A	***art***: art ÷ into productive + acquisitive …
B	***productive***: he may settle in a city and *fabricate* as well as buy these same wares, intending to live by selling them …
C	***acquisitive***: *acquisitive art* ÷ exchange + conquest …
D	***exchange***: *exchange* ÷ conquest + fighting …
E	{*conquest* ÷ fighting +} ***hunting*** …
F	***giving***: one giving and the other …
G	***selling***: selling. The art of selling is divided into two parts,
H	***one's own productions***: the sale of *a man's own productions*;
I	***the work of others***: or exchange of the work of *others*, as the case may be …
J	***retail***: the part of exchange which takes place in the city, being about half of the whole, is termed retailing …
K	***merchant***: the part which exchanges goods of one city for those of another is exchange of the merchant …
L	***food for the body***: *the merchant* is of two kinds, *food for the body* (÷ meat + drinks); and …
M	***food of the soul***: *food of the soul* (music, painting, marionette playing), part is concerned with speech …
N	***play***: and is either for instruction or amusement. One part is termed the art of display + another part …
O	***serious instruction***: is serious instruction which buys + sells learning + knowledge; it has two names …
P	***sale of knowledge of virtue***: one is concerned with speech and the knowledge of virtue,
Q	***sale of other kinds of knowledge***: and the other with the sale of other kinds of knowledge …
R	***sophist***: the trader of a knowledge of virtue is the Sophist.

Table 11.3 The sequence for the definition of the Merchant of Learning in Hippocrates' *Oath*

A	***art***: [ ]
B	***productive***: I *swear by Apollo Physician*, by Asclepius, by Health, by Panacea and by all the gods and goddesses …
C	***acquisitive***: I will carry out … this oath … to hold my *teacher* in this *art* (*technēn*) equal to my parents; to make him …
D	***exchange***: *partner in my livelihood; when he is in need of money to share mine with him; to consider his family* …
E	***hunting***: [ ]
F	***giving***: *as my own brothers, to teach them this art (technēn) if they want to learn* (*mathēsios*) it, *without fee* …
G	***selling***: *or indenture*;
H	***own productions***: *to impart precept, oral and other instruction to my sons, the sons of my teacher*, and to …
I	***the work of others***: *indentured pupils* (*mathētēisi*) who have taken the physician's oath, but to nobody else.
J	***retail***: I will use *treatment* to help the sick according to my ability and judgment, but never with a view …
K	***merchant***: to injury and wrong-doing. … I will help the sick, and abstain from all intentional wrong-doing …
L	***food for the body***: and harm, from abusing the bodies (*somatōn*) of man or woman, bond or free. And …
M	***food of the soul***: whatsoever I see or *hear* in the course of my profession, or outside my profession …
N	***play***: in my *intercourse with men*, if it be what should not be published abroad,
O	***serious***: I will *never divulge, holding such things to be holy secrets*.
P	***knowledge of virtue***: If I carry out this oath, and break it not, *may I gain reputation among men* …
Q	***other kinds of knowledge***: for *my life* and for my *art* (*technēs*);
R	***sophist***: but if I *transgress* it and *forswear* myself, may *the opposite* befall me.

After all three reiterations, we are now in a position to use the Merchant of Learning definition as a template for comparing the sequential order of information in the *Oath*. If both Plato's *Sophist* and the *Oath* conform to the same set of conventions and rules, we should be able to predict the presence in the *Oath* of a sequence of topics that moves in a series through the *art* of *production* to *acquisition* to *exchange*, from *exchange* to *giving* and *selling* one's own productions or those of others in the city or between cities, consisting of goods *for the body* and *of the soul*, the latter of which is concerned with *serious* instruction that involves merchandising *knowledge*. Examination of the shift in topics in the *Oath* demonstrates that the underlying sequence of ideas conforms to this pattern (see Table 11.3).

This first part of the *Oath* deals with the *production* of knowledge of medicine, the *acquisition of knowledge* of this *art* from a teacher, the circumstances under which physicians should provide instruction without fees, and the terms under which they may charge for their teaching. Accordingly, the discourse moves progressively through the classifications for *art*, *production*, *acquisition*, and *exchange* for both *giving* and *selling* forms of knowledge. Whereas the *Sophist* identifies and makes explicit a number of classifications surrounding any one sequence, the *Oath*, by contrast, only touches on those topics that are directly relevant to the ethics of charging fees for the provision of medical training. The parts of the series that do not pertain are passed over in silence. Hence, there is no mention of the class dealing with play, amusements, and entertainments, for the discussion in the *Oath* concerns only the *serious* pursuit of *knowledge*.

Comparing the *Oath* with the template of the definition of the Merchant provides new information concerning the imperative to *do no harm*. There is a distinction between *voluntary* and hence intentional *wrong-doing* and harm versus *involuntary* forms of *harm* which result from mistakes and acts of stupidity. For emphasis, the injunction to *do no harm* is stated initially and then it is repeated once again to reinforce and underscore the importance of this precept.

Comparison of Plato and Hippocrates also allows us to make the connection, through antonymy, to the contrary to *harm* and *wrong-doing* which is *benefits*. Based on the template, it becomes clear that physician's treatments and remedies are placed under the part of merchandising that "sells and exchanges for cash whatever serves the *body* for its support and needs," but also under the kind of *merchandise of the soul*, where *knowledge of virtue* and evil, good and bad, right and wrong, correct and incorrect, is passed from teacher to student primarily by way of verbal instruction, since a part of this topic is said to be concerned with words.

Using the definition from Plato as the lens and blueprint for indexing the information presented in the *Oath* provides the system of classifications that serve as the background context and framework for ordering the topics and ideas. Comparison of these works from two different ancient collections in light of media and information theory highlights the way that new techniques of intertextuality can help to contextualize the information in a text against the larger background of ancient thought and expression.

Results

Comparing the order of the topics in the definition from Plato's *Sophist* with the discourse in Hippocrates' *Oath* brings out a number of regularities in the arrangement of ideas in these works. The sequential order of the topics in the *Oath* corresponds to the order of the definitions in Plato. Thus, the *Oath* combines topics concerned with the *acquisition* and *production* of *knowledge*; *giving* and *selling* one's *art* or offering instruction in *arts* learned from others; as well as *virtuous* and *wrongful* conduct in medicine. As this information is presented, the discourse follows a prescribed and predictable order in the way that the sequence of topics unfolds, indicating that Hippocrates' discourse conforms to the same rules and conventions that are described and explained in Plato.

Showing that the structure of the topics in the Hippocratic *Oath* is consistent with the order of one of the definitions in Plato's *Sophist* indicates that these compositions from two different ancient collections are organized into the parallel sequences that we recognize from the study of other ancient literatures. Since Plato's definition may be identified as an instance of parallelism, mapping the topics and themes in Hippocrates' discourse onto this sequence allows us to connect the information in the *Oath* with the patterns that scholars have identified in other ancient texts and traditions. Like file folders, sequential order indexes more meaning than what appears on the "literal" level of the content of the composition. Specific details are "slotted" into the appropriate place in a sequence that would have served as a familiar, identifiable context to ancient audience members and readers who knew the conventionalized patterns. Thus, the words and phrases in the content vary in different compositions but the overall outline of the topics and ideas in the content remains constant. What appears in the content is therefore a kind of shorthand for more complex dimensions of meaning that inhere in the way that the content is organized into an overall form.

Comparison of repetitions of a serial order between these works highlights the density of the parallels between the two compositions, and begins to give a sense of how sequences frame "networks of associations" that can be uncovered and brought to bear on the interpretation of individual passages. The instructions for the divisions of topics into the classifications explained in Plato's dialogue provide the guidelines—the slots, indexes, or frames of reference—that help the audience or reader track and contextualize the information in the text by providing the background framework in which both texts participate. Scholars have emphasized that the communicative value of works composed in accordance with conventionalized formulas stems not from their "originality" but from the way they use the framework that served as a template for a variety of compositions in this style.

The goal of comparing these works from Plato and Hippocrates in this study was to explain the potential of new techniques for uncovering meanings in foundational source texts and to describe the relevance of this information as a resource for bringing new evidence to bear on current problems and debates. Showing how the ideas in the Hippocratic *Oath* are organized and represented in accordance with the definition of the Merchant of Learning in Plato's *Sophist* provides only a glimpse of the complexity of this ancient medical treatise. Comparative analysis of the two works gives a sense of how new evidence from intertextuality can be utilized to resolve issues of interpretation that have proven intractable due to lack of evidence concerning the meaning and import of words and ideas. It also gives a sense of how information concerning the ideas stored in each of the topics in the series expands with each version of the definition that can be found and compared with the *Oath*. Though it is not possible to cite a number of different texts composed on the line of the Merchant definition here, I would point out as a direction for future research that the passages in the two Platonic dialogues that mention Hippocrates and provide our earliest source of information about the founder of the Greek medical tradition (namely, *Phaedrus* 270c and *Protagoras* 311b), manifest the same sequential pattern. Comparison of these and other compositions with the *Oath* will expand still further our knowledge of this traditional language and the techniques and conventions associated with it. Decoding additional dimensions of meaning encapsulated in the *Oath* will enlarge the base of evidence we can call upon to interpret the text in order to adopt and adapt its principles to contemporary issues.

Conclusion

The ideas expressed in the Platonic and Hippocratic collections have had an unparalleled influence in the history of our Western tradition. The meanings communicated in these ancient Greek texts formed the historical, philosophical, and religious grounding of our traditions and their influence has persisted down through the centuries to this day. The Hippocratic *Oath* is a distinguished classical text that has for centuries served as the keystone of professional ethics in medicine and as the template for all subsequent revisions to ethical codes of conduct. The *Oath* continues to resonate with the public today as the basis of confidence in the professional ethics of physicians and with physicians, nurses, and other healthcare practitioners as a foundation for the ongoing search for meaning in the medical professions.

We return to source texts such as the *Oath* along with the history of commentary on the tradition as part of the continuing quest for new insights concerning perennial questions of meaning and value in medical ethics. Reading the *Oath* in light of Plato's definition brings out added dimensions of meaning concerning the ethics surrounding professional fees, as well as the ethics surrounding actions on the part of the physician that result in harm to the patient.

I have attempted to show how information gained from the study of intertextuality can remove some of the obstacles that have stood in the way of new interpretation of the *Oath*. I have explained how new techniques of textual analysis allow us to study the way information was organized and classified in ancient writings. Intertextuality makes it possible to contextualize material through indexing and cross-referencing of meanings and associations among writings from different ancient texts and collections. I have argued that cross-referencing of information presented in ancient texts provides the insights that can serve as resources for revitalizing our traditions. It is this potential for imagining new terms and possibilities that takes as resources the tools and products of our traditions that makes this approach valuable as an alternative to the discourse styles associated with analytic philosophy.

References

Baker, R. (2002), "On Being a Bioethicist: A Review of John H. Evans, *Playing God? Human Genetic Engineering and the Rationalization of Public Bioethical Debate*," *The American Journal of Bioethics* 2:2, 65–9.

Beauchamp, T.L. and Childress, J.F. (2009), *Principles of Biomedical Ethics*, 6th edition (New York and Oxford: Oxford University Press).

Brodie, T.L. et al. (2006), *The Intertextuality of the Epistles: Explorations of Theory and Practice* (Sheffield: Sheffield Phoenix Press).

Brumbaugh, R.S. (1989), *Platonic Studies of Greek Philosophy: Form, Arts, Gadgets and Hemlock* (Albany, NY: SUNY Press).

Carrick, D. (2001), *Medical Ethics in the Ancient World* (Washington, DC: Georgetown University Press).

Connelly, J.E. (2003), "The Other Side of Professionalism: Doctor-To-Doctor," *Cambridge Quarterly of Healthcare Ethics* 12:2, 178–83.

Douglas, M. (2007), *Thinking in Circles: An Essay on Ring Composition* (New Haven, CT and London: Yale University Press).

Doukas, J. (2003), "Where is the Virtue in Professionalism?" *Cambridge Quarterly of Healthcare Ethics* 12:2, 147–54.

Evans, J.H. (2002), *Playing God: Human Genetic Engineering and the Rationalization of Public Bioethical Debate* (Chicago, IL: University of Chicago Press).

Foley, J.M. (1999), *Homer's Traditional Art* (University Park, PA: The Pennsylvania State University Press).

Garcia, N.E. (1995), "Structure and Style in the Hippocratic Treatise *Prorrheticon 2*," *Clio Medica* 28, 537–54.

Halperin, E.C. (2003), "Address to the Graduates of the Duke University School of Medicine at the Hippocratic Oath Ceremony on May 10, 2003," [website], <http://medschool.duke.edu/modules/som_deanofc/index.php?id=11>.

Havelock, E.A. (1963), *Preface to Plato* (Cambridge, MA and London: The Belknap Press of Harvard University Press).

Hippocrates (1995), *Oath*, Book I. Loeb Classical Library Series, Vol. 147, Revised Edition. W.H.S. Jones (trans.) (Cambridge, MA: Harvard University Press).

Jonsen, A. (1998), *The Birth of Bioethics* (New York: Oxford University Press).

Keenan, J.F. (1999), "Whose Perfection Is It Anyway?: A Virtuous Consideration of Enhancement," *Christian Bioethics* 5:2, 104–20.

Kuczewski, M.G. (2003), "Responding to the Call of Professionalism," *Cambridge Quarterly of Healthcare Ethics* 12:2, 144–5.

Lord, A.B. (1964), *The Singer of Tales* (Cambridge, MA: Harvard University Press).

MacDonald, D. (2003), *Does the New Testament Imitate Homer: Four Cases from the Acts of the Apostles* (New Haven, CT: Yale University Press).

Miles, S.H. (2004), *The Hippocratic Oath and the Ethics of Medicine* (New York: Oxford University Press).

Notomi, N. (1999), *The Unity of Plato's* Sophist*: Between the Sophist and the Philosopher* (Cambridge: Cambridge University Press).

Orr, R.D. et al. (1997), "Use of the Hippocratic Oath: A Review of Twentieth Century Practice and a Content Analysis of Oaths Administered in Medical School in the US and Canada in 1993," *Journal of Clinical Ethics* 8, 374–85.

Parens, E. (ed.) (1998), *Enhancing Human Traits: Ethical and Social Implications* (Washington, DC: Georgetown University Press).

Parry, M. (ed. and trans.) (1971), *The Making of Homeric Verse: The Collected Papers of Milman Parry* (Oxford: Clarendon Press).

Pritzl, K. (1999), "The Significance of Some Structural Features of Plato's *Crito*," *Plato and Platonism: Studies in Philosophy and the History of Philosophy*, Vol. 33. J.M. Van Ophuijsen (ed.) (Washington, DC: Catholic University of America Press).

Romano, C. (2003), "Rescuing the History of Philosophy from Its Analytic Abductors," *The Chronicle of Higher Education Review* [website], (published online 11 July 2003), <http://chronicle.com/free/v49/i44/44b01401.htm>.

Rothman, D.J. (1991), *Strangers at the Bedside: A History of How Law and Bioethics Transformed Medical Decision Making* (New York: Basic Books).

Sommerstein, A.H. (2007), "Introduction," *Horkos: The Oath in Greek Society*, A.H. Sommerstein and J. Fletcher (eds) (Exeter: Bristol Phoenix Press).

Steiner, A. (2007), *Reading Greek Vases* (Cambridge: Cambridge University Press).

Takala, T. (2001), "What Is Wrong with Global Bioethics? On the Limitations of the Four Principles Approach," *Cambridge Quarterly of Healthcare Ethics* 10:1, 72–7.

Thesleff, H. (1999), "Studies in Plato's Two-Level Model," *Commentationes Humanarum Litterarum* 113 (Helsinki: Societas Scientarum Fennica).

van Groningen, B.A. (1960), *La Composition littéraire archaïque grecque* (Noord-Hollandsche Uitg. Mij.).

Vansina, J. (1985), *Oral Tradition as History* (Madison, WI: University of Wisconsin Press).

Whitman, Cedric M. (1958), *Homer and the Heroic Tradition* (Cambridge, MA: Harvard University Press).

Young, E.W.D. (2000), "Physician-Assisted Suicide: Where to Draw the Line?" *Cambridge Quarterly of Healthcare Ethics* 9:3, 407–10.

Zuckert, C.H. (1996), *Postmodern Platos: Nietzsche, Heidegger, Gadamer, Strauss, Derrida* (Chicago, IL and London: University of Chicago Press).

Chapter 12
Sleeping Ethics: Gene, Episteme, and the Body Politic

Deborah Lynn Steinberg

> Behold I tell you a mystery. We shall not all sleep but we shall all be changed, in a moment, in the blinking of an eye, at the last trumpet. The trumpet shall sound. And the dead shall be raised, incorruptible. And we shall be changed. (I Corinthians 15: 51–2)

Introduction

I am not the first person to suggest the utility of science fiction as a source (as well as interesting object) of social theory. It is a genre whose very *raison d'être* involves critical engagement not only with social issues, but with the detailed and complex everyday ways in which a social order may be lived out; the feeling structures that support and are produced by divergent political orders; and the possibilities of (and foreclosures on) individual and collective agency and social change. In this chapter, I would like to consider what science fiction might contribute not only to a critical understanding of particular bioethical issues—in this instance, the convergence of genetics and neoliberal politics—but to a re-imagining of the bioethics field itself.

Along with the other contributors to this collection, I too would suggest that bioethics is at an impasse. While there is certainly no singular approach to bioethical thought, the field has nonetheless come to be dominated by a legalistic preoccupation with regulatory structures, an affective investment in consensus, and an affirmative orientation to scientific innovation. Indeed, at times there seems to be a veritable bioethics mill, directed at "controversy" and perceived "extremity," and aimed less to interrogate critically than to slough off the contestation and uncertainty that can (and I would suggest *should*) attend biotechnological transformations of the social world.

This chapter will examine the "Beggars" trilogy by feminist science fiction writer Nancy Kress, concentrating particularly on the first novel, *Beggars in Spain*. The Beggars novels offer a potent meditation on two particularly salient points of contemporary rupture and cultural contestation: the advent of human genetic engineering, and sleep—or, more specifically, the prospect of a sleepless society. Kress's subject-matter, set in a not-so-distant future USA, is the genetic engineering of a new class of "sleepless"—the ideal worker-citizens of a new cosmopolitan (and post-fossil fuel) world order. My interest here is, in part, the place of science fiction as both a reflection of and a commentary on the feeling-knowledge regimes of a particular cultural moment, what might be termed the *cultural episteme* or, following Foucault's (2002 [1966]) early theorization, the conditions of possibility of knowledge. Kress's works, characteristic of the genre, both anticipate and theorize the tendencies of the social order that produced them. They articulate realism with excess and the absurd, insight with counterintuitive devices of plot, asking us not only to consider, but in a sense to "live," at times *reductio ad absurdum*, the underpinning logics and futural tendencies embedded in current scientific and political practices. Sleeplessness, in the Kress works, offers a symbolic apotheosis—an ultimate convergence—of real contemporary trends toward a 24/7 society and of real social transformations generated not only by new techniques of genetic manipulation, but the genetification of the social field itself. The Beggars world offers, as we shall see, an allegory of class transformation and embodied distinction in the wake of technological and biopolitical revolution. The novels foreground cultural ambivalences that are distinctly bioethical, elaborating both dystopic and utopic projective fantasies about bodies at the interstices of discourse, technology, and social order. In so doing, the Beggars fantasy leads us to the centre of the "crisis of bioethics" itself, described elsewhere in and throughout this volume.

In forging this analysis, I aim to contribute to the bioethics field in two ways. First, I want to engage with bioethics as a genre of representation and a framework of engagement, as well as a field of knowledge. In this context, I aim to incorporate an element into a bioethical critical standpoint that is not usually part of the discourse—that is, the question of feelings. I want to ask what happens to bioethical discourse when it is concerned with what might be termed the "feeling regimes" or "feeling structures" of knowledge, body practices, modes of governance, and science. An analysis of science fiction offers a useful (though of course not the only) way into such a consideration. This is in part because of the necessary and explicit articulation of feeling and knowledge that characterizes narrative as opposed to traditional academic genres of writing or regulatory modes of discourse.

Second, I wish to look at a particular example of science fiction fantasy to consider the ways in which it both re-presents and critically assesses contemporary body-political anxieties and scientific trends. Here I treat the Kress works as an affectively infused meditation on the confluence of neoliberal body politics and genetic engineering. The novels, I shall argue, by their strategic counterintuitive understandings of the body, suggest the intrinsically destructive dimensions of both neoliberalism and genetics—indeed, showing that each is an artefact of the other. At the same time, the Kress works also elaborate the phantasmatic, seductive underpinnings of this confluence: the desires (and the denials) in play, desires anchored in both *commonsense* and *common-emotion*—those unremarked upon "already knowns" and preferred affective orientations that constitute everyday life. It is this insight that allows us to leap from the fictional to the real, to consider the world we live in from an affectively inflected bioethical standpoint and thereby to problematize not only what disturbs, but also what is comfortable, consoling. This is a bioethics that is not primarily oriented to consensus building, or to a simply affirmative, even if regulatory, approach to scientific innovation. Rather, it suggests a bioethics that has something of the character of McClintock's idea of a science predicated on a "feeling for the organism" (see Fox Keller 1984)—and by corollary, as a feeling enterprise.

Behold I Tell You a Mystery

Over the course of the early- to mid-1990s, Nancy Kress published the "Beggars" trilogy, beginning with *Beggars in Spain* in 1993, *Beggars and Choosers* in 1994, and *Beggars Ride* in1996. This trilogy emerged in a context of a burgeoning of dedicated publication of feminist science fiction. It took its place alongside a plethora of fictionalized and scholarly assessments of genetics, of competing bio-ethics, of competing speculative social orders, and indeed of competing feminist paradigms. In both contexts, the relationship of the political to the embodied, and of feeling to knowledge, provided the foundations of what Haran (2003) has termed the "utopian impulse" of feminist theory itself. As we shall see, the core themes of the Kress trilogy anticipated and continue to have contemporaneous bioethical resonance at a number of levels. The focus on sleep and sleeplessness provides a pointed metaphor for a society in which 24/7 awakeness is technologically possible. This literary device refers implicitly to a contemporary social condition in which we increasingly see 24/7 expectations placed on the functioning of social institutions and human bodies. The ethical values embedded in "sleeplessness" and the instrumental manipulation of human beings through genetics play into two linked popular and bioethical anxieties: on the one hand, the boundaries of *humanness* and on the other, the obligations of *humaneness*. Both are troubled themes that have stood at the heart of science fiction explorations, applied to the speculative consequences of scientific hubris, rampant capitalism, and authoritarian governmentality. They are points of ethical meditation, highlighting questions of social responsibility, political dissent, and the possibilities of justice and transformation.

Beggars in Spain

Beggars in Spain opens with a scene that takes place in an IVF-genetics clinic set in a not-so-distant future USA. Roger Camden, an extraordinarily successful business tycoon (described as a "data-atoll investor") and, himself, a brutal embodiment of hyper-productivity, is negotiating to produce a daughter with the genetic enhancement of sleeplessness, a trait that is part of a secret experiment. His wife Elizabeth, who sits with him, is a cowed, sullen, and yet resistant figure who we later learn has a drinking problem directly as a response to Roger's ruthlessness and his inexhaustible drive. Indeed, Roger is, himself, virtually sleepless (and regards this as his highest virtue). By accident, Elizabeth conceives twins, one enhanced through the IVF-genetic process and one, naturally. The twins are Leisha and Alice—sleepless and sleeper, respectively. This sets up two counterpoints of intimate tension that are followed through the rest of the novel (and also, in increasingly complex forms, throughout the trilogy): firstly, tensions between Roger and Elizabeth which emblematize a clash of gendered neoliberal values—the imperialist machismo of enterprise and acceleration (culture) versus the passive and entropic properties of domesticity (nature); and secondly, the competing femininities of Leisha and Alice, embodying the contrasting values of *fast time* versus *slow time* and troubling the intersecting questions of what is human and what is humane.

We are further told that the social world in which this experiment to genetically engineer sleeplessness takes place is one already transformed by "Y-energy," which has replaced fossil fuels. Y-energy is a form of cheap, ubiquitous, and limitless energy invented by Kenzo Yagai. While the novel never specifies the particulars of Y-energy production, we are given to understand that it is essentially the realized achievement of a counterintuitive proposition: the possibility of perpetual motion. This Y-energy driven society has also been transformed by "Yagaism," a political philosophy of meritocratic social order where individual excellence and industriousness are the basis of the social contract—itself understood in marketized terms as "trade." Both Y-energy and Yagaism constitute a new world order in which the utilitarian and anti-entropic values of neoliberalism, articulated as a collectivist philosophy, reach their apogee (and perhaps their own undoing).

The birth of Leisha and the other sleepless children presages a radical rupture in a world in which genetic enhancement has already been assimilated as a normative practice in the service of social privilege (and "good" social order). The appearance of the sleepless heralds what unfolds as a dramatic transformation of class hierarchy and a new form of racialized distinction. The sleepless themselves are posited as unusually beautiful (with few exceptions), possessing an intelligence beyond the range of "natural" norms and as preternaturally industrious. As the plot unfolds, it further emerges that the sleepless are extraordinarily bodily efficient—sleeplessness means that they virtually do not age. Sleeplessness furthermore turns out to be a dominant genetic trait, thus creating a new "natural order" as sleepless adults have sleepless children and constitute an increasingly separate people with a distinct culture accruing directly from the sleepless biological trait. The sleepless, moreover, exactly embody the ideals of Yagaism. They are perpetual productive motion with virtually no material cost or embodied friction. They are embodied paradigms of individual excellence: innovative and supremely industrious and innately imbued with ideal affect—being unflaggingly sociable, positive, and fulfilled in service.

As the novel proceeds, a new world order is produced with distinctions among the Sleepless; the "donkeys"—those who are genetically enhanced but not sleepless, who monopolize most of the labour (a professional order of labour as robotics take care of the drudgery); and the "Beggars" (also referred to as "Livers"), the genetically unenhanced majority who do no work at all, but live a life of "low" hedonistic pursuits, with an overweening sense of entitlement and who, in Yagaist terms, offer nothing in the contractual trade of a meritocratic civil society. Amidst this new order, troubled (and troubling) figures appear, most notably Jennifer Sharifi, a "flawed sleepless" who emblematizes the irreconcilable tensions and hostilities brewing within the new order. As we shall see, Jennifer comes to stand as an ambivalent ethical commentary on the potentialities and foreclosures of neoliberal political economies. Her paranoia and fanaticism signal an underpinning disquietude, a fatal flaw both of desire and disaster.

We Shall Not All Sleep

> Ong Smiled. "Appearance factors are the easiest to achieve, as I'm sure you already know" …
> "Good enough," Camden said. "The full array of corrections for any potential gene-linked health problem, of course."
> "Of course," Dr Ong said …
> "And," Camden said, "no need to sleep." (Kress 1993, 4)

In her 2002 study, Elizabeth Ettorre discussed the ways in which values of capital (human, social, economic) accrue to genetics and genetic modification. This represents a long-standing theme of feminist and other critical assessments of genetic science, including historical analyses of its antecedent developments within nineteenth- and twentieth-century eugenics.[1] The value of capital (positive or negative) attaches not only to attributed properties of bodies (genetic traits, lineages, relationships), but also to the scientific, economic, and political enterprises surrounding genetic practices, as well as to the growing hegemony of genetic ideas and ideologies. This theme is prominently articulated in the Beggars trilogy. As evidenced in the passage above, taken from the stage-setting scene at the start of *Beggars in Spain*, this is a futural USA in which genetic enhancements (and genetics *as* enhancement) are both achieved and normative. Ong's "of course" evokes genetic modification not only as a taken for granted everyday underpinning of social life, but also as a compact of understanding between two men, united both by superordinate social position as well as knowledges (both know what is *not*, as well as what *is*, widely known). The exchange between Ong and Camden invokes seductive utopian tropes characteristic not only of genetic engineering themed science fiction, but also of the public relations often attached to genetics itself (see, for example: Haran et al. 2007). These are the notions that genetic modification can beautify the body surface, even as it can improve the elegant

1 See Kirkup et al. 1999 and Steinberg 1997 for summary discussion of the key periods of feminist debate on reproductive and genetic engineering that form the immediate theoretical context of the Kress works.

efficiency of an organism. That such precision is possible—though perhaps not ethical—constitutes much of the hype that has surrounded genetic science. Such notions, one might argue, stand at the fulcrum between seductive, marketized fictions and projective fact.

Genetic capital in the Beggars world, furthermore, is part of a circular economy that is foundational to modern (including late-modern) capitalism: it is the purchase of the already well-off and privileged, and it produces new indices of privilege. Interestingly, the genetic modification enterprise in itself is posited as a comfortable extension of the political economic values of the contemporary capitalist world. It is a projective future in which the tensions and debates about genetics have been resolved and successfully assimilated: Ong's "of course" signifying a commonsense understanding not only of the distance we have come from such times, but of the "unjustified" paranoia that characterized the troubled early reception of genetic modification practices. In the Beggars world, genetic modification is the *status quo*, introducing new embellishments, yes, but offering no breach within the social order. It is the engineering of the specific trait of sleeplessness that is offered as the point not only of rupture, but of radical schism.

Embodied Capital and Entropic Life

> "Without that energy expenditure [REM sleep], nonsleep cerebrums save the wear-and-tear and do better at coordinating real-life input, thus greater intelligence and problem solving … suppress REM sleep and people don't get depressed. The nonsleep kids are cheerful, outgoing … joyous" …
> "At what cost?" Mrs Camden said. She held her neck rigid, but the corners of her jaw worked.
> "No cost. No negative side effects at all." (Dr Susan Melling and Elizabeth Camden in Kress 1993, 12–13)

The Beggars world is premised on a set of interestingly counter-intuitive reversals concerning the functioning of the body and the entropic effects of time and energy expenditure. Entropy describes the process whereby useful energy is transmuted into non-usable form. It is, in other words, the process of decay, decline, disarray, and disengagement. Ageing is entropy. Stress is entropic. Friction is the guarantor that there will be no possibility of perpetual motion. In the Beggars world, the functions of sleep and sleeplessness are both reversed and, significantly, articulated through a distinctly neoliberal moral discourse concerning the nexus of bodies, work, and value. From the first to the final book, the hegemonic view of sleep (which is both problematized and romanticized simultaneously), is constituted as a failing. It is posited in scientific terms as the literal basis for and direct cause of mortality. It is understood pervasively as the wasting of energy, the using up of the body, both in terms of industry (the body unavailable for productive work) and in terms of the very viability of the organism. Sleep, in other words, is the ultimate entropic trait of the living world. Sleep is also understood as that which is inelegant and ugly about the body: the signifier and material harbinger of the body's propensity to decline, to social disengagement, to parasitism—sleep, as we are repeatedly told, is the Beggars' trait. As suggested in the above passage, and a sentiment that is reiterated by various characters throughout the trilogy, the sleeper is, by reason of this trait, predisposed to inferior intellect, to entropic, destructive emotions, and to compromised social and economic utility.

The sleepless body, by contrast, is constituted as anti-entropic. Sleeplessness is presented as the literal—and importantly, a profoundly *desired*—embodiment of the values not only of industry but of neoliberal governmentality, both in terms of physical efficiency and affective orientation. The sleepless, it is oft repeated, are by nature industrious, invested in service, and optimistic. They are naturally excellent, superior, and embody materializations of a conjoined economic and moral utility that supersedes the merely enhanced. The sleepless are offered as exemplars both of a nostalgically individualistic, Protestant, middle-class work ethic and an imperialistic liberalism of contemporary forms of what may perhaps be usefully termed "cosmopolitan globalisation" (Johnson and Steinberg 2004). The sleepless, moreover, are constructed as frictionless, both in terms of bodily function and affectively. They, like Y-energy, emblematize one of the most potent fantasies of modern life: the possibility of inexhaustible self-renewal. Both are figurations that stand in as consoling phantasmatic projections—and as impossible symbolic resolutions—to the profound contemporaneous crises that have accrued to the inevitable drying up of a fossil-fuel-driven political economy. As self-renewing resources, sleepless and Y-energy, both, embody the surface fantasy[2] of perpetual motion and the powerful normotic[3] phantasy, central to religious discourses not limited to Western forms, that life itself may be transubstantiated, transformed, absolutely known, and live on eternally.

And the Dead Shall Be Raised

Beggars in Spain can be read as a parable of class revolution, and one that is constituted on and through a racialized field. Marx (and Marxist thought) has theorized the ways in which industrial capitalism became the bedrock of a radical

2 "Fantasy" is used here in the denotative sense of (more or less conscious) imaginative projection. I use the psychoanalytic term "phantasy" to refer to unconscious, inchoate desires and fears that can underpin such projections.

3 See Bollas 1987 for discussion of "normotic" in the psychoanalytic context. "Normotic illness" as, in essence, the transformation of the self into an ideal object, a virtual automaton of "normality," totalizingly invested in facts, utility, knowability, and rational control. Taken as a cultural description, a "normotic phantasy" might describe the invested repudiation of what is subjective (feeling, the body) in favour of an idealized ultimate rationality. As such, it can be suggested that normotic phantasy constitutes the cultural "unconscious" of modernity and modern science, with their principled idealization of rational utilitarianism, objectivity (the repudiation of feeling and body), and law.

reconfiguration of the social order. Thompson (1991), for example, has argued that the industrialization of labour and early capitalist forms of exchange saw the invention both of the working class as alienated labour and of a new middle class who owned the means of production and profited from the labour of others. The narrative structure of the Beggars trilogy follows the dominant narrative structure of such historical accounts of class formation and the rise of Victorian modernity and Victorian values. Indeed, the sleepless can be seen, in this light, as paradigmatic modern workers and citizens. At the same time, Kress's projective fantasy of a genetic modification for sleeplessness is also understood to be inassimilable into the modernist values and social order that produced it. In the first part of *Beggars in Spain*, the rupture is ominous and apocalyptic:

> Leisha, you're a different kind of person entirely. More evolutionarily fit, not only to survive but to prevail. Those other objects of hatred you cite—they were all powerless in their societies. They occupied inferior positions … Every Sleepless is making superb grades, none have psychological problems, all are healthy and most of you aren't even adults yet. How much hatred do you think you're going to encounter once you hit the high-stakes world of finance and business and scare endowed chairs and national politics? (Stuart Sutter [Leisha's "sleeper" college boyfriend] in Kress 1993, 51)

The first half of the novel witnesses the Sleepless subjected to Nuremburg styled laws, excluding them from all manner of sport, work, and community. They are persecuted, subjected to physical attacks, and treated as mutant, repudiated Others—their perceived monstrosity to the sleeper majority based on and articulated through a distinctly racialized repertoire of envy. Indeed, sleeplessness as a biogenetic trait comes to stand in for and refer to the panoply of reviled Others that have accrued to modern racial taxonomizations. Interestingly, though only given a passing reference—the overwhelming majority of characters at the centre of the initial narrative are white, with the notable exception of Jennifer Sharifi—the Beggars world is posited as a post-racist world. This is as an extension of a more generalized egalitarianism that is attributed not only to international relations but, in many respects, to gender relations. The markedly and conventionally unequal relationship between Roger and Elizabeth in this context signifies both the residual tendencies of a previous (pre-genetified) order and, at the same time, the latent (masculine-imperialist) tendencies of a post-genetics world.

As Haran (2003) has noted, references to National Socialism and its holocaustic racial ideology are a common thread in the dystopian currents of post- (and in some cases contemporaneous with[4]) Second World War science fiction. The hatred to which the Sleepless are subjected is not only cast in this light, but the engineering of sleeplessness itself is construed as unleashing and revivifying tensions of the previous racial order. Interestingly, Kress explores the intersubjective relations

4 See for example: Burdekin 1985 [1937].

of racial hatred though the metaphor of *genetic* difference. In both contexts, racial hatred is understood as an intrinsic tendency that directly accrues to and follows from racial distinction. There is an implication that genetic science has undermined the scientific-biological validity of "race" (in its modern taxonomic forms)—hence the post-racism of a genetified world—while at the same time having the power to (re)introduce it, this time in an empirically "valid" form. That what is engineered (sleeplessness) is counterintuitive to all that is currently known about biology and entropy, sets up a compellingly ambivalent assessment of the underpinning politics and social implications of genetic science. It is in this "Nuremburg" period, as I shall discuss below, that a schism among the Sleepless is produced and the most profound dystopic elements of the narrative (and the theoretical analysis it forges) is set out.

Fast Time

The latter half of *Beggars in Spain* witnesses a radical shift in the social order and the emergence of a new *status quo*. The explicitly classed languages of the new structures emerging from the assimilation of sleeplessness are interesting to consider:

> The United States was a three tiered society now: the have-nots, who by the mysterious hedonistic opiate of the Philosophy of Genuine Living had become the recipients of the gift of leisure. Livers, eighty percent of the population, had shed the work ethic for a gaudy populous version of the older aristocratic ethic: the fortunate do not have to work. Above them—or below—were the donkeys, genetically enhanced sleepers who ran the economy and the political machinery, as dictated by, and in exchange for, the lordly votes of the new leisure class. Donkeys managed, their robots labored. Finally, the Sleepless, nearly all of whom were invisible in Sanctuary anyway, were disregarded by Livers, if not by donkeys. All of it, the entire trefoil organization—id, ego, and superego, some wit had labelled it sardonically—was underwritten by cheap ubiquitous Y-energy. (Kress 1993, 238)

The obviously Marxian references invoked here (populism, aristocratic ethic, leisure, opiate of the masses) places the new society both within and in contrast to the class categories of (post)industrial capitalism. If genetic modification is a marker of middle-class distinction, sleeplessness is the trait that embodies the new middle-class ego-ideal as well as its new aristocracy—its superego. While a schismatic hierarchical ordering of social life remains intact (and familiarly so), the character of classed existence has radically shifted. Leisure linked with plenty, once a marker of privilege, becomes a marker of dispossession; hence, a "new poverty," but this time of utility—the "Livers"/"Beggars" are a "useless," infantilized, and parasitic majority. They embody the underpinning trajectories of life defined by consumption, in a radical breach from the means and mode of production. No longer alienated bodies of toil for the profit of others, they are the excessive bodies of gross consumption and infantile regression at the expense of others. Powered by ubiquitous self-renewing energy (both Y- and sleepless), the situation of the "Liver"/Beggar is a destitution defined by plenty. The remade working class do not work but anodize themselves with bread and circuses and an opiate mythology that they are better off than donkeys, who do or manage nearly all the work.

The resonances of this portrait with many aspects of contemporary life are unmistakable. We are in the midst of just such a transformation of labouring life, with the monopolization of work, rather than leisure, increasingly serving as a marker of middle-class status and a day-to-day reality. Even if bodies do still inconveniently sleep, the advent of 24/7 life has a clear technological reality, based materially in new digital communications, but also conscripted as a cultural ideal increasingly ascribed to all aspects of civil society, blurring boundaries between public and private, between night and day, between action and its contemplation. The neoliberal effect, invested in perpetually climbing standards of merit and excellence, in the superordinate value competition and global markets, and in inexhaustibility as both a premise and an ideal that can be attributed to our resources, is increasingly a normative mode of institutional rationalization, applied as much to public services and educational reform as to business, as much to modes of institutional governance as to personal habits in the privacy of the home.[5] In the Beggars narrative, the beautiful body of Leisha, her triumph of brilliance and empathy, is the emotive lynchpin of this bioethical projection, and of its utopian purchase. She is at once a familiar fetish and a paradigmatically compelling ego-ideal. Yet there is also a darker undercurrent here, subtly elaborated in the counterintuitive propositions of Y- and sleepless energy. This is an undercurrent that bespeaks the realities of bodies as, in actual fact, *exhaustible* resources, of the exhaustibility of all resources that support life and of "exhaustibility" as a characteristic of life itself. These are realities that, by their very nature, can have no purchase, no place, no means to realize a neoliberal utopia. An economy of finite and declining energy inevitably attaches both to political ecology and to the entropic properties of living bodies. The neoliberal ethic is, thus, one that the body will always fail. At the same time, the Beggars trilogy's emphasis on the superlative elegance of genetically enhanced and sleepless bodies highlights and, indeed, invests in the profound seductions of what is intrinsically an impossible ethic. Recombinant genetics emerges, at one and the same time, as a realist referent to ground a transcendent fantasy and as a magical phantasm, by which means a materially impossible social and bodily renaissance will be accomplished. In the Beggars world, both sleeplessness and genetic enhancement stand in as reciprocal metaphors and as intertwined phantasmatic projections, narcissistic and normotic—or what Freud described as the "phantasies of action."[6]

5 For extended discussion of these transformations as they have played out in the British context, see Johnson and Steinberg 2004.

6 The psychoanalytic concept, "phantasy of action" refers to the projective recovery of the phallus (power in the social world).

Incorruptible

> Jennifer disturbed her. Not for the obvious reasons she disturbed Tony and Richard and Jack: the long dark hair, the tall, slim body in shorts and halter. Jennifer didn't laugh. Leisha had never met a sleepless who didn't laugh, nor one who said so little, with such deliberate casualness. (Kress 1993, 43)

As I have noted above, the trait of sleeplessness connotes a classed ideal of embodied utility, but at the same time, particularly set out in the first half of *Beggars in Spain*, it emblematizes a rearticulated racial order in which genetics emerges as a "new-racism" (see Barker 1983). In the Beggars world, the superhuman can stand in, simultaneously, for both ideal and repudiated. The dramatic tension arising from the ambivalent effects of genetification, generally, and the modification of sleeplessness, specifically, emerges as a rupture, not only between sleepless and sleeper, but *within* the sleepless population. This is emblematized in the contrast and ultimate contestation between Leisha Camden and Jennifer Sharifi. Leisha is the humanized, idealized sleepless, who maintains as primary her relationship with her twin, non-enhanced, sister Alice, and with sleepers. She establishes herself as avatar both for justice for sleepers, as well as for the benign communalist potentialities (as she believes unshakeably) of Yagaism. The notion that sleepers are "Beggars" (the view of the majority of sleepless) she only half believes. As the narrative progresses, Leisha finds and trusts not only the essential humanity of "Beggars," but also, particularly through her bond with Alice, the value of this humanity as "trade." Leisha is also blonde, slender, and beautiful, the feminized embodiment of a distinctly American order of values and object of desire. As a pivotal figure, she also signifies a transformed gender order in which "equality" (albeit ambivalently) reconciles and assimilates conventional feminine beauty ideals with (phallic) social power.

Jennifer Sharifi emerges as both counterpoint and nemesis, not only of Leisha, but of sleeper humanity itself. She is "dark"—the product of a liaison between an Arab potentate and a Western beauty. Affectively dehumanized, Jennifer is relentless and utterly without humour. She is a fanatical figure, who founds the defensive and paranoid Sanctuary—a closed, survivalist, and terrorist as well as communalist community of sleepless. Moreover, Jennifer's fanaticism is constituted as a hybrid of Islamic militantism (she is both devotional in prayer and speaks continually of a "holy war" with sleepers) and an extreme neo-Calvinism that repudiates anything less than absolute excellence and perpetual motion, whether of body or of labour or of affective bonds. Both the figuration of Jennifer and of Sanctuary itself make explicit reference to the tensions of the Cold War as well as to its more recent (post-Cold War) variant, which pits Islamic religious fundamentalism against the neoliberal West (while at the same time, demonstrating their reciprocal imbrication).

Sanctuary is a society defined by both paranoia and repudiation. It is, in Kristeva's (1992) terms, melancholic. Kristeva explains melancholia as the affective and psychic effect of a paranoid schizoid spiral: that is, a spiral in which the Other (and Otherness within the self) is always abjected as monstrous. Sanctuary, like Jennifer, maintains the meritocratic values of Yagaism, paradoxically valorizing and yet rejecting its individualism, and forms what might be read as a communalist, if not communist, society that wages a cold (and eventually "hot") war against Leisha and her few supporters who wish to maintain trade with sleepers.

> [W]hat obligation do we have to those so weak they don't have anything to trade with us? We're already going to give more than we get; do we have to do it when we get nothing at all? Do we have to take care of their deformed and handicapped and sick and lazy and shiftless with the products of our work? (Tony Indivino, who is soon to be murdered—martyred—by sleepers, speaking to Leisha on the eve of the creation of Sanctuary, in Kress 1993, 39–40)

The Sanctuary community eventually moves off-planet and, on the basis of their superordinate economic utility—derived explicitly from the trait of sleeplessness—attempt to secede from the United States by means of a threat (and intent) to release an unparalleled biological weapon. Jennifer's perception of the sleepless as at one and the same time endangered and exploited, but biologically superior and entitled, fuels an escalating paranoia and militancy. Eventually (as Kristeva suggests is the quintessential spiral of the paranoid schizoid position), the abjection of the monstrous outsider (the sleepers) is turned inward, as Jennifer begins to purge Sanctuary of injured or dissenting sleepless, murdering the former and exiling the latter—including her own "supersleepless" granddaughter Miranda. It is ultimately Miranda who wrests Sanctuary (and the hostage USA) from the grip of Jennifer's paranoia and radical extremism.

It is interesting to consider the ambivalent figuration of Jennifer. She can be read, on the one hand, as a biologically flawed sleepless. As suggested in the passage cited above, this is indeed how Leisha perceives her. And Kress ultimately repudiates Jennifer on this basis, as the Beggars series maintains its empathetic and idealized construction of Leisha, who remains humane and heroic throughout; and indeed, all the more so when she herself is eventually assassinated by another fanatical figure (this time anti-sleepless) in *Beggars and Choosers*. On the other hand, even as she is cast manifestly as Leisha's alter-ego, Jennifer also latently figures the alternative trajectory of the same trait. In this sense, Jennifer figures as the deeper reality not only of the sleepless characteristic, but of both sleeplessness and genetification as twin (and inextricably linked) biopolitical ethics. Thus, contained within its seductive phantasies, the Beggars narrative nonetheless suggests that intersecting class and racialized hierarchies are foundational to and logical consequences of both a genetified and neoliberal social order. In turn, the twin drives of both neoliberalism and genetics—epitomized in the (metaphoric) trait of sleeplessness—set the preconditions for paranoid affectivities and resurgent conditions of cold war. *Beggars in Spain* thus offers a commentary on the underpinning paranoid schizoid conditions of late modernity, following its dystopian political and conceptual trajectories, but also highlighting its profound seductions.

And We Shall Be Changed

> The body can be *read* as a metaphor for the story …. (Sargisson 1996, 148; original emphasis)

Kress's work provides a salient case in point for the power of science fiction, both as object of and as resource for social theory. In the first instance, the Beggars trilogy depicts a constellation of bioethical ruptures and anxieties (and, indeed, rather prophetically anticipates others) in the wake of revolutions in both genetics and the technologies of labouring life. Here ambivalences surrounding issues of de/humanization, the attrition of humane liveability, and the relationships of political governance, social injustice, and science are pointedly articulated not only as body-political questions, but also, in so doing, as epistemic-*affective* questions. The narrativized form itself allows Kress to infuse feminist theoretical debate on science, culture, and politics with an emotional sensibility. This allows readers to grasp not only the blurred boundaries between dystopian and utopian futures (genetified and neoliberal), but also their phantasmatic purchase.

Through the metaphor of sleeplessness, the works offer a complex critical reflection on the epistemic-affective (knowledge-feeling) underpinnings of neoliberal (as well as foundationalist and reactionary) politics *per se*. *Beggars in Spain* provides a pointed allegory not only of "sleepless" values as an embodied, technological, and political-economic aspiration, but as emergent from and a basis for a distinctive social order. Kress offers the sleepless body as both immortalizing and stabilizing against its obverse—the sleeping body as destructive and entropic. The counterintuitive character of these constructions provides the dystopic undercurrent that means that the seductive new order remains fantastical, notwithstanding the realist conventions of plot and characterization that would seem to place sleeplessness in a realm of futural fact. At the same time, the seductions of sleeplessness are diffused into normative assumptions not only of the plot, but of the wider cultural episteme surrounding the gene: the projective fantasies that genetics can and will produce beautiful, disease-free bodies—leaving only the (rather rhetorical) question of whether it *should* produce such bodies. This fantasy (and the answer to this question) is consolidated in the figure of Leisha—the beautiful, empathetic, and heroic centre of the narrative, who, in her unconditional humanity, human*izes* the dehumanizing tendencies of both sleeplessness and technocratic utilitarianism. Leisha is, interestingly, persuasively—however, counter-intuitively—the humane ideal and product of what Kress's novels suggest are a foundationally dehumanizing science and a social order intrinsically bent towards the paranoid and totalitarian.

The complex counterpositioning of the themes of humanness/humaneness in the Kress works thus mirrors the ambivalent dystopic tendencies of the late-capitalist work ethic in and of itself, and of its associated imperatives to bodily repudiation and transformation. In both the metaphor of sleep and the elaborated references to recombinant genetics and a transformed (post-fossil fuel) energy base, Kress elaborates the ways in which late-capitalist values are simultaneously affective, that is, imbricated in imperatives of feeling, as well as materially embedded in structures of action and modes of exchange. Indeed, the question of "trade," offered up simultaneously as a site of social contract, a desired cultural ideal, a crisis of knower as well as of knowledge, and an ethical affective stance, locates the analytic currents of the trilogy at a "real world" time of epistemic as well as political and economic transformation and rupture. The conjunction of magic and realism in the narrative treatment of technology (genetics and fuel production) paints a disturbing (and compelling) portrait of the ways in which improbabilities, and indeed impossibilities, can become plausible objects (ends and/or means) of phantasmatic projection and belief. If the neoliberal ideal can only be realized by bodies in perpetual motion and technologies that functionally defy (and eradicate) the essentially entropic character of life itself, then the Beggars world both obscures and yet tells us something of the self-deluding character of our attachment to sciences as well as modes of governance that, on closer scrutiny, prove to be based in no more than consoling fantasy.

Finally, it is not incidental that social injustices and the possibilities of their redemption articulate im/plausibly over bodies. The Beggars world invokes a dangerous and powerfully ambivalent bioethic in which the body presages an immanent social world, and is also an artefact—disquieting in each instance—of both utopian and dystopian desire. These are dissonances arising not simply out of spectacular technological or social ruptures, but out of what is (already) normative, and the ways in which what apparently disturbs, also fits. In this way, the Beggars allegory sheds some light not simply on what would seem to threaten comfortable lives, but on the comfort that is, and can be, powerfully, normatively, taken in destructive things.

Kress's works do not offer us a simple way out of the bioethical impasse they depict. But in the portrait of that impasse as a vivid and profound tension of feeling as well as knowledge and social praxis, there is perhaps an immanent alternative. This potential may arguably arise as a latent tendency of the science fiction genre itself, with its intersection of allusive speculation and projective identification applied to socio-ethical critique. As science fiction, Kress's works clearly are not simply a thought experiment, but a *thought-feeling* experiment that enables us to apprehend the profound dissonances and dystopic underpinnings of both biotechnology and neoliberal "revolutions." Sleepless values are profoundly embedded in both, presaging potentially catastrophic material consequences of which the using up of bodies unto death is only one.

References

Barr, M.S. (2000), *Future Females: The Next Generation: New Voices and Velocities in Feminist Science Fiction Criticism* (Lanham, MD: Rowman and Littlefield Publishers).

Barr, M.S. (2006), *Lost in Space: Probing Feminist Science Fiction and Beyond* (Chapel Hill, NC: University of North Carolina Press).
Benjamin, J. (1988), *The Bonds of Love: Psychoanalysis, Feminism and the Problems of Domination* (New York: Pantheon).
Bollas, C. (1987), *The Shadow of the Object: Psychoanalysis of the Unthought Known* (London: Free Association Books).
Burdekin, K. (1985 [1937]), *Swastika Night* (London: Lawrence and Wishart).
Butler, J. (1993), "Endangered/Endangering: Schematic Racism and White Paranoia," in R. Gooding-Williams (ed.), *Reading Rodney King: Reading Urban Uprising* (New York: Routledge), 15–23.
Crosby, J.C. (2000), *Cauldron of Changes: Feminist Spirituality in Fantastic Fiction* (Jefferson, NC: McFarland and Co.).
Ettorre, E. (2002), *Reproductive Genetics, Gender and the Body* (London: Routledge).
Ettorre, E. (2006), "Re-Shaping the Space Between Bodies and Culture: Embodying the Biomedicalised Body," *Sociology of Health and Illness* 20:4, 548–55.
Ettorre, E. (2007), "Genetics, Gender and an Embodied Ethics of Reproduction", paper presented at CESAGen Seminar, Lancaster University, March.
Foucault, M. (2002 [1966]), *The Order of Things* (London: Routledge).
Fox Keller, E. (1984), *A Feeling for the Organism: The Life and Work of Barbara McClintock* (New York: W.H. Freeman).
Franklin, S. (2007), *Dolly Mixtures: The Remaking of Genealogy* (Durham, NC: Duke University Press).
Haran, J. (2003), "Re-Visioning Feminist Futures: Literature as Social Theory", PhD Thesis, University of Warwick.
Haran, J. (2004), "Theorizing (Hetero)sexuality and (Fe)male Dominance," *Extrapolation* 45:1 (spring), 89–102.
Haran, J. et al. (2007), *Human Cloning in the Media* (London: Routledge).
Haraway, D.J. (1989), *Primate Visions: Gender, Race and Nature in the World of Modern Science* (London: Verso).
Haraway, D.J. (1991), *Simians, Cyborgs and Women: The Reinvention of Nature* (London: Free Association Books).
Haraway, D.J. (1997), *Modest Witness @ Second Millennium: FemaleMan Meets OncoMouse* (New York: Routledge).
Hellekson, K. (2000), "Toward a Taxonomy of the Alternate History Genre," *Extrapolation* 41:3 (fall), 248–58.
Johnson, R. and Steinberg, D.L. (eds) (2004), *Blairism and the War of Persuasion: Labour's Passive Revolution* (London: Lawrence and Wishart).
Jordanova, L. (1986), *Languages of Nature: Critical Essays on Science and Literature* (London: Free Association Book).
Kirkup, G. et al. (eds.) (1999), *The Gendered Cyborg: A Reader* (London: Routledge).
Kranko, C. (2002), "What-if-ing the Titans: Nancy Kress's Dialogic Beggars Trilogy," *Extrapolations* 43:2 (summer), 131–63.

Kress, N. (1993), *Beggars in Spain* (New York: HarperCollins).
Kress, N. (1994), *Beggars and Choosers* (New York: Tom Doherty Associates).
Kress, N. (1996), *Beggars Ride* (New York: Tom Doherty Associates).
Kristeva, J. (1992), *Black Sun: Depression and Melancholia*, L.S. Roudiez (trans.) (New York: Columbia University Press).
Larbalestier, J. (2006), *Daughters of Earth: Feminist Science Fiction in the Twentieth Century* (Middletown, CT: Wesleyan University Press).
Lefanu, S. (1988), *In the Chinks of the World Machine: Feminism and Science Fiction* (London: The Women's Press).
Little, J.A. (2007), *Feminist Philosophy and Science: Utopias and Dystopias* (Amherst, NY: Prometheus Books).
McDowell, L. and Pringle, R. (eds) (1992), *Defining Women: Social Institutions and Gender Divisions* (London: Polity).
Plumber, K. (1995), *Telling Sexual Stories: Power, Change and Social Worlds* (London: Routledge).
Sargisson, L. (1996), *Contemporary Feminist Utopianism* (London: Routledge).
Schiebinger, L. (1993), *Nature's Body: Gender in the Making of Science* (Boston, MA: Beacon Press).
Sontag, S. (1991), *Illness as Metaphor [1977] / AIDS and its Metaphors [1988]* (London: Penguin).
Spannier, B.B. (1995), *Im/Partial Science: Gender Ideology in Molecular Biology* (Bloomington, IN: Indiana University Press).
Steinberg, D.L. (1997), *Bodies in Glass* (Manchester: Manchester University Press).
Taylor, B. (1993), "Unconsciousness and Society: The Sociology of Sleep," *International Journal of Politics, Culture and Society* 6:3, 463–71.
Thompson, E.P. (1991), *The Making of the English Working Class* (London: Penguin).
Tobach, E. and Rosoff, B. (1994), *Challenging Racism and Sexism: Alternatives to Genetic Explanations* (New York: The Feminist Press).
Turney, J. (1998), *Frankenstein's Footsteps: Science, Genetics and Popular Culture* (New Haven, CT: Yale University Press).
Van Dijck, J. (1998), *Imagenation: Popular Images of Genetics* (Basingstoke: Macmillan).
Williams, S. (2005), *Sleep and Society: Sociological Ventures into the (Un)known* (New York: Taylor and Francis).

Chapter 13

The Last Temptation of Marion Woodman: The Anorexic Remainder in *Bone: Dying Into Life*

David L. Clark

I

More than a decade after its publication, we have only begun the task of reading Marion Woodman's cancer narrative, *Bone: Dying into Life* (2000). The fact that a fuller understanding of the journal selections collected under that vivid title is still in its infancy should perhaps come as no surprise, since Woodman herself opens the book by warning against reading it too quickly. What risk is evoked here? When time is of the essence, as it surely is amid the experience of the mortal illness that the book chronicles, why is "speed" necessarily the enemy of consciousness (xii)? Among many other things, *Bone* is a labour of love—both an account of Woodman's profound love for her husband, Ross, whose Afterword graces the book, and a memory of her struggle to "surrender" to the amorous embrace of Sophia, the demanding but finally benevolent goddess of consciousness who forms "the still point" (ix) of her life and work. But the book *is* a labour, the first-hand record of an agonistic subject-in-process, the outcome of which is unknown and unknowable—even if there are voices in *Bone*, as I want to argue, that suggest otherwise and that clamour for a punctual form of knowledge where none may be had. All that is certain is that today, happily, in the shadow of her cancer, Marion Woodman thrives—not in spite but because of the travail of soul and body that she describes in *Bone*. She often characterizes this labour as a form of parturition or giving birth to herself, although these metaphors of reproduction vie uneasily in the text with figures of disavowal, loss, and emaciation. This ambivalently executed work includes the creation of *Bone* itself, whose pangs of remembrance and imagination are enacted on every page. Like its author, the text is a case of dying into a life that is marked in advance by the violence and conflict of its origins.

We need to trace these mortal and mortifying marks if we are to understand the book at all; to read *Bone* closely and slowly, just as Woodman bids us in her prefatory remarks, will mean first of all resisting the temptation to erase these signs of struggle and incompleteness in the name of what is perhaps too quickly or too triumphantly called "life." Woodman is dying into *life* … but nothing could be less certain, less available to thought than the nature of this newly won existence. To this day, Woodman loves, teaches, and writes. She is alive, but as the title of her book puts to us, that quickened condition remains complexly interwoven with death and with forms of irreducible loss for which there may be no recompense. *Bone* is difficult to read because the radically reconfigured life that it describes and incarnates—the flesh made word, so to speak—is arduous: at its most far-reaching and self-searching moments, and there are many of these, *Bone* evokes a form of living that is not a thing or a substance that could be touched or brought to the light of consciousness, but a way of being-in-the-world, a resoluteness towards an ungraspable future that the mortally ill subject endures at the moment that it is summoned to keep watch over death. The vigilant "life" into which Woodman dies, or rather, is "dying," is not so much a place or destination as it is a time, or a timeliness, which she repeatedly captures in the words of Hamlet: "the readiness is all."

But ready for what? That may well be the wrong question, since it threatens to make the uniqueness of the moment of sheer facility that thrives at the heart of *Bone* answerable to something particular, as if one knew with a kind of visionary illumination and certainty not only *that* which was coming but also the clear direction of the path leading towards it. We might remember that Hamlet's phrase, "the readiness is all," does not mean that he moves from indecision to decision; it is rather a question of progressing *from* the abstention from decision (which is just as much a decision) *to* the more radical condition of in-decision through which all new decisions must pass if they are genuinely to be new. It would be fairer to the nuances of Woodman's text to say not "ready for something" but more starkly, "being-*ready*," dwelling in a state of tensed anticipation, by turns joyous and fearful, for the *arrivant*, for the *coming* of who knows what. Precisely what one must be ready for is not a query that needs to be answered in advance: the readiness is *all*. Somehow the experience of cancer induces this productively unstable condition in Woodman, even if there are moments in *Bone*—to which I want to draw readers' attention—in which metaphors and myths of certitude threaten to tempt her away from the wisdom of Hamlet. The most difficult thing of all, it turns out, is not the cancer that attacks Woodman's uterus or the treatment that ravages her body, but choosing in freedom to live without absolute surety—which is to say, in the book's Keatsian idiom, *dying into life*. As she argues, cancer opens the way for her "to be strong enough to surrender certainty. To leap into the mystery" (233). Readiness is therefore not passivity but rather an agile alertness, an active reluctance either to reach anxiously after fact or consent to the assurance of the given; it is not a state of self-possession so much as a species of willing dis-possession, a relinquishing of the need always to possess oneself and thus to know ahead of time what one's future and what one's future self will look like. This explains the uncanny rightness of the scene with which *Bone* concludes: Woodman is swept away by the irrepressible sound of the Dutchmens' tubas, and although her heart pounds and her spine cracks and her husband looks on in astonished horror, she casts herself into the unknown, at once unsure *and* preternaturally calm—as if coming to the realization that the jump is not the means by which to get from one place to the next but is itself the destination.

If Woodman's mortal illness is a "gift" (xv), it is a gift of honouring radical uncertainty; it is a gathering up of the courage to reject the consolations to be found in the idealizations, abstractions, and projections that in effect relieve the subject of the agony (but also the pleasure) of its responsibilities and decisions. A great part of *Bone*, especially its most pressingly affective moments, comes in the form of a prayer to Sophia—and we now see why. For prayer can only authentically *be* prayer if it is made in the midst of incertitude, in the profound openness to the unknown. As the French philosopher Jacques Derrida argues,

> This suspension of certainty is part of prayer .... If I knew or were simply expecting an answer, that would be the end of prayer. That would be an order .... No, I expect nothing like that. I assume that I must give up any expectation, any certainty, as the one, or the more than one, to whom I address my prayer, if this is still a prayer. (2005, 231)

The subtlest form of the Demon Lover with whom Woodman must wrestle in *Bone* is the trickster who would transform prayer into its parodic semblance—"an order," a determinate plan or myth or even metaphor, in which Woodman had surrendered not certainty but her freedom to decide either for certainty or uncertainty, death or life. At the point that *Bone* becomes programmatic, at the point that it declares itself most sure, it threatens to become nothing more than an elaborate version of "A Patient's Guide to Radiation Therapy" (100)—the name of the withered and withering instruction manual that Woodman indeed folds into the narrative of her book, as if to inoculate itself with the very kind of idealizing and emaciating discourse that it does not wish to become. A particular determinable faith in a particular determinate promise: that is the danger of religiosity with which *Bone* flirts, and at those points, I want to suggest, it is half in love not with dying into life but with its unsafe mimic—with easeful death, and thus with living *for* death. "With cancer," Woodman says in the book's opening sentences, "I discovered how much dying it takes to get here" (xi)—*here* being that no man's land of decision and responsibility where, precisely, there are no absolutely obvious instructions, no assured path or "patient's guide" leading one safely or predictably from *here* to *there*, from the sorrow of the actual to the reassurances of what Woodman calls the "archetypal dimensions" (113) of existence. It is instead a state of radical freedom: "I am alive," Woodman announces at the book's conclusion. "I am free ... to live ... to die" (241), she says, pacing her declaration with ellipses that figure forth the blank contingency of decision, the momentary absence of all plans, programmes, and metaphors that lies at the heart of every determination that makes a claim to freedom.

With Woodman the stakes are typically high, and because of that the book in which they are raised obliges its most attentive readers to proceed with caution. For various reasons, however, not everyone is or can be so circumspect. Not everyone is willing or able to follow the winding path that is Woodman's ongoing journey of consciousness and something other than consciousness. Yet this is not the difficulty to which Woodman first draws our attention in the book. In her Foreword she characterizes *Bone* as hard-going not because of the wrenching scenes that are to follow—some of which even her husband Ross finds impossible to read—or because of the sobering realization that death is not opposed to life but the very matrix in which life and freedom have meaning. The problem that initially concerns Woodman is that her readers will find it difficult to make sense of the book's idiosyncratic narrative form, and in particular the peculiar co-existence of different verbal and visual languages in one textual space. To be sure, the body of *Bone* is itself already a heterogeneous text, its sometimes wild excursions into the psyche's undiscovered countries barely kept in check by the journal entry dates that implacably sound off through the narrative. These dates are the chronological stitching-points that knit the fabric of this story together, and in effect prevent it from pulling itself into pieces, so ferocious is the mortal struggle at its core. But this is only part of what makes the volume "complex" (xii), as Woodman says. For the journal entries comprising the bulk of the narrative compete and cooperate with an elaborate out-work: photographs, illustrations, and images, as well as fragments drawn from poems and scattered psychological and philosophical writings in various hands. All of these materials function as a gloss on the text and form its elaborate "margin" (xii)—or rather one of its margins. What worries Woodman is how her readers will negotiate both these borders and the emotional and intellectual hinterlands that they mark. We are never sure if these extra-textual voices and perspectives are avatars of the author, externalizations of her inner life, or whether in their otherness they speak for and out of spaces of alterity by which Woodman is herself haunted—"new images," as she says, "that I don't yet comprehend" (xii). Do the marginal remarks confirm and amplify what is being said in the body of the narrative, distilling what is being experienced into memorable epigrams and summaries? Or do they allegorize that body, spiriting away its complex local densities with answers and lessons that are *grafted* onto the book's central narrative from a wholly different place?

"If the rumblings in the margins seem disruptive to the text, then you, as reader, need not be slowed down," Woodman counsels: "Skip them" (xii). Why dwell at all on this question of haste—and in a text that elsewhere avows an ambiguous faith in "the speed of bone" (221)? Why suggest to readers that the gloss itself should be glossed? I think that this is Woodman's quiet way of calling attention to the fact that the book is replete with borders, and that a great part of reading her work involves the question of how to traverse its verges of thought and feeling. That the material on the margins is more significant than Woodman at first seems willing to admit is evident in her quick change of heart about the matter. Contradicting her initial advice to her readers, she tells us that by passing over the text's margins too quickly we risk repudiating *Bone*'s most urgent details. "We are now moving at a pace that is dissolving the world into an abstraction before *we can take it in*," Woodman writes, her buried metaphor of ingestion reminding us of the connections that obtain between slow reading and eating slowly, on the one hand, and the fast life and an indifference to sustenance, on the other. "If the marginalia slows you down, it is doing what I intended, knowing what it has done for me" (xii; emphasis added). This is a book with which to tarry, then, and not one whose insights can be taken up or cast off without remainder.

As if to ensure that we work hard at reading *Bone*, it is a text that is replete with margins, many more than the already complicated partitions dividing Woodman's journal entries from their glosses. Literary criticism in the shadow of deconstruction has taught us that the difference *between* the body of a work and its glosses almost always repeats and reproduces differences *within* each field. It is those interior partitions, perhaps less legible than the boundaries dividing Woodman's autobiographical voice from the voices of the others that she draws into her circle, to which I want principally to attend. It may be that Woodman's focus on the text's obvious, formal divisions displaces—hides, but also remembers—the analogous strata unsettling the integrity of the body of the book, and throwing into question some of its more strident claims for wholeness. In other words, the formal split between *Bone*'s body and marginalia is expected to bear away evidence of more substantial self-divisions rippling through the text. To say the least, these differences call for a *slow reading*. Friedrich Nietzsche demanded such deliberation when it came to reading writing that mattered—not the only point in *Bone* in which Woodman's work resonates with that of the German philosopher whom she otherwise derides as ushering in a world without god and without sacred books (see, for instance: Nietzsche 1997, 6).

This is the sort of interpretation that I want to bring to bear here, making tentative steps towards parsing the intricacies of Woodman's illness narrative, this, by dwelling less on its large features—its insistent arc from disaster to triumph, crucifixion to resurrection, or death to life. If we read *Bone* entirely from Sophia's perspective, everything about Woodman's psychic life is answerable to the lucidity of consciousness. But what would it mean to reverse the perspective—turn the telescope around, as it were—and to see Sophia from the point of view of the localized eddies that swirl inside *Bone*'s overall narrative and that trouble the Apollonian surety about its author's metamorphosis that is evoked by its very subtitle? What mutinous remnants haunt this extraordinary story of health and illness, loss and recompense, mortality and divinity, disrupting the economies of spirit that reconcile these terms in elegant dialectical "spirals" around Sophia's "still point"? A slow reading is a way of being in the world that ratifies the presence of these leavings in our lives, and affirms their productive and restless place amid our tempting dreams of untrammelled integrity and purposiveness. These are dreams that Woodman's book pursues, but not without a palpable degree of ambivalence. Far from being a well-wrought urn, unequivocally confident in its findings, *Bone* is a text that is riven with self-differences—and in this way it earns the right to say, as it does in its opening sentence, that it is a "book about living, not dying" (xi).

II

Sophia is the name that Woodman uses to describe the dissenting work that she conducts on behalf of the "feminine," which is the wisdom of the ages that she marshals to resist the predations of abstraction and idealization—the seductive yet suicidally destructive impulses that she identifies with the "masculine" and for which she blames modernity's sorrowful inability to bring living and dying into a meaningful convocation. These impulses, she has observed throughout her writings, form and deform the culture at large, but *Bone* is unique for exploring the extraordinary degree to which they have continued to shape her own psychic life. Among other things, Sophia means authentically *embodied* life, life lived in a manner that apprehends and prizes the subtle knot of spirit and flesh that is, as Woodman says, every person's "birthright" (168). How does one come to see and grasp this "patrimony" and make it one's own? The "body-soul work" that is a mainstay of Woodman's practice as an analyst and as a teacher has been largely devoted to nurturing this ennobling and healing task in others. The objective is not so much a decisive breakout to a wholly different universe—for where or what could that transcendent place be?—as a circuitous *return* to that universe's otherwise obscured and wounded heart. To dedicate and to re-dedicate oneself to the labour of consciousness *is* this movement of circling recollection; Sophia is therefore not a single location towards which all consciousnesses move (which would make her indistinguishable from the Christian God Woodman abandons in childhood) but, as it were, the curvature of psychic space in which the soul is given the opportunity to fashion itself.

Bone is a testament to the project of Marion Woodman's own soul-making. This is a project that was always already underway in her life but it takes the trauma of her cancer and the immanent prospect of her death to give its centrality to her life a new imperative—as if she were confronting its demands and intuiting its significances for the first time. This is the "gift" of her experience with illness, the rich but unhappy endowment that comes her way unexpectedly and without declaring itself as such. As Plato teaches, resolute attention to and concern with death (*meletē thanatou*) is what awakens the self to itself and to the need to gather up its parts into a meaningful whole. He suggests that true thinking is in essence nothing more than this act of vital self-possession before the prospect of one's death. In the words of the Czech philosopher and human rights activist, Jan Patočka (whose work Jacques Derrida reads so closely in his book, *The Gift of Death*), "the concern of the soul is inseparable from the concern for death which becomes authentic concern for life; … life is born from this event of looking death in the face" (in Derrida 1995, 16). Looking back at Woodman's *oeuvre* from the vantage-point of *Bone*, I am not sure whether all of her work isn't *mortified* in this way, a testimony to the possibilities of dying into life whose antecedents can be traced to Socrates's argument in the *Phaedo*. What makes *Bone* stand out among Woodman's other published writings, however, is the frankness with which it admits to the need for her to pursue this reparative and constitutive work in her own life—and thus for the healer to heal herself. As she confides in her journal entries, helping others recognize their "covenant with Sophia" (14)—and thus to live a more fully realized life—had somehow led her to disregard the importance of reaffirming the same compact in herself. This irresponsible distraction from what Woodman calls her "own truth" (17) is counted as one of the causes of her cancer, and so the difficult path back to consciousness begins there, in her sacrum, where the disease appears literally and metaphorically. Like Apollo in Keats's *Hyperion*, the process of dying into life is characterized as the advent of a new dawn. The dense opacity of her tumour forms the dark background against which Woodman sets the clarifying powers of her evolving consciousness. Under the blaze of its ultimately incontestable light, she comes to discern the patterns that organize her existence and that give meaning to the anguish of her illness.

Woodman is the first to admit that a great part of herself resisted this illumination, but the overall psychological momentum of *Bone* is irrefutably one from unconsciousness to consciousness, repression to self-transparency. It is the light that enables her to parse the obscurities of the world and therefore to transform it into a truly liveable place; "consciousness makes the difference" (12), as she says, between being an ego that submits to fate, and an ego that cooperates with destiny. Step by step, Woodman brings into view not only the inner significance of her cancer but also, more powerfully, the ways in which her illness forms a part—indeed a crucially important part—of a larger voyage of consciousness begun when she was a child. "I am seeing the archetypal dimensions that have forced me towards wholeness against my will," Woodman observes; "I see the progression of spirals through which I have moved upward and downward, higher into spirit, deeper into grounding .... What an incredible map I seem to have followed!" (113). In her account of the radiation chamber, Woodman affords us a glimpse of what it means to dwell within the darkest depths of the vale of soul-making; but *Bone* does not find its centre there. Instead, in moments that surprise Woodman as much as they offer profound reassurance, she finds herself occupying a vantage point on her own life that is nothing if not divine—a placeless place from which Woodman glimpses both the centre and the circumference, the local details and the large design, the still point and the spirals around which the widening gyres of her life are oriented.

It is only because of the incandescent light of consciousness that Woodman is able to apprehend her experience with cancer not only as the traumatic destruction of the body but as the prelude towards a subtler and more fully realized mode of embodied life: as Woodman says in the opening words of *Bone*, the "shattering" effect of her illness is the means by which she assumes a path to "wholeness." There are many moments in *Bone* in which this unity is not a state to be desired but a deed to be celebrated; indeed, the book *as* a book, as a crafted story that gathers together the strands of Woodman's life and weaves them into a meaningful whole, stands as both a figure for and testament to this accomplishment. Its articulate achievement contrasts with the ragged cry of pain that it also subsumes within its covers. In the details of the narrative, we see how the light of consciousness brings much-needed clearness to being-ill, this, primarily, by locating Woodman's experience with cancer amid a larger significance that would be all but invisible to ordinary sight. Going into her surgery, Woodman has the first intimations of this design: "[M]aybe this is the sacrifice of my feminine organs to prepare me for the next step—to release me from all physical mothering," she muses, "to release me into a new vibration in my body" (17). Through cognate narratives of purposiveness, the senselessness of disease is compelled to yield sense: the cancer is "a lesson to be learned" (5); it is the means by which her body makes itself into an "instrument" (105) that forces her to come to consciousness. For a month after the radiation treatment, there is nothing—the blank space in Woodman's diary entries speaks volumes. Then the narrative of the book starts up again, and even in her disoriented state—"still not sure who has emerged," she confides to her journal—Woodman finds much needed consolation in the outlines of an archetypal "map" of the territory ahead: "felt the crucifixion this year, and the tomb, and Easter Sunday" (132), she writes, transforming bare survival into redemption and resurrection. In a testament that makes the highest possible claims for the powers of metaphor (for Woodman, they are in the end responsible for healing what the physicians cannot cure), we are invited to take these consolatory figures seriously.

The self-achieving consciousness is monumentalized in *Bone* as a courageous convocation with Sophia. Under these mythic conditions, the remnants which resist consciousness or inhibit the apprehension of the divine marriage of soul and body can be figured as perverse. Indeed, not to accede to Sophia's light is experienced as a form of weakness, even cowardliness and apostasy. When Woodman balks at giving herself wholly over to alternative therapies that have been urged upon her by others, for example, she feels answerable to Sophia's all-seeing eyes. "I need to acknowledge that in my December 12 session with Jean I could not get by the *ifs*, and therefore could not surrender to the wisdom of the limbic system, as Jean encouraged me to do .... Fear is still stronger than faith. Forgive me, Sophia" (82). Here and elsewhere in *Bone* Woodman describes her continuing attachment to conventional medicine in terms of trepidation, irresponsibility, and perfidy—as faults requiring a kind of confession to a superior power. It is in moments like these that we see that the incandescence of consciousness not only positively illuminates the ultimate purposiveness of the nature of things; it also negatively brings a normative gaze to bear on the heart's reluctance to give itself too quickly over to that design. The aura of impotence and failure that attends Woodman's self-castigations reminds us that the claims *Bone* makes for light and clarity in the face of death are not only Apollonian but also residually masculinist inasmuch as they associate perfectly understandable hesitations with "fear," and strength with acts of heroic self-possession. But facing death need not necessarily be described in these judgmental terms as a test of the psyche's willingness and ability to triumph over doubt and self-difference. As the cultural theorist Gillian Rose wrote prior to her own cancer death, it was philosophers like Martin Heidegger who taught us to believe that "being-toward-death" was properly a matter of attaining "'a supreme lucidity and hence a supreme virility.'" Against Heidegger, and, indeed, against a tradition of life-writing going back to Plato, Rose opposes the very different thought of Emmanuel Levinas, for whom the proximity of death is "'foreign to all light'" and "'absolutely unknowable'" (Rose 1996, 133). Levinas is not interested in the subject who comes into a form of stringent clarity by steeling itself for death; it is the mortality and suffering of the *other*—and this includes the other that is also oneself—which has precedence in human life, and which deprives the self of its pretensions to mastery (see, for instance: Levinas 1998).

Levinas invites us to revalue the alterities that lie beyond and before consciousness, and to treasure their traces as evidence of our radical singularity, mortality, and unknowability. For him, we are never more ourselves than when we are most vulnerable, and thus calling out to the other for justice and responsibility. In Heidegger, by contrast, the potent philosophical subject seeks total self-sufficiency through heroic self-assertion and the disavowal of the other. In a way that has complex resonances with Woodman's project, Levinas characterizes this ascetic way of being-in-the-world as a refusal either to eat or to demonstrate a need to eat: "*Dasein* in Heidegger is never hungry," he writes (Levinas 1969, 134).[1] Committed to the radiance of Sophia and the labour of consciousness, however, Woodman's book approaches Levinas's insight into the anorexic remainder haunting philosophical idealisms about facing death with caution. In her hands, what refuses to be brought into the light of day is more often banished to a deeper darkness; hence the degree to which *Bone*'s narrative is moved along not only by inclusive affirmations but also by sharp disavowals. For example, Woodman characterizes her surgery as "the letting go of something that is finished in order to move into new life" (58). Moving forward, her primary task is to make sure that this renunciation penetrates to the profoundest part of herself; and she adds: "How then to let go? How to be sure at the unconscious level that I am letting go?" (58), as if the searchlight of consciousness could sweep into the farthest corners of the psyche. On the eve of entering the radiation chamber, Woodman's resoluteness is again expressed in the form of disavowals: "Your task right now is to let the old thinking go, flush the toilet, accept the love, walk free" (124). On the Christmas Eve following her radiation therapy, she revels in a vision of the wholeness of the nature of things: "God/Goddess in every living thing—the totality of the universe" (218). But in the next sentence, we see that this totality is at best a qualified one, for it is constituted by the refusal of part of itself: "The old questions won't matter; the old answers will be obsolete" (218). When Woodman receives the diagnosis of a metastasized cancer from Dr Thomas, she prays to Sophia for, among other things, "the steadfastness to reject sentimentality" (184). As Woodman repeatedly says, the voyage of consciousness is for her a voyage of ongoing reduction, of bravely purging what is deemed to be inessential and burdensome. "Simplify. Get rid of all conflict" (205): these are the categorical imperatives of her newly

1 "*Dasein*" is the term Heidegger uses to name the barest structure of the being of human being.

embodied life, a life of light, lightness, transparency … and above all, *evacuation*: "the letting go—the clearing" (28).

But is this sort of voiding simplification possible, or, for that matter, self-evidently desirable? In one of the book's most affecting moments, Woodman recalls how her mother, on the threshold of her death, lets go of her beloved daughter. Unable to say goodbye to Woodman in person, she leaves a fragment from Shakespeare to speak on her behalf. Written out in her "beautiful handwriting," the scene her mother chooses is from *Julius Caesar*: "If we do meet again, why, we shall smile," Brutus says, bidding farewell to Cassius; "If not, why then, this parting was well made" (58). Does it matter that Woodman's mother casts their separation as one between two virile but imaginary men? In the world of actual mothers and daughters, are partings ever "well made"? Through Woodman's eyes we see what it feels like to be the remnant, the one who is let go, and from that reversed perspective it is obvious that the cut, as "beautiful" as it is, and perhaps because it is so "well made," is dissatisfying because it unfolds with otherworldly perfection. Compelled to play the role of the remainder, Woodman objects and pushes back: "I wanted you to die my way," she recalls; "God had another way" (58). So much is said in this cry from the heart: to be sure, there is anger at losing control over her mother's life, a sense of being pre-empted both by her death and by the way in which she said good-bye; but there is inconsolable grief too, not only for the loss but also for the incalculability and inaccessibility of that loss, the sorrowful realization that the mother's departure from Woodman's life cannot be economized into something that is "well-made." For can the psyche ever "simply" have done with any part of itself, much less a part of itself to which it is so deeply attached that only the extremity of a mortal illness can loosen those binds? Perhaps it is the prospect of death that prompts these fantasies of cleanly perfect divisions and reorganizations of life. Or is this faith in the purgative powers of renunciation itself an idealism of the sort that Judith Butler (1993, 27–55), Jacques Derrida (1989, 1–43), and others have associated with fantasies of achieved mourning work—work in which the psyche imagines that it can, through the heroic effort of repudiation, part with its losses without ever looking back? Is it the case that all partings are melancholically incomplete, but some forget this messy and discomforting fact, and become triumphantly mournful? These questions seem worth asking of a text which is so palpably haunted by what *remains*—beginning with the book itself, whose effect is vividly, permanently, and publically to *remember* what its author deems worthy of being abandoned and forgotten. That the book was written at all puts to us that at the very least Woodman is unwilling to disavow her disavowals, the result being that she remains connected, psychically speaking, to the very things that she has given up. She avows them, but in the negative form of renouncing them. The look forward to what she calls her "new life" is literally written in the form of a sustained look back at the "old."

Many other left-overs trouble the book's strident demands to let go: the marginal materials that Woodman at first disdains ("Skip them," she says, as if they were a meal that she could avoid), but then acknowledges as an important part of the body of her book; the physical and psychic spaces from which Woodman's cancer was cut and burned, all absent presences forming and deforming her life; the lingering effects of the radiation on her body and spirit, including the literal and metaphorical scars she bears; the memories of her dead friend Mary, whose anguish at being alone before death Woodman remembers in order to forget (67); the sounds of the "groaning" and "weeping" patients and family members that waft unbidden and unstoppably into her head as she lies in her "radiation tank" (131), all the intimations of otherness haunting the edges of her consciousness; the loss of her beloved brother, Fraser Boa, the grief for whom, as Woodman herself admits, lies locked up in her own flesh and thus the object of a melancholic return rather than a mournful having-done-with (7). Consider too the break with the oncologist, Dr Thomas, which happens at a crucial turning point in the course of the recovery from her illness. Of that split Woodman tells us emphatically that she "hold[s] no resentment, no anger" (205). Yet she chooses to reproduce her formal letter of discharge to Thomas in its entirety, thereby preserving the renunciation of the physician even if the physician himself is renounced. And then there is the striking image of herself as her own remains, her "body going back to dust." "Think of our compost heap in which earth does go back to earth" (184), she writes in her journal, folding metaphors drawn from the burial service into more familial and domestic terms. Up until this point in the book, the move to the beautiful new house on Sydenham Street in London, Ontario has figured forth the birth of Woodman's embodied psyche; not surprisingly, given the logic of sacrifice that governs the book's narrative, this move is accompanied by a decisive disavowal: "only essentials going to the new house," she insists: "Move into the new life. That is where it is to happen. High ceilings, light, a garden, fresh air, fresh sunlight, new hope" (28–9). But Sydenham, like the psyche for which it is a metaphor, is not only this scene of space and illumination, for we learn that out back, away from the light, the home's cast-offs ferment in the darkness and also make their claims on Woodman's thoughts. For a strange moment, Woodman allows that the protected home is also a kind of cemetery or bone-yard, exposed to an otherness for which there is no conscious apprehension: "This is not metaphor," Woodman flatly says; "so be it" (184). Although untranslatable into the idiom of the archetype, the "compost" nevertheless asserts its rightful place in the nature of things.

The tensions surrounding the irreducible remainder that limns consciousness without necessarily being drawn into its light become perhaps most apparent around Woodman's characterization of the surgery to remove her "carcinoma of the endometrium" (15). "My baby was born by Caesarean section and disposed of," she writes, self-consciously rejecting the diagnostic terminology of the physicians, "—but a baby, nonetheless, that forever changed my life" (167). Woodman has just told us that the "metaphorical connection between birth and death is very strong in [her] … psyche" (167), perhaps to prepare us for this strange way to imagine the nature and fate of her cancer. But it is worth noting here how even Woodman's language strains to accommodate what it has been being asked to explain metaphorically: the growth in her uterus must be cut away, all traces annihilated if she is to survive her illness. But at the same moment as Woodman speaks of "disposing" of the cancer, it is refashioned as a spectral "baby" who is figuratively speaking dead to the precise extent that it remains alive to Woodman's memory. The literal act of having-done with the tumour competes with the figural translation of that act into a violent giving-birth; yet the cancer remains, to the extent that it resists its too easy sublimation into the form of a "baby," even one that is stillborn. Nothing could more powerfully call for being cast off than the cancer, yet Woodman experiences that saving rejection as an abortion that allows her to recuperate her loss as a loss of *life*—albeit a monstrous and fatally parasitic life, without coherence and quite possibly at the far side of the recuperative powers of metaphor. In the end, the cancer surgery that forms the literal ground for these elaborate figures insists itself, this, by throwing into relief the macabre overreaching of Woodman's metaphors. Bordering on the hallucinatory, these figures possess consolatory power for Woodman, but from the readers' perspective they call attention to the hyperbolic demands that Woodman's archetypal understanding places on her illness—and to the ways in which her illness can resist those demands, bringing the edifice of metaphor crashing down to earth. Of the cancer we might indeed also say, "This is not metaphor. So be it."

Woodman often characterizes her disavowals as a stripping down, "letting irrelevant matter go …. Lightening up, simplifying in order to concentrate on essentials" (112). Fleshless "bone" is the book's metaphor *par excellence* for this emaciated purity. But one cannot read these figures of refinement and deprivation (and refinement *as* deprivation) and not also see the striking similarity between the principle means by which Woodman renews her covenant with Sophia and much less felicitous forms of renunciation that are explored in the text. For isn't the psyche that takes pride and pleasure in "lightening up" and "letting go" not also in some spectral sense an anorexic psyche? Does the fiercely reiterated desire to buoy herself up through a process of divestiture not mimic a more archaic lust operating in Woodman's psyche, the thing of darkness that she struggles to acknowledge as her own? Is the path of unburdening simplification—a path that is undertaken, precisely, in the name of turning from "old eating patterns, old patterns of relationship" (40)—not evidence of the survival of these patterns, a repetition of the addiction to perfection, albeit in a finer tone? "When I *was* anorexic," Woodman tells us, "I always felt that starvation brought me close to God. It brought me close to death, a Demon Lover, whose radiance lured my senses into a life so exquisite I yearned to escape gross matter" (62; emphasis added). By safely locating this condition of disavowal in the past, Woodman repudiates the will to repudiate, lightening herself of the burden of the craving for lightness that once controlled her life. But is the irrefutable lucidity of consciousness, the clarity that it offers to Woodman in her darkest hour, not itself a form of this seductive "radiance"? As she puts it, "Starvation is a metaphor for getting out of an impossible situation—death to the old and maybe hope for the new" (81). In its local context, Woodman is thinking both of herself as a younger woman and that aspect of her present self which, in agreeing to undergo the killingly destructive radiation treatment, "colludes" with the desire to withdraw from life. But does this account of starvation not also exactly describe the process of dying *into* life—the move from the "impossible situation" of the cancer diagnosis and treatment, through a period punctuated by increasingly demanding renunciations ("death to the old"), all in expectation of "hope for the new"?

This is a difficult and counterintuitive thought, to be sure, but provoked by a book that brims with such possibilities and that does nothing but encourage them in its readers. An anorexic remainder haunts Woodman's myth of feminine consciousness as its dark semblance. We see this most clearly near the book's conclusion. On New Year's Day, 1995, Woodman feels "caught between two worlds, trying to move into new imagery, still not knowing what's in the bones in my back" (221). Then, a flash of certainty and a flood of images: "One thing I do know: I am no longer ashamed of having been anorexic. I yearned for lightness; I still yearn for lightness. Lightness is freedom—freedom from the heaviness of too much stuff, too many words, too heavy a pull toward inertia …. I yearned for bone—the lightness of bone, the stark reality of bone, the speed of bone, the beauty of bone" (221–2). It would take a great deal properly to unpack the complexities of this admission, but for the purposes of this argument it is important to emphasize not only Woodman's unexpected turn towards embracing—rather than forsaking—her anorexic impulses, but also the unblushing surefootedness with which she makes this turn. With respect to her anorexic desires, she is here more like a woman who seeks the thing she loves, than one who flees from something she dreads. Elsewhere in the book, Woodman prides herself in the hard-won consciousness that anorexia means falling prey to the seductions of the Demon Lover, "the pathological idealism" that "continues to murder the feminine that cherishes life" (216). But on New Year's Day comes a clarity about the nature of that clarity, a consciousness not about the seductive powers of the Demon Lover but about the consciousness that makes those powers visible. "[B]one … bone … bone … bone": the self-conscious tolling of the title of the book puts to us how Woodman herself grasps the uncanny resemblance between the yearning for lightness that is anorexia and the cherishing of the feminine that is the covenant with Sophia. As Woodman tells us in the next sentence, honouring the "feminine, right here and now in my body, my bone" is inevitably caught up in the labour of "letting the weight of possessions go" (222). The greatest threat to consciousness is that in its ferocious quest to unburden itself it falls over into the idealization and wasting abstraction that it abhors. For the dark side of taking on the beauty and speed and lightness of bone in the name of escaping what feels like inertia can also mean the *skeletalization* of the psyche. The very title of Woodman's book inadvertently remembers that discomforting possibility.

"Let your last remnants of your yearning for God-like perfection go," Woodman notes towards the end of her book, calling for a final and therefore monumentally decisive act of renunciation. But does a fully-embodied life lie on the other side of that perfect release … or does death? In the name of what, if not another kind of ascetic purity, is this summons made? What but another way of being in the world whose rarity and worth is predicated on the disavowal of those elements that are deemed to be a contagion? All disavowals in *Bone* have in a sense been a prelude to the casting off of these "last remnants," the disposal of all that remains—or is imagined to remain—between Woodman's partly unconscious earlier life and the authentically realized existence that awaits her in the face of death. "Cherish your imperfect humanity," she continues: "Die into life" (207–8). Insofar as the call to consciousness is also an expression of this "yearning" for "perfection," Woodman here finds herself at a profound limit. *For the very act of disavowing the seductive desire for flawlessness re-inscribes the arc of that desire anew.* The "last remnant" is last in the sense of being irreducible because it is produced and reproduced by Woodman's impulse to lighten herself of its weight.

Perhaps it is no accident that this is the moment when Woodman most pointedly recalls the origins of her book's subtitle in Keats's poetic fragment, *Hyperion*. As she says, "I hope I can 'with fierce convulse / Die into life'" (207). We should recall that in the third, uncompleted book of *Hyperion*, Apollo, the young sun god, attempts, like Woodman, to come into consciousness with the assistance of the goddess of memory, Mnemosyne. Apollo's new life is obscurely connected not to the disavowal of the past but to its conservation. At the moment that Apollo passes from a twilight state of hiddenness into brilliant visibility, he suffers pangs that evoke childbirth even as they conjure up death—a tortured transitional moment that naturally speaks to Woodman and explains why these lines in Keats are ones to which she returns several times in her book. But what is not remembered about the Keats passage also haunts her use of it. For *Hyperion* breaks off at this point, and was abandoned by the poet, as if in writing these words down something unexpected had dawned upon him. Has Apollo and the creator-poet for which he is an idealistic figure in fact ascended to a higher mode of being? Keats is not altogether confident in the answer to that question, as ferociously pressing as it is to him on this, the eve of his own mortal illness and in the shadow of his brother's death. The poet-creator struggles to be born, and to divest himself of the dreamy naiveté of the pastoral in which he had once found comfort, however illusory; but at the point of that parturition a terrible doubt falls across his path, a sense that his own declaration of authenticity rings false, tolling him back to his sole self. What is this virile "life" into which he so grandly aspires to die? In turning to the classical language of *Hyperion* Keats exchanges the language of the pastoral for that of epic. But is this necessarily the progress towards enlightenment that it feels at that moment to be? Or has he simply moved from one mythical universe to another, exchanging abstractions but describing this exchange as the triumph of life, the violent leap *from* a dead (because lifeless) world *to* a living one that dies? The fact that the poem breaks off at this point is perhaps the most palpable answer that Keats could give—it is the way the poem abstains from answering; and in that self-fracturing gesture, *Hyperion* signals an inconclusive attachment to the world of Apollonian light towards which it turns so expectantly. Keats's speaker lays claim to dying into life, but then shudders to a halt, the poem ceasing at the precise moment that it appears to begin, or rather to begin anew.

Keats is a crucial part of the secular scripture informing Woodman's thinking; along with Shakespeare and the Bible, it is his work that she carries with her into the inferno of the radiation chamber. In what ways does *Bone: Dying into Life*, whose title directs us to this crisis point in Keats's life and work, also register a similar crisis—but protect itself from this crisis by remembering it in the form of someone else's words? For I do think that a part of Woodman is wary of the claims made for this life into which she dies, especially insofar as that life demands an ascesis that is structurally indistinguishable from the anorexia of her earlier self, a life which imagines itself as having purged from its subtle body the "last remnant." More than any other Romantic poet, perhaps, Keats resisted the tendency to be blinded by his idealisms, including those most tempting of idealisms—the ones that appear to offer a foolproof escape from idealism. Woodman's allegiance to Keats is, I think, a secret fealty to that difficult insight, even if she appears to take the poet's faith in a wrenching transformation without remainder at face value. Elsewhere in the book there are significant signs, however, that Woodman senses the difference between claiming and actually showing that the enlightened state of the covenant with Sophia is unquestionably superior. Wrestling with whether to take the full course of radiation therapy, for instance, Woodman resists giving herself over to "the power of that machine and the perfectionist mind that controls it" (73). Her friend Pauline objects to that objection, probing the deepest presuppositions of Woodman's stance. You see a killing perfectionism in the biomedical technology of the medical regime, Pauline points out; but isn't your faith in the healing powers of consciousness itself a perfectionism, and thus no less murderously indifferent to life? "'You know,' she said, 'idealization can be a lack of femininity. If you idealize to the point of blinding yourself to what may save your life, that is not being on the side of life, the positive side of the feminine. Blindness is negative'" (73). Woodman's response to the corrosive powers of Pauline's insight is at best noncommittal, and the conversation quickly turns from Woodman's psyche to the psyches of other unnamed "women" (74). But this deflection does nothing to reduce the significance of the interrogation at the hands of Pauline, who is, after all, an avatar of Woodman, an other who speaks for an alterity that thrives within Woodman herself—and thrives to the point that she is given a role in the narrative of *Bone*. Another way of saying this is that if the first person voice in *Bone*—identified as Marion—speaks for an abiding faith in the feminine, she does not and cannot speak for the book as a whole, which, in the form of Pauline, contains a critique of itself. Pauline models a "feminist" consciousness whose principle target is the frightening prospect of a "feminism" that will risk death to be on the side of life.

That "feminism" is surely what Woodman elsewhere calls a "projection." And as she tells us, when it comes to "muster[ing] every ounce of Spiritual Warrior in myself to defend my feminine feelings and values" there are "No projections allowed!" (62). What is revealing is that this declaration of the need to unburden herself of projections—more "yearning for the lightness of bone"—is made at the conclusion of the one journal entry in which Woodman most calls attention not only to their operation but also to the ways in which they pre-empt experience as much as they give shape and meaning to it. For Woodman has here recalled a trip that Ross makes to New York during the course of her illness; as she claims, even her loving husband must for a time be renounced, "moved off" (62), lest she be distracted from the true path of consciousness. The notion that Ross could in fact be disposed of, even momentarily, seems fantastically unlikely, a fact confirmed by Woodman's own journal entries which re-inscribe his metaphorical presence in his literal absence. While in New York Ross sees *Angels in America*, Tony Kushner's Pulitzer Prize winning play about HIV/AIDS—one of the few occasions in *Bone* in which Woodman acknowledges the rich world of illness narratives that informs her own story. Woodman does not see the play herself, and hears of its details only second-hand, through her husband's reporting of them. But the narrative structure of the journal entry in which this occasion is remembered is very telling, for *before* any of Ross's perceptions of the play are even mentioned, Woodman rewrites the play so that it becomes an allegory of the struggle to reaffirm the covenant with Sophia. Ross has told her that "The Great Work begins" is the play's evocative last line, but rather than considering how, in its own context, this turn of phrase grows out the play for which it effects closure, it triggers in her a surge of interpretive labour that drains Kushner's story of its own details and replaces them with a story that sounds uncannily like the story that *Bone* is telling. "The Great Work that is beginning is the realization of the feminine as the bridge between God and humankind," she writes, proceeding to give a brief but detailed analysis of the play's archetypal dimensions. *Bone* overwrites *Angels in America*, and for the moment that superimposition is given the full weight of Woodman's authority as an analyst. Only at the end of this move on the play does Woodman pause, noting—albeit tentatively—that what she has been saying with such confidence may not be fair to Kushner's vision: "But I'm not sure that's what *Angels in America* is about," she concedes.

A week later, in a different journal entry, Woodman returns to the matter of the play, where she more frankly admits that her views about its details were "straight idealization" (70).

> Ross saw a Nietzschean world, a world where there is no god, no sacred book. We are on our own. We have to improvise and do what we can for ourselves. "The Great Work" is the invention of ourselves, even as the play is an invention of ourselves. And as for the angel, she flies on pulleys that we can see, an impoverished homemade creature.

"So much for that projection!," Woodman writes, but "At least I brought to consciousness what I think 'The Great Work' is" (70). Woodman acknowledges that she has simplified and abstracted the play but recuperates her self-conscious surprise at so fundamentally mistaking its content by reassuring herself that even in error she continues on the path of consciousness. But in context, this seems like a half-hearted justification, especially when set against the more passionate account of the play that Ross provides. Whatever Woodman *says* has happened, these two journal entries tell a somewhat different story. We are most often told that grasping the archetypal dimensions of reality is a matter of holding the illuminating mirror of consciousness up to the nature of things; but here we see not so much a mirror at work, as a lamp, and, as it were, catch Woodman in the act of projecting upon reality what may only be true only in her own imagination. For it is Woodman who is improvising here, not the supposedly deprived characters moving about Kushner's stage, and it is Woodman who self-consciously draws our attention to it. In other words, we are afforded the opportunity to see in Woodman what she eventually sees and regrets in Kushner's play, namely the possibility that what feels like a universal truth, more evidence of how "God organizes our lives" (61), is in fact "an invention of ourselves."

For a brief moment, it is as if the curtain is raised on the work of consciousness and revealed to be a projection—not an account of the nature of things but a device that is "homemade" and that "flies on pulleys." Is *Bone* itself not such a device? In these journal entries about Kushner are we not given a chance to observe the machinery of consciousness, the push and pull of the book's own pulleys? Woodman barely contains that realization about the work of consciousness by associating it with what she dismisses as "a Nietzschean world," a world she experiences as "impoverished." Yet in admitting that her interpretation of Kushner's play is an "idealization" and a "projection," Woodman also tacitly concedes that the myth of consciousness is not without its own impoverishment. *Angels in America*, or rather, Ross's "Nietzschean" view of it, stands as a figure for all that resists the idealizing designs that *Bone* has on reality—that is, as another instance of an irreducible remainder, a remainder, moreover, that is allowed in the second journal entry to "splutter back into life" after having been relegated to the margins by the forcefulness of Woodman's glossing powers. I am not so sure that the notion that, in this world, "We are on our own," and that "We have to improvise and do what we can for ourselves," is nearly as far from Woodman's project of soul-making as her dismissal of it as "Nietzschean" suggests. Woodman wants to dispose of that surprising connection between her book and Kushner's play by locating the latter in a universe of nihilist abstraction, but the fact that it is also a universe that is identified with and filtered through Ross—who haunts the book—reminds us that the world of *Angels* is closer to Woodman's psyche than at first might appear. The threatening if counterintuitive proximity of *Angels* to *Bone* would help explain the preemptive way in which Woodman attempts to assimilate Kushner's universe to her own, only to end up conceding the violence of that move.

What is revealing is that between the two journal entries concerning *Angels*, Woodman circles back to the question of "projections." It is as if in the days between simplifying the play and realizing the violence of that simplification, Woodman is prompted to consider the role of other idealizations in her life and work. We know that the book is about to suffer a seismic shift because Woodman cites Susan

Sontag's *Illness as Metaphor* in the margins: "Nothing is more punitive than to give a disease a meaning—the meaning being invariably a moralistic one .... The disease itself becomes a metaphor" (67). In many respects *Bone* is written *against* Sontag's influential reflection on the representation of disease—particularly cancer narratives—since it is an exploration of metaphor as a source of healing rather than as a fund of stigmatization. But for a moment Woodman pauses to reconsider this faith, and to allow for the possibility that the work that she is doing in the name of consciousness (which is work whose primary goal is to give meaning to illness, her own and others') also risks moralizing it, fitting it to normative frameworks that coarsen human experience even as it claims to alleviate suffering. Woodman responds to Sontag's observation with a list of "punitive" metaphors by which her own illness has been characterized:

> "It's the father complex, kills the mother, tears out the womb." Or "It's the Negative Mother imprinted on your cells driving you to death." Or "Endometrial cancer is found to have a hereditary factor." Or "You never gave up your grief for Fraser. Your grief is destroying you." Or "Tear things to shreds. Let your rage go." Or "The cancer personality gives all to others and keeps nothing for itself, and when it has given all, it gives more." (68)

What is astonishing about these competing narratives of illness, these different ways of bringing cancer to the bar of consciousness, is that not one is without relevance to Woodman's own project of soul-making. Yet they are dismissed as aggressive denials of her life rather than lucid explanations of her encounter with death. "Projections! Projections!," she exclaims, in a journal entry that is remarkable for being one of the few instances in *Bone* in which Woodman allows herself outwardly to express a flash of anger. As projections, they are improvisations that say much more about the projectors' "love of death" than the ill person's need to live. These are the myths and stories for which the ill subject is cruelly "sacrificed," as Woodman says, but it seems important to say they are also idealizations that *Bone* elsewhere affirms and explores to one degree or another. All of these dismissed stories of Woodman's cancer are also stories that *Bone* tells, even if they are characterized here as explanations of her illness that have been violently imposed upon her by others: the family history of cancer, the melancholic attachment to Fraser, the depletions that she suffers for playing the maternal role with her patients and students, each of these epidemiologies Woodman must also acknowledge as her own. And as she suggests, things get complicated when the sick subject does the most embarrassing thing: rather than dying according to plan, she "splutters back into life" (68)! Woodman is herself an instance of that messy excess, inasmuch as she here demurs the projections for which she is also responsible for putting into play in *Bone*. The projections that she castigates are at once hers and not-hers, familiar and unfamiliar; this is an indeterminacy for which *Bone* seems uneasily prepared, not least because it remembers that Woodman's life is larger than the designs that would explain it. In his contribution to a volume honouring his wife's writings, Ross Woodman observes that "Marion's life and work resides not in the construction of a masculine system, but in the feminine deferral of it" (2005: 79). Yet Woodman's renunciating gesture threatens at points to take on elements of the masculine system it would rather let go—especially its asceticism, and its faith in a higher orderliness. What saves it from becoming what it beholds are these moments of self-difference, the internal margins where the book interrogates its most passionately held assumptions. Embracing the uncertainty of its own future readings by writing against herself, Woodman refuses the last temptation, the temptation to be seduced by the anorexic requirements of her own system. These are the moments in which her text "splutters back into life."

We have only begun to read Marion Woodman's *Bone: Dying into Life*.

Acknowledgements

A longer version of this chapter was first published in *Spring: A Journal of Archetype and Culture* 72:1 (2005), 131–58.

References

Butler, J. (1993), *Bodies That Matter: On the Discursive Limits of "Sex"* (New York: Routledge).

Derrida, J. (1989), "Mnemosyne," in *Memoires: For Paul de Man*, C. Lindsay et al. (trans.) (New York: Columbia University Press).

Derrida, J. (1995), *The Gift of Death*, D. Wills (trans.) (Chicago, IL: University of Chicago Press).

Derrida, J. (2005), "Epoché and Faith: An Interview with Jacques Derrida," in Y. Sherwood and K. Hart (eds), *Derrida and Religion: Other Testaments* (New York: Routledge).

Levinas, E. (1969), *Totality and Infinity: An Essay on Exteriority*, A. Lingis (trans.) (Pittsburgh, PA: Duquesne University Press).

Levinas, E. (1998), *Otherwise Than Being; or Beyond Essence*, A. Lingis (trans.) (Pittsburgh, PA: Duquesne University Press).

Nietzsche, F. (1997), *Daybreak: Thoughts on the Prejudices of Morality*, M. Clark and B. Leiter (trans.) (eds) (Cambridge: Cambridge University Press).

Rose, G. (1996), *Mourning Becomes the Law: Philosophy and Representation* (Cambridge: Cambridge University Press).

Woodman, M. (2000), *Bone: Dying into Life* (New York: Viking).

Woodman, R.G. (2005), "Marion Woodman's 'Vale of Soul-Making,'" *Spring: A Journal of Archetype and Culture* 72:1, 43–85.

Index